Informatik aktuell

Herausgegeben
im Auftrag der Gesellschaft für Informatik (GI)

Andreas Maier · Thomas M. Deserno
Heinz Handels · Klaus H. Maier-Hein
Christoph Palm · Thomas Tolxdorff
Herausgeber

Bildverarbeitung für die Medizin 2018

Algorithmen – Systeme – Anwendungen

Proceedings des Workshops
vom 11. bis 13. März 2018 in Erlangen

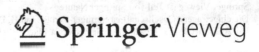

Herausgeber

Andreas Maier
Friedrich-Alexander-Universität
Erlangen-Nürnberg
Lehrstuhl für Mustererkennung (Informatik 5)
Martensstr. 3, 91058 Erlangen

Thomas M. Deserno, geb. Lehmann
Technische Universität Braunschweig
und Medizinische Hochschule Hannover
Peter L. Reichertz Institut für Medizinische
Informatik
Mühlenpfordtstr. 23, 38106 Braunschweig

Heinz Handels
Universität zu Lübeck
Institut für Medizinische Informatik
Ratzeburger Allee 160, 23562 Lübeck

Klaus H. Maier-Hein, geb. Fritzsche
Deutsches Krebsforschungszentrum
Medizinische Bildverarbeitung E230
Im Neuenheimer Feld 581, 69120 Heidelberg

Christoph Palm
Ostbayerische Technische Hochschule
Regensburg
Regensburg Medical Image Computing (ReMIC)
Galgenbergstr. 32, 93053 Regensburg

Thomas Tolxdorff
Charité – Universitätsmedizin Berlin
Institut für Medizinische Informatik
Hindenburgdamm 30, 12200 Berlin

ISSN 1431-472X
Informatik aktuell
ISBN 978-3-662-56536-0   ISBN 978-3-662-56537-7   (eBook)
https://doi.org/10.1007/978-3-662-56537-7

Die Deutsche Nationalbibliothek verzeichnet diese Publikation in der Deutschen Nationalbibliografie; detaillierte bibliografische Daten sind im Internet über http://dnb.d-nb.de abrufbar.

CR Subject Classification (1998): A.0, H.3, I.4, I.5, J.3, H.3.1, I.2.10, I.3.3, I.3.5, I.3.7, I.3.8, I.6.3

Springer Vieweg

© Springer-Verlag GmbH Deutschland 2018, korrigierte Publication 2018

Gedruckt auf säurefreiem und chlorfrei gebleichtem Papier

Springer Vieweg ist Teil von Springer Nature
Die eingetragene Gesellschaft ist Springer-Verlag GmbH, DE
Die Anschrift der Gesellschaft ist: Heidelberger Platz 3, 14197 Berlin, Germany

Die Original-Version des Buches wurde korrigiert. Ein Erratum finden Sie unter https://doi.org/10.1007/978-3-662-56537-7_97

Bildverarbeitung für die Medizin 2018

Veranstalter

LfM   Lehrstuhl für Mustererkennung
Friedrich-Alexander-Universität Erlangen-Nürnberg

Unterstützende Fachgesellschaften

BVMI   Berufsverband Medizinischer Informatiker
CURAC   Deutsche Gesellschaft für Computer- und Roboterassistierte
Chirurgie
DAGM   Deutsche Arbeitsgemeinschaft für Mustererkennung
DGBMT   Fachgruppe Medizinische Informatik der
Deutschen Gesellschaft für Biomedizinische Technik im
Verband Deutscher Elektrotechniker
GI   Gesellschaft für Informatik - Fachbereich Informatik
in den Lebenswissenschaften
GMDS   Gesellschaft für Medizinische Informatik,
Biometrie und Epidemiologie
IEEE   Joint Chapter Engineering in Medicine and Biology,
German Section

Tagungsvorsitz

Prof. Dr.-Ing. Andreas Maier
Lehrstuhl für Mustererkennung, FAU

Dr. Stefanie Demirci
Technische Universität München

Dr. Tobias Heimann
Siemens Healthcare GmbH, Erlangen

Tagungssekretariat

Siming Bayer und Weilin Fu
Lehrstuhl für Mustererkennung, FAU Erlangen-Nürnberg
Postanschrift: 91058 Erlangen
Lieferanschrift: Martensstraße 3
Telefon: +49 9131 85 27826
Email: bvm-orga@dkfz-heidelberg.de
Web: http://bvm-workshop.org

Lokales BVM-Komitee

Prof. Dr.-Ing Andreas Maier
Christoph Luckner
Siming Bayer
Weilin Fu
u.v.m.

Verteilte BVM-Organisation

Prof. Dr. Thomas M. Deserno, Sven Neumann, Aleksej Hecht, Aaron Wiora
Technische Universität Braunschweig (Tagungsband)

Prof. Dr. Heinz Handels, Dr. Jan-Hinrich Wrage
Universität zu Lübeck (Beitragsbegutachtung)

Prof. Dr. Andreas Maier
Friedrich-Alexander-Universität Erlangen-Nürnberg (Sponsoring)

Priv.-Doz. Dr. Klaus H. Maier-Hein, Jens Petersen
Deutsches Krebsforschungszentrum Heidelberg (Anmeldung)

Prof. Dr. Christoph Palm, Dr. Alexander Leis, Leonhard Klausmann
OHT Regensburg (Internetpräsenz, Newsletter)

Prof. Dr. Thomas Tolxdorff, Dr. Thorsten Schaaf
Charité – Universitätsmedizin Berlin (Internetpräsenz)

Programmkomitee

Priv.-Doz. Dr. Jürgen Braun, Charité-Universitätsmedizin Berlin
Prof. Dr. Thorsten Buzug, Universität zu Lübeck
Dr. Stefanie Demirci, Technische Universität München
Prof. Dr. Thomas Deserno, Technische Universität Braunschweig
Prof. Dr. Hartmut Dickhaus, Universität Heidelberg
Dr. Jan Ehrhardt, Universität zu Lübeck
Dr. Ralf Floca, DKFZ Heidelberg
Dr. Nils Forkert, University of Calgary, Canada
Prof. Horst Hahn, Fraunhofer MEVIS Bremen
Prof. Dr. Heinz Handels, Universität zu Lübeck
Dr. Tobias Heimann, Siemens Healthcare GmbH Erlangen
Prof. Dr. Matthias Heinrich, Universität zu Lübeck
Prof. Ron Kikinis, MD, Harvard Medical School Boston USA
Prof. Dr. Andreas Maier, Universität Erlangen
Priv.-Doz. Dr. Klaus Maier-Hein, DKFZ Heidelberg
Prof. Dr. Lena Maier-Hein, DKFZ Heidelberg
Dr. Andre Mastmeyer, Universität zu Lübeck
Prof. Dr. Hans-Peter Meinzer, DKFZ Heidelberg
Prof. Dr. Dorit Merhof, RWTH Aachen
Prof. Jan Modersitzki, Fraunhofer MEVIS, Lübeck
Prof. Dr. Heinrich Müller, Technische Universität Dortmund
Prof. Dr. Nassir Navab, Technische Universität München
Dr. Marco Nolden, DKFZ Heidelberg
Prof. Dr. Christoph Palm, OTH Regensburg
Prof. Dr. Bernhard Preim, Universität Magdeburg
Priv.-Doz. Dr. Karl Rohr, Universität Heidelberg
Priv.-Doz. Dr. Dennis Säring, FH Wedel
Dr. Sylvia Saalfeld, Universität Maarburg
Prof. Dr. Heinz-Peter Schlemmer, DKFZ Heidelberg
Dr. Stefanie Speidel, Helmholtz-Zentrum Dresend-Rossendorf
Prof. Dr. Thomas Tolxdorff, Charité-Universitätsmedizin Berlin
Prof. Dr. Klaus Tönnies, Universität Magdeburg
Dr. Gudrun Wagenknecht, Forschungszentrum Jülich
Dr. René Werner, UKE Hamburg
Dr. Stefan Wesarg, Fraunhofer IGD Darmstadt
Priv.-Doz. Dr. Thomas Wittenberg, Fraunhofer IIS, Erlangen
Prof. Dr. Ivo Wolf, HS Mannheim
Priv.-Doz. Dr. Stefan Wörz, Universität Heidelberg

X

Sponsoren des Workshops BVM 2018

Die BVM wäre ohne die finanzielle Unterstützung der Industrie in ihrer so erfolgreichen Konzeption nicht durchführbar. Deshalb freuen wir uns sehr über langjährige kontinuierliche Unterstützung mancher Firmen sowie auch über das neue Engagement anderer.

Chili GmbH
Friedrich-Ebert-Str. 2, D-69221 Dossenheim
http://www.chili-radiology.com

Haption GmbH
Dennewartstr. 25, 52068 Aachen
http://www.haption.de

Sepp.med GmbH
Gewerbering 9, D-91314 Röttenbach
http://www.seppmed.de

Siemens Healthcare GmbH
Henkestr. 127, D-91052 Erlangen
http://www.healthcare.siemens.de

Springer Springer-Verlag GmbH
Tiergarten Strasse 17, D-69121 Heidelberg
http://www.springer.com

Ziehm Imaging GmbH
Donaustraße 31, D-90451 Nürnberg
https://ziehm.com.de

Preisträger des BVM-Workshops 2017 in Lübeck

BVM-Preis 2017 für die beste wissenschaftliche Arbeit (1. Platz)

Xiaolin Huang (FAU Erlangen-Nürnberg)
mit *Yan Xia, Yixing Huang, Joachim Hornegger, Andreas Maier*
Overexposure Correction by Mixed One-Bit Compressive Sensing for C-Arm CT

BVM-Preis 2017 für die beste wissenschaftliche Arbeit (2. Platz)

Robert Mendel (OTH Regensburg)
mit *Alanna Ebigbo, Andreas Probst, Helmut Messmann, Christoph Palm*
Barrett's Esophagus Analysis using Convolutional Neural Networks

BVM-Preis 2017 für die beste wissenschaftliche Arbeit (3. Platz)

Monique Meuschke (Otto-von-Guericke Universität Magdeburg)
mit *Wito Engelke, Oliver Beuing, Bernhard Preim, Kai Lawonn*
Automatic Viewpoint Selection for Exploration of Time-Dependent Cerebral Aneurysm Data

BVM-Preis 2017 für den besten Vortrag

Tanja Kurzendorfer (FAU Erlangen-Nürnberg)
mit *Alexander Brost, Christoph Forman, Michaela Schmidt, Christoph Tillmanns, Andreas Maier* (Friedrich-Alexander Universität Erlangen-Nürnberg)
Fully Automatic Segmentation of Papillary Muscles in 3D LGE-MRI

BVM-Preis 2017 für die beste Posterpräsentation

Matthias Wilms (Universität zu Lübeck)
mit *Heinz Handels, Jan Ehrhardt*
Patch-based Learning of Shape, Appearance, and Motion Models from Few Training Samples by Low-Rank Matrix Completion

BVM-Award für eine herausragende Promotion (geteilt)

Sandy Engelhardt (DKFZ Heidelberg)
Computer-Assisted Quantitative Mitral Valve Surgery

BVM-Award für eine herausragende Promotion (geteilt)

Florian Bernar (University of Luxembourg)
Novel Methods for Multi-Shape Analysis

Vorwort

In der computergestützten Verarbeitung und automatischen Analyse medizinischer Bilddaten werden momentan erhebliche Fortschritte erzielt und die Grenzen des Machbaren sichtlich erweitert. Der Workshop *Bildverarbeitung für die Medizin (BVM)* bietet ein Forum zur Präsentation und Diskussion der neuesten Algorithmen, Systeme und Anwendungen in diesem Bereich. Ziel ist sowohl die Vertiefung der Interaktion zwischen Wissenschaftlern, Industrie und Anwendern als auch die explizite Einbeziehung von Nachwuchswissenschaftler, die über ihre Bachelor-, Master-, Promotions- und Habilitationsprojekte berichten. Die BVM konnte sich durch erfolgreiche Veranstaltungen in Aachen, Berlin, Erlangen, Freiburg, Hamburg, Heidelberg, Leipzig, Lübeck und München als zentrales interdisziplinäres Forum etablieren.

Für den diesjährigen Workshop konnten neben den spannenden Beiträgen der Teilnehmer vier hochinteressante eingeladene Vorträge gewonnen werden:

- Professor Jan Baumbach, Technische Universität München, zum Thema *Systems Medicine - The next generation of computer-assisted medicine.*

- Professor Philippe Cattin, Center for Medical Image Analysis & Navigation, Universität Basel, zum Thema *Reinventing Bone Surgery: From Planning to Execution of Hard-Tissue Cut.*

- Dr. Zeike Taylor, University of Sheffield, zum Thema *From mechanistic to data-driven models for surgical planning, guidance, and simulation.*

- Professor Alejandro Frangi, University of Sheffield, zum Thema *Precision Imaging: from population imaging analytics to in silico clinical trial.*

Dieses Jahr feiert der BVM Clinical Track seine Premiere. Wir freuen uns, dass wir 10 herausragende Publikationen präsentieren können. Darunter Einreichungen vom Massachusetts Institute of Technology, dem New England Eye Center und Johns Hopkins University. Weiterhin konnten wir noch folgende hochkarätige Redner gewinnen:

- Professor Christoph Bert, Universitätsklinikum Erlangen

- Professor Arnd Dörfler, Universitätsklinikum Erlangen

- Professor Robert Klopfleisch, Freie Universität Berlin.

Aus insgesamt 84 Einreichungen, davon 60 Originalarbeiten und 24 Abstacts, wurden 28 Vorträge, 44 Poster und sechs Softwaredemonstrationen angenommen. Die besten Arbeiten werden auch in diesem Jahr mit wertvollen BVM-Preisen ausgezeichnet. Die Webseite des Workshops findet sich unter

XIV

http://www.bvm-workshop.org

An dieser Stelle möchten wir allen, die bei den umfangreichen Vorbereitungen
zum Gelingen des Workshops beigetragen haben, unseren herzlichen Dank für ihr
Engagement bei der Organisation des Workshops aussprechen: den Referenten
der Gastvorträge, den Autoren der Beiträge, den Referenten der Tutorien, den In-
dustrierepräsentanten, dem Programmkomitee, den Fachgesellschaften, den Mit-
gliedern des BVM-Organisationsteams und allen Mitarbeitern des Lehrstuhls für
Mustererkennung der Friedrich-Alexander-Universität Erlangen-Nürnberg.

Wir wünschen allen Teilnehmerinnen und Teilnehmern des Workshops BVM
2018 spannende neue Kontakte und inspirierende Eindrücke aus der Welt der
medizinischen Bildverarbeitung.

Januar 2018
Andreas Maier (Erlangen)
Thomas Deserno (Braunschweig)
Heinz Handels (Lübeck)
Klaus Maier-Hain (Heidelberg)
Christoph Palm (Regensburg)
Thomas Tolxdorff (Berlin)

Inhaltsverzeichnis

Die fortlaufende Nummer am linken Seitenrand entspricht den Beitragsnummern, wie sie im endgültigen Programm des Workshops zu finden sind. Dabei steht V für Vortrag, P für Poster und S für Softwaredemonstration.

Eingeladene Vorträge

Tutorials

Clinical Track

Medical Descriptors & Measurement

Medical Image Segmentation

Interventional & Multimodal Imaging

Computer-Aided Diagnosis

Poster Medical Imaging

Poster Medizinische Bildverarbeitung

Poster Learning & Segmentation

Software Demo

Cell Imaging & Digital Pathology

Vessel Imaging & Analysis

Medical Image Reconstruction

Medical Image Enhancement

Autorenverzeichnis

Systems Medicine
The Next Generation of Computer-assisted Precision Medicine

Jan Baumbach

Chair of Experimental Bioinformatics, Technical University of Munich, Germany
jan.baumbach@wzw.tum.de

Recent advances in modern OMICS technology allow measuring the expression of all kinds of biological entities (genes, proteins, metabolites, miRNAs, etc.) at low cost and in high-throughput. Computational challenges for analyzing such big data emerge, ranging from the low signal to noise ratio to high model complexity, which render simple statistical questions arbitrarily complicated. We will discuss several bioinformatics tools for de-isolating biological networks and multiple OMICS data types: de novo pathway enrichment, in vitro high-throughput screening (HTS) data integration, time-course network enrichment, cancer subtyping, and breath analysis. Using Huntington's disease patients' expression data we will employ a guilt-by-association approach to illuminate the power of molecular networks to identify novel disease mechanisms. We will then extend this principle to study HTS data gained from large-scale drug screens, siRNA knockdown and CRISPR/CAS9 knock-out screens, as well as microRNA screens. In addition, we will show how to unravel temporal systems-level response patterns using whole-genome time-series gene expression profiles of lung cells after Influenza infection. We discuss how this kind of computational network biology has strong potential to enable precision medicine by classifying breast cancer subtypes utilizing complex combo-features gained from combining networks with multiple OMICS data. Finally, we will show how modern image analysis technology can be used for non-invasive precision medicine by profiling metabolic patterns in human breath from COPD and lung cancer patients.

Reinventing Bone Surgery
From Planning to Execution of a Hard-Tissue Cut

Philippe Cattin

Center for Medical Image Analysis & Navigation (CIAN) University of Basel,
Switzerland
philippe.cattin@unibas.ch

Cutting bones is one of the oldest medical procedures performed to human patients. Thanks to the high mineral content of bone we have archaeological evidence of skull trepanation dating back more than 10.000 years. Despite the rapid development of surgical instruments over the last 200 years, the fundamental mechanism of bone cutting has not changed ever since.

In this talk, 1 will show you how researchers of the flagship proJect MIRACLE (Minimally Invasive Robot-Assisted Computer-guided Laserosteotomtry) are working on laser technology to reinvent bone surgery. The MIRACLE project not only reinvents the way hard tissues are being cut but also works on novel concepts to plan and visualize these surgical interventions in virtual and augmented reality environments.

From Mechanistic to Data-driven Models for Surgical Planning, Guidance and Simulation

Zeike A. Taylor

Fraunhofer Institut IIS Erlangen, Germany
z.a.taylor@sheffield.ac.uk

Biomechanical and biophysical models are key tools in many applications of surgical planning and optimisation, surgical guidance, and interactive simulation for training and rehearsal. The most robust and accurate models usually are those based on the relevant equations of continuum mechanics (solid, fluid, thermal, etc.), and which are generally solved with numerical methods such as FEM. Given high quality patient-specific inputs, these can enable accurate prediction of, e.g., deformations of soft tissues, flow patterns in blood vessels, energy delivery profiles around ablation devices, etc. Two main difficulties arise, however: 1) computation times can be prohibitive, especially from the point of view of clinical deployment; and 2) the requisite "high quality patient-specific inputsmay simply not be available. To address these issues, our group and collaborators are beginning to explore how data-driven approaches can be used as surrogates for full mechanistic models, both to achieve faster computation, and to either mitigate the effects of parameter uncertainty or at least better characterise its effect. We believe that by exploiting the huge advances in machine learning and related areas experienced in recent years, entirely new classes of flexible, fast, and reliable simulation techniques can be achieved. Results achieved so far to this end will be described.

Precision Imaging
From Population Imaging Analytics to In-silico Clinical Trials

Alejandro Frangi

Centre for Computational Imaging & Simulation Technologies in Biomedicine,
University of Sheffield, The United Kingdom
a.frangi@sheffield.ac.uk

Medical image computing is witnessing exciting times. Specifically to this talk, new opportunities and challenges have emerged with the growing availability of large population imaging repositories being collected in the UK, USA, Canada, Germany, and The Netherlands, to name Just a few.

Against this backdrop, we are interested specifically in developing new methods for and applications of Precision imaging to maximally exploit the wealth of information behind large imaging repositories and associated meta data. Precision imaging is not a new discipline per se but rather a distinct emphasis in medical imaging and image computing borne at the crossroads between, and unifying the efforts behind mechanistic and phenomenological model-based imaging and image computing. Precision imaging fundamentally recognizes the need for both data-driven and hypothesis-driven approaches to image analysis and image-based modeling.

The exponential rate at which data availability is growing will rapidly outpace the exponential growth rate of available computational resources and is never sufficiently abundant to deal with the combinatorial complexity intrinsic to many disease mechanisms. As described by Helbing, this implies the problem of "dark data", i.e. the share of data we cannot process is increasing with time. Consequently, we must know what data to process and how which requires science. Anderson's vision of big data (i.e., assuming we will not need theory and science anymore) is unlikely to prevail. Artificial intelligence will unlikely change this situation fundamentally.

Precision lmaging captures three main directions in the effort to deal with the information deluge in imaging sciences, and thus achieve wisdom from data, information, and knowledge. Precision lmaging is finally characterized by being descriptive, predictive and integrative about the imaged obJect. This paper provides abrief and personal perspective on how the field has evolved, summarizes and formalizes our vision of precision imaging for precision medicine, and highlights connections with past research and current trends in the field.

Deep Learning Fundamentals

Katharina Breininger, Vincent Christlein, Tobias Würfl, Andreas Maier

Pattern Recognition Lab, Friedrich-Alexander-Universität, Erlangen, Germany
katharina.breininger@fau.de

Deep learning has received a lot of attention in the machine learning community. Successful applications from speech recognition or computer vision are already part of our daily life. Much effort has been devoted to transferring this success to medical image computing. Therefore, neural networks have become an essential research direction. The first half of this tutorial is designed to familiarize participants with neural networks. The second half presents the transition from neural networks to deep learning.

The building blocks of classical neural networks, such as the multi-layer perceptron, activations and loss functions, are explained. Furthermore, the concepts of gradient-based learning and backpropagation to calculate the gradients are introduced.

The second part of the tutorial covers the elements of convolutional neural networks, around which most successful deep learning applications revolve. Special attention is devoted to regularization techniques, which are essential to state-of-the-art performance. Best practices and exemplary architectures conclude the tutorial.

Advanced Deep Learning Methods

Paul Jäger, Fabian Isensee, Jens Petersen, David Zimmerer, Jakob Wasserthal, Klaus H. Maier-Hein

Division of Medical Image Computing, German Cancer Research Center (DKFZ), Heidelberg, Germany
p.jaeger@dkfz-heidelberg.de

The remarkable rise of deep learning has led to an overwhelming amount of new papers coming up by the week. This tutorial intents to filter out the research most relevant for the medical image computing (MIC) community and present it in a structured and understandable form. It is composed of five parts: Classification, Segmentation, Detection, Generative Models and Semi- Supervised Learning. Each part starts off with a thorough motivation, shows exemplary use cases related to MIC, provides a brief model overview and describes the current state-of-the-art methods in the respective area. Basic knowledge about Neural Networks as covered by the "Deep Learning Fundamentals" tutorial is recommended.

Innovation Generation, Disruption and Exponential Technologies in Medical Imaging

Michael Friebe

Catheter Technologies and Image Guided Therapies, OvGU
michael.friebe@ovgu.de

Healthcare in general and medical imaging in particular will change dramatically in the next 20 years with the emergence of artificial intelligence (including machine and deep learning), 3D printing, personalized diagnosis and therapies, shift from therapy to prevention, and many related delivery and economic changes. Huge opportunities are present in developed, emerging and developing nations, each with completely different needs and infrastructural environments, and with a completely different reimbursement system. The tutorial will prepare the attendees for the changes that will likely come up in the coming years and subsequently focus on recognizing the need for a change in our development and innovation process, that must focus on digitization and connectivity, small footprint, robustness, and low cost, and with that explore alternative financing methods. Due to the regulatory processes in place and the ever increasing complexity of getting products into the market there could also be lots of opportunities for reverse innovation. The lecture will also present the product and technology approach and some recent examples of the chair of catheter technologies and image guided therapies that focus on joint product developments between clinicians and engineers leading to the question of what are good versus bad value propositions for medical technology / imaging products? Following questions will be addressed:

- What actually is innovation and can meaningful innovation generation for healthcare products and services be learned?
- What are good versus bad value propositions for medical technology / imaging products?
- What likely impact will exponential technologies have on healthcare delivery / medical imaging in the next 20 years?
- What entrepreneurial opportunities will develop because of that and how do we prepare ourselves for that?
- What is reverse innovation and how can all benefit from that?

Endoscopy

Thomas Wittenberg

Fraunhofer Institut IIS Erlangen
wbg@iis.fraunhofer.de

In the last 40 years progress in the field of diagnostic and interventional endoscopy (gastroenterology and laparoscopy) have been made, mainly driven through new technical developments from various areas of medical technologies such as optics, micro-mechanics, electronics, robotics, informatics, and image processing. These advances allow soft and gentle minimal-invasive access and interventions in all hollow organs, including the abdomen, stomach, large and small intestines, joints a was well nasal cavities. To accelerate the development and application of such diagnostic and therapeutic possibilities in all fields of endoscopy a understanding of the available technological possibilities is necessary. In this short tutorial, we will give an overview about the following topics:

- Brief history and introduction to endoscopes
- Components of endoscopy systems (Illumination, sensors, instruments, ...)
- Types of endoscopes (rigid, flexible, capsule, stereo)
- Examples for clinical application of diagnostic and interventional endoscopy
- Endoscopy and robotic interventions
- Endoscopy based challenges for image processing
- Future developments

As part of the tutorial we will provide a hands-on demonstration for some endoscopy procedures including colonoscopy and laparoscopy training systems.

Abstract: Digitale Pathologie für mobile Endgeräte

Hannah Büchner[1], Ingmar Gergel[2]

[1]Hochschule Mannheim, mbits imaging GmbH
[2]Deutsches Krebsforschungszentrum, mbits imaging GmbH
hannahbuechner@mbits.info

Digitalisierung spielt im heutigen Zeitalter, besonders in der Medizin, eine entscheidende Rolle. Neben der Radiologie, welche bereits digitalisiert ist, gibt es auch in anderen Fachdisziplinen eine Umstellung bisheriger Workflows. So hat sich auch in den letzten Jahren die digitale Pathologie weiterentwickelt. Anstatt mit einem konventionellen Mikroskop die Glasobjektträger zu betrachten, werden diese zunehmend digitalisiert. Für die Anwendung in der klinischen Routine gibt es aktuell einige Herausforderungen. Einerseits existiert noch kein Standard für ein einheitliches Bildformat, vergleichbar zu DICOM in der Radiologie. Andererseits werden die virtuellen Schnitte durch die verschiedenen Auflösungsstufen sehr groß (bis zu 30 GB), weshalb für die Übertragung ein stabiles Breitbandnetz notwendig ist. Des Weiteren sind derzeit für den Bereitschaftsdienst in der Pathologie keine performanten, mobilen Lösungen für den ortsunabhängigen Zugriff verfügbar.

Im Rahmen einer Bachelorarbeit wurde ein Prototyp entwickelt, welcher ermöglicht, dass verschiedene Dateiformate (.svs, .svslide, .scn, .vms, .vmu, .ndpi, .mrxs, .bif, .tif, .tiff) verarbeitet und standortunabhängig sowohl inner- als auch außerhalb der Arbeitszeiten zur Verfügung stellt. Dieser Prototyp wurde in die Software mRay (CE-zertifiziertes Medizinprodukt IIb) integriert. Um die meisten Bildformate zu unterstützen, wird die OpenSlide-Bibliothek (Open-Source) verwendet. Die eingelesenen Bildinformationen werden in eine eigene Pyramiden-Datenstruktur, bestehend aus mehreren in Bildkacheln eingeteilte Auflösungsebenen, überführt. Um die Speicherplatz-Problematik zu adressieren, werden die Bildkacheln mit verschiedenen Heuristiken (Luminanz, Biomarker) bewertet, sodass relevante Bildareale vorab geladen werden. Dank der Bildkachelung ist es außerdem möglich sehr große Bilder schrittweise zu übertragen und am mobilen Endgerät zu visualisieren.

Vorläufige Ergebnisse zeigen, dass durch die entwickelten Heuristiken und das Vorabladen der volle Funktionsumfang auch mit einer schlechten und keiner Netzwerkverbindung (offline) gewährleistet ist.

Ziel der Arbeit ist es, die digitale Pathologie nicht nur im Bereich von Konsultationen (Schnellschnitt) und Konferenzen, sondern auch in der Lehre durch den mobilen Zugriff zu unterstützen. Es gilt weiterhin zu evaluieren, inwiefern die interdisziplinäre Zusammenarbeit bei Konferenzen durch die Visualisierung mehrerer Bildtypen (MRT, CT, H&E-gefärbte Schnitte) zu einer Verbesserung in der Patientenbehandlung insgesamt führen kann.

Abstract: Digital Cytomorphology

Deep Learning on an Image Data Set of Cell Morphologies in Acute Myeloid Leukemia

Christian Matek[1,2], Carsten Marr[1], Karsten Spiekermann[2]

[1]Institute of Computational Biology, Helmholtz Center Munich, German Research Center for Environmental Health, Neuherberg, Germany
[2]Department of Internal Medicine III, University Hospital Munich, Ludwig-Maximilians-University Munich - Campus Großhadern, Munich, Germany
c.matek@med.uni-muenchen.de

Examination of Leukocyte cytomorphology using light microscopy, a method dating back to the nineteenth century, remains an important cornerstone in present-day Leukemia diagnostics.

In contrast to other laboratory tests, cytomorphological examination has so far defied automation and to this day is usually performed by trained human examiners. Hence, the diagnostic yield of that method is highly operator-dependent and hard to correlate quantitatively with other diagnostic modalities or clinical data.

We digitised a set of 100 blood smears without pathological findings and 80 blood smears taken from patients with different stages of Acute Myeloid Leukemia (AML) from the University Hospital of Munich Laboratory for Leukemia Diagnostics during 2014-2016.

All blood smears come from routine diagnostics, were stained using Pappenheim's stain and scanned at 100-fold magnification and oil immersion with a digital microscope - scanner. Finally, at least 100 Leukocytes per smear were classified into a 20-category scheme by trained cytomorphology examiners.

This dataset is used for training and validation of a convolutional neural network in order to allow independent recognition of malignant and non-malignant cell populations relevant in AML diagnostics.

We review the technical strengths and challenges of the digital image acquisition and examination process from the perspective of the routine clinical workflow. We furthermore show first results of the training and validation process of the convolutional neural network and assess the performance of that methodology as applied to our cell classification problem.

Abstract: First Approaches Towards Automatic Detection of Microaneurysms in OCTA Images

Lennart Husvogt[1,2,3], A. Yasin Alibhai[2], Eric Moult[3], James G. Fujimoto[3], Nadia Waheed[2], Andreas Maier[1]

[1]Pattern Recognition Lab, Friedrich-Alexander-Universität Erlangen-Nürnberg
[2]New England Eye Center, Tufts Medical Center, Boston, MA, USA
[3]Biomedical Optical Imaging and Biophotonics Group, Massachusetts Institute of Technology, Cambridge, MA, USA
lennart.husvogt@fau.de

We investigated automatic detection of micro aneurysms in optical coherence tomo-graphy angiography. Data of two patients was gathered at the New England Eye Center. Patients with diabetic retinopathy were imaged on an Optovue Avanti device. In order to do automatic detection, we trained a classifier for general image detection tasks using the Weka Trainable Segmentation Plugin [1] that is included into the CONRAD software package [2]. For demonstration purposes, we trained a Random Forest Classifier on a single training image with 92.416 training samples. For feature extraction Gaussian Blur, Sobel Filter, Hessian, Difference of Gaussians, and Membrane Projections were chosen. The trained forest comprised 200 trees. For verification, a second case was processed and the output probability of the classifier was overlaid. Training data and the resulting overlay are depicted in Fig. 1.

The results look promising. All micro aneurysms of the second patient are detected. Interestingly, such results could be obtained using only a single patient

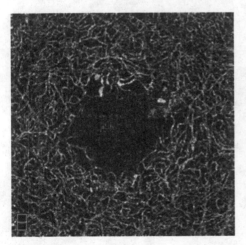
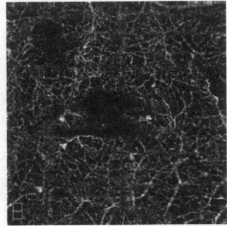

Fig. 1. The training image is shown on the left-hand side. Using only this single image for training micro aneurysms, we could obtain the segmentation result on the right-hand side that contains all relevant micro aneurysms.

as training and traditional learning methods. In future work, we will perform quantitative evaluation using several subjects and explore the utility of the different feature descriptors. To the best of our knowledge, this is the first paper on automatic detection on micro aneurysms in OCTA data.

References

1. Arganda-Carreras I, Kaynig V, Schindelin J, et al. Trainable weka segmentation: a machine learning tool for microscopy image segmentation. Neuroscience. 2014; p. 73–80.
2. Maier A, Hofmann H, Berger M, et al. CONRAD: a software framework for cone-beam imaging in radiology. Med Phys. 2013;40(11).

Abstract: Automatic Malignancy Estimation for Pulmonary Nodules from CT Images

Katrin Mentl, Rimon Saffoury, Andreas Maier

Pattern Recognition Lab, Friedrich-Alexander University of Erlangen-NÃ¼rnberg
katrin.mentl@fau.de

Early detection of lung cancer is crucial to increase the chance of cure. As lung cancer often manifests itself in the presence of malignant pulmonary nodules, the assessment of such is of high clinical importance. Lung cancer screening is primarily performed using diagnostic imaging modalities such as CT, while invasive methods such as biopsy are used as a last resort to confirm diagnosis.

Various prediction models that are based on both patient (e.g., age, smoking status) and radiological features (e.g., nodule's type) have been suggested. However, the manual extraction of the essential radiological characteristics from CT scans is a cumbersome and time-consuming task, which is, moreover, subject to inter-observer variation.

To overcome these limitations, we propose a pipeline which automatically extracts relevant features from a CT baseline scan and outputs a malignancy probability score based on established prediction models such as the Mayo Clinic model. The following radiological features are extracted: presence of emphysema, nodule's diameter, nodule's type and presence of spiculation. The presence of emphysema is classified based on the ratio of low attenuation areas to the lung volume, while the other features mainly depend on the automatic lung nodule segmentation. The nodule type, i.e. solid, part solid or non-solid is determined using a two-step classification scheme and the presence of spiculation is detected with a SVM classifier.

We evaluated our segmentation approach on over 1,000 nodules and reached a low mean absolute error of around 1 mm. We achieved high accuracies across all classification tasks and promising performance on the investigated prediction models. Thus, we propose to consider the system as decision support in routine clinical practice.

Amplitude of brain signals classify hunger status based on machine learning in resting-state fMRI

Arkan Al-Zubaidi[1], Alfred Mertins[2], Marcus Heldmann[1],
Kamila Jauch-Chara[3], Thomas F. Münte[1]

[1]Department of Neurology, University of Lübeck
[2]Institute for Signal Processing, University of Lübeck
[3]Department of Psychiatry, University of Kiel
arkan.al-zubaidi@neuro.uni-luebeck.de

Resting-state fMRI (rs-fMRI) is a method of functional brain imaging that allows the task-free exploration of the intrinsic functional connectivity in humans. Since central nervous pathways regulate food intake and eating behavior, it is assumed that changes in the homeostatic state have an impact on the connectivity patterns of rs-fMRI. Here, we compare the accuracy of three data-driven approaches in classifying two metabolic states (hunger vs. satiety) depending on the observed rs-fMRI fluctuations. These methods assess local and global functional connectivity as well as amplitude (intensity) fluctuations of neural signals: First, regional homogeneity (ReHo), which describes the synchronization of time series of a given voxel and its nearest neighbors. Second, the degree of centrality (DC), which measures the number of connections of a voxel to all the other voxels above a certain threshold. Third, the fractional amplitude of low-frequency fluctuation (fALFF), which measures voxel-wise signal amplitude. After extracting the associated connectivity parameters of 90 brain regions for each method, we use features selection algorithms with the objective function of linear support vector machine classifier and permutation tests to investigate which method and which brain regions differentiate best between hungry and satiety. Our results indicate that the fALFF method is more accurate than ReHo and DC in capturing the changes of the resting brain during states of hunger and satiety. This opens up the possibility to use this measure to characterize certain states (e.g., sleep stages) or disease conditions (e.g., mitochondrial encephalopathy).

Die Original-Version des Kapitels wurde korrigiert. Ein Erratum finden Sie unter
https://doi.org/10.1007/978-3-662-56537-7_98

Abstract: Assessment of Segmentation Dependence in Macroscopic Lung Cavity Extraction

Asmaa Khdeir[1,2,*], Tobias Geimer[1,2,3,*], Shuqing Chen[1], Eric Goppert[1], Maximilian Dankbar[1], Christoph Bert[2,3], Andreas Maier[1,3]

[1]Pattern Recognition Lab, Friedrich-Alexander-Universität Erlangen-Nürnberg
[2]Department of Radiation Oncology, Universitätsklinikum Erlangen, FAU Er-N
[3]Erlangen Graduate School in Advanced Optical Technologies, FAU Er-N
*Both authors contributed equally.
asmaa.k.khdeir@fau.de

Training of respiratory motion models and population-based patient phantoms of the lung often requires the definition of the entire lung cavity region in the 4D-CT. To ease the workload of clinical experts, automatic selection is highly desirable. Many lung cavity extraction methods rely on a pre-segmented lung volume. We propose a simple yet fully automatic pipeline that preserves the 3D shape of the lung while also incorporating the chest wall and diaphragm, both of which carry significant respiratory information.

The proposed pipeline consists of three main parts: First, a convex-hull algorithm provides a mesh representation encompassing the lung region in continuous world coordinates. Second, raycasting w.r.t. the original dimensions returns a voxelized binary volume, and third, morphological operation includes the desired parts of the diaphragm and chest wall.

For seven 3D-CT patient datasets in end-inhale respiratory state, we evaluated the pipelines robustness against the chosen segmentation method by comparing three different initial segmentations: 1) An intensity-based method using adaptive thresholding, 2) a registration-based atlas segmentation, and 3) segmentation by a 3D fully convolutional neural network.

A dice-score increase of up to 0.167 and average pair-wise sensitivity of 91.2 % and specificity of 98.7 % show that the pipeline is reasonably robust against varying initial segmentations, indicating that a simple intensity-based method provides similar results to complex deep-learning approaches. The resulting lung cavity can find use in population models of internal organ structures or serve as a cropping mask for the ground truth of motion models.

Abstract: Percutaneous Pelvis Fixation Using the Camera-augmented C-arm

First Successes in Ex Vivo Deployment

Mathias Unberath[1,*], Javad Fotouhi[1,*], Emerson Tucker[1,*], Alex Johnson[2], Greg Osgood[2], Nassir Navab[1,3]

[1]Computer Aided Medical Procedures, Johns Hopkins University, Baltimore, USA
[2]Department for Orthopedic Surgery, Johns Hopkins Hospital, Baltimore, USA
[3]Computer Aided Medical Procedures, Technische Universität München, München
*These authors have contributed equally.
unberath@jhu.edu

Today, percutaneous techniques are widely accepted for treatment of bone fractures in spine and pelvis. These techniques are enabled by modern imaging technology, such as mobile C-arm X-ray machines, and allow for substantial reductions in blood loss, collateral tissue damage, and overall surgery duration [1]. While minimally invasive surgery is beneficial for the patient, it increases the task load for the surgeon. The main challenge is the mental alignment of patient and medical instruments to the intra-operative X-ray images [2]. This task is particularly complicated for fractures of complex anatomies, such as superior pubic ramus fractures.

Treatment of undisplaced superior pubic ramus fractures requires several K-wire placements. While advancing the K-wire through the bone, X-ray images from various perspectives are acquired to constantly validate the trajectory, as misplacement of the K-wire could cause severe damage to the external iliac artery and vein. It is not unusual that a single K-wire placement takes up to ten minutes. To assist the surgeon in understanding the spatial relations of the K-wires with respect to the anatomy, we previously proposed an augmented reality visualization system that fused live 3D information acquired using an RGBD camera attached to the C-arm with pre-operative CT volumes of the patient. This system, the so-called camera-augmented C-arm (CAMC), was successfully evaluated in simulacra motivating further efforts to deploy the system in clinical practice [3].

In this clinical track contribution, we will briefly review the CAMC system and how it benefits wire placement in complicated anatomies, report preliminary successes in deploying this technology to ex vivo procedures, and conclude with directions for future work and further improvements of our system.

References

1. Gras F, Marintschev I, Wilharm A, et al. 2D-fluoroscopic navigated percutaneous screw fixation of pelvic ring injuries-a case series. BMC Musculoskelet Disord. 2010;11(1):153.

2. Qian L, Unberath M, Yu K, et al. Towards virtual monitors for image guided interventions-real-time streaming to optical see-through head-mounted displays. arXiv preprint arXiv:171000808. 2017.
3. Tucker E, Fotouhi J, Lee SC, et al. Towards clinical translation of augmented orthopedic surgery: from pre-op CT to intra-op X-ray via RGBD sensing. Proc SPIE; p. accepted.

Abstract: Augmented Reality im Operationssaal

Stephan Vedder

Universität Heidelberg, mbits imaging GmbH
vedder@mbits.info

Die Integration präoperativer Bilddaten in den Arbeitsablauf im Operationssaal ist eine Herausforderung, die mit immer leistungsfähigeren Bildgebungsverfahren an Dringlichkeit gewinnt. Sie steht unter der Randbedingung, Bildinformationen kontextspezifisch ohne Störung des Eingriffs bereitzustellen.

Experimentelle Augmented-Reality-Techniken, bei denen präoperative Daten auf 2D-Live-Kamerabilder gerendert werden, leiden daran, dass die Erfassung der Lage des Patienten komplexe Trackingsysteme, sowie multimodale Marker erfordert, die zwischen Bildgebung und Eingriff tage- oder wochenlang am Patienten verbleiben müssen.

Durch die Nutzung einer Tiefenkamera, ergibt sich die Möglichkeit für eine markerlose Registrierung. Anhand der gewonnenen Tiefeninformationen lässt sich eine Transformation durch Surface Matching Algorithmen bestimmen. Dazu werden die von der Tiefenkamera erzeugten Tiefendaten mit den Volumendaten einer prä- oder intraoperativen Bildgebung registriert. Anhand der berechneten Transformation ist eine passgenaue Darstellung der Bilddaten auf das reguläre Kamerabild möglich.

In dieser Arbeit wurde für die Erfassung von Farb- und Tiefenbild eine Intel Realsense Kamera verwendet. Damit das Tiefenbild für den Matching Vorgang nutzbar wird, muss daraus in mehreren Vorverarbeitungsschritten eine Punktwolke berechnet werden. Für den Matching Vorgang wurden mehrere Matching Algorithmen getestet und verglichen. Dabei konnte festgestellt werden, dass die Fast Point Feature Histogramme in Kombination mit einem RANSAC Algorithmus die besten Ergebnisse hinsichtlich Performanz und Genauigkeit liefert. Auf einem durchschnittlichen Laptop können bereits mehr als 3 Registrierungen pro Sekunde bei hoher Genauigkeit berechnet werden (weniger als 5mm Translationsfehler bei einem rauschfreien Tiefenbild). Da der Matching Vorgang sehr rechenintensiv ist, kann nicht für jeden Videoframe eine Transformation berechnet werden. Um nichtsdestoweniger eine gute Darstellung zu erhalten, werden die berechneten Ergebnisse durch einen Kalman-Filter geglättet. Des Weiteren ist die Darstellung des Volumens in Echtzeit ebenfalls eine anspruchsvolle Aufgabe, weshalb dieser Vorgang optimiert wurde. Dazu wird das Volumen über Vorverarbeitung auf der GPU genau auf den benötigten Bereich beschränkt.

Es ist geplant, dass eingesetzte System im Rahmen der Eingriffsplanung in der minimal invasiven Nierentumorentfernung zu evaluieren. Ziel dieser Evaluation wird die Machbarkeit einer Zugangsplanung mit dem vorgestellten AR-System sein.

Abstract: Efficient Labeling of Optical Coherence Tomography Angiography Data using Eye Tracking

Lennart Husvogt[1,2,3], Eric Moult[2], Nadia Waheed[3], James G. Fujimoto[2], Andreas Maier[1]

[1]Pattern Recognition Lab, Friedrich-Alexander-Universität Erlangen-Nürnberg
[2]Biomedical Optical Imaging and Biophotonics Group, Massachusetts Institute of Technology, Cambridge, MA, USA
[3]New England Eye Center, Tufts Medical Center, Boston, MA, USA
lennart.husvogt@fau.de

We implemented an approach for the efficient labeling of structural and angiographic optical coherence tomography (OCT) data using eye tracking. OCT is a non-invasive imaging technology, which provides volumetric data from scattering tissues in micrometer resolution. Due to its widespread use and non-invasiveness, clinicians acquire large amounts of volumetric ophthalmic data on a daily basis. The amount of these data provides a good basis for the use of machine learning algorithms for the detection and monitoring of ophthalmic diseases and their progression. However, a challenge lies in the lack of annotation. Manual labeling of volumetric data in high resolutions is a time-consuming process. Our approach is to employ eye tracking to label larger scale pathology, such as choroidal neo-vascularization, macular edema and geographic atrophy in

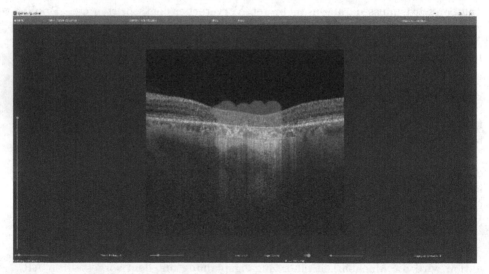

Fig. 1. Cross-sectional view of OCT data with area affected by geographic atrophy highlighted in green.

ophthalmic data. Our approach trades off pixel perfect slow labeling with faster labeling of larger regions affected by disease.

We use a commercially available GP3 eye tracker by Gazepoint [1]. The eye tracker tracks the user's eyes and triangulates the fixation point on a computer display. Cross-sections of ophthalmic data are enlarged and displayed on a screen and the user can scroll through the volumetric data. The user can look at areas affected by disease and push a button to label. Input is handled through either a keyboard or a game controller. Structural and angiography data can be displayed separately or combined by overlaying the angiography channel onto the structural channel. This allows using both channels for labeling simultaneously. Diseases such as age-related macular degeneration show prominent changes in both structure and vasculature of the affected eyes.

References

1. Gazepoint.   GP3   eye   tracker.   Accessed: 2017-11-20. https://www.gazept.com/product/gazepoint-gp3-eye-tracker/.

Abstract: Leveraging Open Source Software to Close Translational Gaps in Medical Image Computing

Jens Petersen[1,2], Sabine Heiland[1], Marti Bendszus[1], Jürgen Debus[3],
Marco Nolden[2], Caspar J. Goch[2], Klaus H. Maier-Hein[2]

[1]Dept. of Neuroradiology, Heidelberg University Hospital, Heidelberg, Germany
[2]Div. of Medical Image Computing, DKFZ, Heidelberg, Germany
[3]Dept. of Radiation Oncology, Heidelberg University Hospital, Heidelberg, Germany
jens.petersen@dkfz.de

Many imaging biomarkers (IBs) fail clinical translation. The main reason is not a lack of utility, but translational gaps [1] during validation and qualification. One important problem in this context is the landscape of existing IT systems in the clinical environment. Systems are highly heterogeneous and proprietary, causing significant translational challenges that are often purely infrastructural in nature.

We present a novel infrastructural solution that aims to facilitate the translation of state-of-the-art medical image computing research. The system was designed to fulfill a number of properties we deem essential for successful adoption: 1) It operates parallel to clinical routine and does not interfere with traditional diagnostics. 2) It is based entirely on existing open-source software and can be implemented without additional cost. 3) Deployment of novel tools requires minimal effort and does not require algorithmic knowledge from clinicians. 4) Intellectual property is protected as image data remains within the clinic and methods and models are exchanged in the form of Docker images with compiled routines. Additional benefits include scalability, both to other computing resources and to other clinical partners, and high comparability between algorithms/IBs, as they are tested in the same environment.

As a proof of concept, we applied the system to the problem of automatic segmentation and volumetry of complex brain tumors, a well-researched topic that has yet to make an impact in clinical routine. A prototype is currently being used at the Department of Neuroradiology at Heidelberg University Hospital. Segmentation algorithms can be seamlessly deployed on live clinical data, resulting in volumetric measurements that are used for standardized volumetric assessment in clinical research.

References

1. O'Connor JPB, Aboagye EO, Adams JE, et al. Imaging biomarker roadmap for cancer studies. Nat Rev Clin Oncol. 2017;14(3):169–186.

3D-CNNs for Deep Binary Descriptor Learning in Medical Volume Data

Max Blendowski, Mattias P. Heinrich

Institute of Medical Informatics, University of Lübeck
blendowski@imi.uni-luebeck.de

Abstract. Deep convolutional neural networks achieve impressive results in many computer vision tasks not least because of their representation learning abilities. The translation of these findings to the medical domain with large volumetric data e.g. CT scans with typically $\geq 10^6$ voxels is an important area of research. In particular for medical image registration, a standard analysis task, the supervised learning of expressive regional representations based on local greyvalue information is of importance to define a similarity metric. By providing discriminant binary features modern architectures can leverage special operations to compute hamming distance based similarity metrics. In this contribution we devise a 3D-Convolutional Neural Network (CNN) that can efficiently extract binary descriptors for Hamming distance-based metrics. We adopt the recently introduced Binary Tree Architectures and train a model using paired data with known correspondences. We employ a triplet objective term and extend the hinge loss with additional penalties for non-binary entries. The learned descriptors are shown to outperform state-of-the-art hand-crafted features on challenging COPD 3D-CT datasets and demonstrate their robustness for retrieval tasks under compression factors of ≈ 2000.

1 Introduction

Deep Convolutional Neural Networks (DCNNs) have obtained new breakthrough achievements on a variety of computer vision (CV) tasks. Currently, research has predominantly focused on image domains with two spatial dimensions (2D images). Developing strategies to adapt these concepts to 3D medical images such as computed tomography (CT) and magnetic resonance imaging (MRI) remains an open question, which we aim to address for correspondence retrieval tasks in this work.

The recent trend towards very deep networks with 100+ layers (e.g. ResNet, [1]) are hard to translate into the medical domain where volumetric data consumes much more memory. Image registration is an important task in the medical environment and heavily dependends on expressive local image descriptors. Here, the use of feature learning through CNNs instead of relying on handcrafted descriptor designs has great potential.

In this work, we investigate and modify a recently introduced architecture named Binary Tree Architecture [2] within the context of supervised binary decriptor learning.

We extend the Binary Tree Convolution Block Structure, that showed convincing results on 2D classification tasks with a considerably smaller number of parameters and therefore constitutes a promising foundation for 3D CNNs, by residual connections. In addition, we propose a new loss function that encourages binary output values and allows us to obtain robust and discriminant local binary descriptors for 3D lung CT images.

2   Related work

Handcrafted descriptors like the binary robust independent elementary features (BRIEF, [3]) were developed to efficiently compare image regions based on a Hamming distance, which combines the XOR- and POPCNT-operations and is computationally very efficient. The concept of patch-based local self-similarity, another descriptor design, was successfully introduced into 3D medical image processing with the binary self-similarity context decriptor (SSC) by [4] - which later serves as a benchmark.

Learning descriptors using DCNNs has clear advantages as demonstrated e.g. in [5]. However, related work in metric learning for medical images [6] is limited by requiring aligned images and has addressed the use of memory-efficient binary descriptors only in the 2D case [7]. To overcome these shortcomings, our work explores the learning of binary descriptors based on only sparse correspondences of few landmarks, which can be directly used in existing frameworks for feature-based alignment.

So far, very little research has tackled representation learning in 3D medical images and no standard choices for pretrained networks that could be employed for transfer learning have yet emerged. Existing 3D-CNN approaches e.g. for lung nodule detection [8] show promising results. Nevertheless, their training goal differs from our correspondence finding task and does not aim for binary representations. Although there are CNN-based 2D approaches for image registration like FlowNet [9], generating 3D displacement fields for medical 3D images is an even more challenging task. Yet, methods like the 2D DeepFlow algorithm [10] show that two-step approaches – composed of a separate descriptor extraction followed by a discrete flow field computation – can successfully be employed.

Considering the difficulty to generate discriminative binary 3D descriptors in the first place, we leave their straightforward integration into existing discrete registration frameworks for future work. In this work, we focus on the design, training and evaluation of a new CNN architecture, which automatically extracts binary descriptors in 3D volumes.

3   Materials and methods

Our method is illustrated in Fig. 1 (top). The overall design comprises a two-stream architecture. While the features in the upper path undergo more detailed transformations, the lower path acts as injection of minimally modified raw input data to deeper network layers. Therefore, we employ two max-pooling layers with spatial kernel sizes and strides according to the downsampling layers in the upper stream and a convolution with kernel size 1 followed by batch normalization to acquire the correct number of channels for the addition of both streams. The feature transformations before the addition in the upper path comprise a first Extended Binary Tree Block in between two downsampling blocks.

Fig. 1 (bottom) shows the architecture of an Extended Binary Tree (EBT) Block. The dashed box contains the originally proposed design by [2]. Their main motivations for this binary tree design are (i) an increase of the expressive capacity of DNNs and (ii) tackling the vanishing gradient problem. Based on the theoretical findings of [11], stating that the expressive capacity of DNNs grows exponentially in terms of depth and only polynomially with regard to the width, it is beneficial to stack many layers with small width. In EBTs the parameter growth is even smaller, since the width is continuously decreasing by a factor of 0.5 for each level of the binary tree. However, with increasing depth DNNs become harder to train, due to vanishing gradients. This encourages the concatenation of features obtained at different layers in the binary tree architecture to enable gradient flow along shorter pathways during backward steps. In order to further improve the gradients' backpropagation, we extend the original Binary Tree Architecture (BTA) with residual connections inspired by the

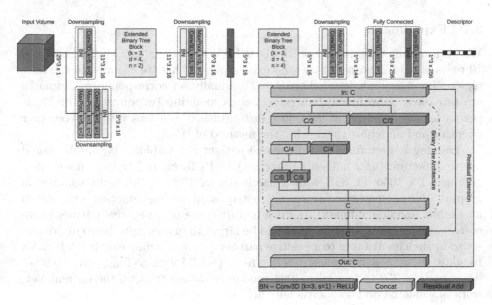

Fig. 1. Multistream-3D-CNN-Architecture and Extended Binary Tree Block.

ResNet design [1]. We therefore obtain the final output of an EBT module by $\mathbf{Y} := f_{BTA}(\mathbf{X}; \mathcal{W}) + \mathbf{X}$. The input tensor $\mathbf{X}$ and the output $\mathbf{Y}$ of an EBT block have the same dimensionality, as all intermediate features.

The computation of $f_{BTA}(\mathbf{X}; \mathcal{W})$ is fundamental for our network. This core architecture is defined by three parameters: the kernel size k, the tree depth d and the number of channels C. The root of an BTA block is the input tensor $\mathbf{X}$ itself, here denoted as $\mathbf{X}_{0,\text{left}}$. At each tree level k two mapping functions $f_{k,left}$ and $f_{k,right}$ are applied to the predeceding level's left child $\mathbf{X}_{k-1,\text{left}}$. These mapping functions both consist of a commonly used sequence: BatchNorm, convolutions filters with 3x3x3 kernels and ReLU activation. Both functions output tensors $\mathbf{X}_{k,\text{left}} = f_{k,left}(\mathbf{X}_{k-1,\text{left}}; \mathcal{W}_{k,left})$ and $\mathbf{X}_{k,\text{right}} = f_{k,right}(\mathbf{X}_{k-1,\text{left}}; \mathcal{W}_{k,right})$ with unaltered spatial dimensions but having $\frac{C}{2^k}$ channels. Finally, all right feature tensors from each level and the left feature tensor of the last level are concatenated to obtain $f_{BTA}(\mathbf{X}; \mathcal{W}) = \text{concat}(\mathbf{X}_{1,\text{right}}, ..., \mathbf{X}_{d,\text{right}}, \mathbf{X}_{d,\text{left}})$.

In our architecture we use EBT modules in the upper two-stream path of the network and after the streams are merged.

Our aim is to learn binary descriptor vectors. Therefore we use the hyperbolic tangent activation function instead of ReLU for the final fully connected layers, in order to restrict the range to $[-1, 1]$. This simplifies the adaption to the valid output set $\{-1, 1\}$, which is achieved by applying the sign function elementwise on the network's output. However, direct quantisation leads to a drastic drop in retrieval performance. We tackle this problem by incorporating an extra loss term operating on the resulting vector $\mathbf{b}$ as proposed in [11]. For each entry its absolute distance to 1 is penalized $L_{quant} = \sum_{i=1}^{bits} \||\mathbf{b}_i| - 1\|_1$

3.1 Experiments

We perform our experiments on the DIR-LAB COPD dataset [12]. It contains 10 pairs of 3D CT scans (inhale and exhale phase) that we cropped to the lung region. For every inhale-exhale pair 300 manually set corresponding landmarks are provided. Additionally, we extract corresponding keypoints in both scans per patient by detecting at least 3000 distinguished positions with the Foerstner operator and matching them using the method of [13].

Training is performed in a leave-one-patient-out fashion. We implemented our architecture (0.22 million parameters) in PyTorch and train a model on a Nvidia GTX 1050 Ti 4GB with a batch size of 128 for 25^3 input volumes in around 1.5h per patient. We employ a triplet hinge loss function - i.e. given an anchor (inhale landmark) its Euclidian distance to a negative partner (non-corresponding exhale landmark) should be larger than a margin (here empirically set to 5) than its distance to a positive partner (corresponding exhale landmark). In addition, we penalise values differing from $\{-1, 1\}$ with $\alpha \cdot L_{quant}$ ($\alpha = 0.005$). After each of 250 epochs with 4096 randomly drawn triplets, the current network is validated on two additionally held out datasets. Parameter updates are performed with the Adam optimizer and exponentially decreasing learning rates from 0.003 to 0.0001. The number of consecutive EBT modules ($n = 2, n = 4$)

used in our architecture was found empirically. Our network compresses the greyvalue information of 25^3 volumes with 32bit float values into 256bit descriptors, i.e. by a factor of ≈ 2000. Computing the 300 inhale and around 3000-9000 exhale descriptors per patient together with the kNN search takes less than 5 seconds.

4   Results

For each patient, we evaluate the descriptor retrieval performance for the 300 manually set landmarks of the inhale phase. To demonstrate the robustness of the learned representation, we investigate if the correct corresponding exhale landmark can be found inside the next k-nearest neighbours (kNN) from the set of all landmarks and keypoints in the exhale phase. The kNN are determined by Hamming distances. Fig. 2 (left) shows the mean retrieval performance of our trained descriptors (blue) in comparison the benchmark SSC descriptor [4] (red) quantising 48 patch-distances to the same number of bits (256). E.g. the retrieval rate @k=10 improved from 43% (SSC) to 74% (ours). However, without the usage of the quantisation loss the rate @k=10 drops to ~60%. Fig. 2 (right) demonstrates the evolution of descriptor entries towards a binary distribution due to the additional loss term.

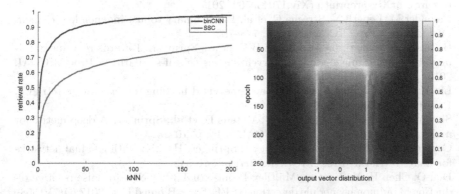

Fig. 2. l: Retrieval rate: Ours vs. SSC; r: Normalized CNN output value distribution.

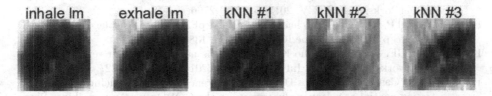

Fig. 3. (slices from left to right) inhale landmark, corresponding target exhale landmark, top 3 kNN search results; corresponding landmark found at kNN#1.

5 Discussion

In our experiments we demonstrate that our network architecture is able to produce descriptors readily usable for landmark retrieval tasks even in the presence of highly non-rigid deformations usually occurring due to breathing-induced lung motion. Our learned descriptors clearly outperform the handcrafted SSC features by a large margin, encouraging further research towards an incorporation of this method into discrete medical image registration frameworks - to this end leveraging a fully convolutional architecture for dense descriptor computations. Finally, our proposed extended binary tree modules could well be employed for other tasks since they are straightforward to implement and exhibit sufficient expressive capacity while using a moderate number of parameters.

Acknowledgement. This work was supported by the German Research Foundation (DFG) under grant number 320997906 (HE 7364/2-1).

References

1. He K, Zhang X, Ren S, et al. Deep residual learning for image recognition. Proc ICCV. 2016; p. 770–778.
2. Zhang Y, Ozay M, Li S, et al. Truncating wide networks using binary tree architectures. arXiv preprint arXiv:170400509. 2017.
3. Calonder M, Lepetit V, Strecha C, et al. Brief: binary robust independent elementary features. Proc ECCV. 2010; p. 778–792.
4. Heinrich MP, Jenkinson M, Papie z BW, et al.; Springer. Towards realtime multimodal fusion for image-guided interventions using self-similarities. Proc MICCAI. 2013; p. 187–194.
5. Liu H, Wang R, Shan S, et al. Deep supervised hashing for fast image retrieval. Proc ICCV. 2016; p. 2064–2072.
6. Simonovsky M, Gutiérrez-Becker B, Mateus D, et al.; Springer. A deep metric for multimodal registration. Proc MICCAI. 2016; p. 10–18.
7. Conjeti S, Roy AG, Katouzian A, et al.; Springer. Hashing with residual networks for image retrieval. Proc MICCAI. 2017; p. 541–549.
8. Dou Q, Chen H, Yu L, et al. Multilevel contextual 3-D CNNs for false positive reduction in pulmonary nodule detection. IEEE Trans Biomed Eng. 2017;64(7):1558–1567.
9. Dosovitskiy A, Fischer P, Ilg E, et al. Flownet: Learning optical flow with convolutional networks. Proc ICCV. 2015; p. 2758–2766.
10. Weinzaepfel P, Revaud J, Harchaoui Z, et al. DeepFlow: Large displacement optical flow with deep matching. Proc ICCV. 2013; p. 1385–1392.
11. Montufar GF, Pascanu R, Cho K, et al. On the number of linear regions of deep neural networks. Adv Neural Inf Process Syst. 2014; p. 2924–2932.
12. Castillo R, Castillo E, Fuentes D, et al. A reference dataset for deformable image registration spatial accuracy evaluation using the COPDgene study archive. Phys Med Biol. 2013;58(9):2861.
13. Heinrich MP, Handels H, Simpson IJ; Springer. Estimating large lung motion in COPD patients by symmetric regularised correspondence fields. Proc MICCAI. 2015; p. 338–345.

Detecting and Measuring Surface Area of Skin Lesions

Houman Mirzaalian-Dastjerdi[1,2], Dominique Töpfer[2], Michael Bangemann[3], Andreas Maier[1]

[1]Department of Computer Science 5, University of Erlangen-Nürnberg
[2]Softgate GmbH, Erlangen
[6]Praxisnetz Nürnberg Süd e.V.
houman.mirzaalian@fau.de

Abstract. The treatment of skin lesions of various kinds is a common task in clinical routine. Apart from wound care, the assessment of treatment efficacy plays an important role. Fully manual measurements and documentation of the healing process can be very cumbersome and imprecise. Existing technical solutions often require the user to delineate the lesion manually and rarely provide information on measurement precision or accuracy. We propose a method for segmenting and measuring lesions using a single image. Surface area of lesions on bent surfaces is estimated based on a paper ruler. Only roughly outlining the region of interest is required. Wound segmention evaluation was performed on 10 images, resulting in an accuracy of 0.98 ± 0.02. For surface measuring evaluation on 40 phantom images we found an absolute error of $0.32 \pm 0.27\,\mathrm{cm}^2$ and a relative error of $5.2 \pm 4.3\,\%$.

1 Introduction

Due to the prevalence of diseases such as diabetes, pressure ulcers etc., dealing with skin lesions is a common and frequent task in clinical routine. For monitoring treatment efficacy it is important to be able to measure the area of the skin lesion precisely. As pure manual methods (measuring width and height and approximating the shape by a rectangle or ellipse) are imprecise and cumbersome, a great deal of effort has gone into developing (semi-)automated techniques. In [1], a transparent grid film is placed on the lesion and its contour is marked manually. This allows for a more precise determination of the surface area, however, it is also time-consuming and due to direct contact of the film with the lesion, it may hurt the patient. Modern techniques such as laser scanners are requiring costly additional equipment [2]. That is why photographic techniques have gained more and more attention. In addition to already commercially available tools using manual delineation, there have been recent attempts to make use of 3D reconstructions from multiple images. The 3D model provides geometric information for measuring [3, 4]. The aim of this work is to investigate an easy, fast and low cost segmentation tool with high measurement accuracy. We propose a new method for both lesion segmentation and surface measurement based

29

on a single image taken with a commercial handheld digital camera or smartphone. From only one image, less information can be obtained than from a 3D model, especially in case of the wound being on a curved surface. For helping to estimate the local scale of the image even for curved surfaces, a flexible paper ruler is used.

2   Material and methods

Our approach comprises two main steps, wound segmentation and lesion surface area calculation. As only a single image is used, some conditions must be met during image acquisition for keeping the measurement error as low as possible. 1) The camera shall be perpendicular to the wound surface. 2) The wound shall be located in the center of the image (for minimizing lens distortion). 3) The ruler has to be placed parallel to the largest wound diameter as close as possible to it. Ideally, it should also reflect the curvature of the surface.

2.1   Wound segmentation

The user needs to provide a region of interest (ROI) including only wound and skin by drawing a contour (Fig. 1(a)). For classifying the pixels in the ROI into the classes skin and wound, a Random Forest (RF) classifier has been trained. Feature vectors were generated by applying a filter bank consisting of Gaussian, Difference of Gaussian, Sobel and Hessian filter using different values for the standard deviation.

The output of the RF is a probability map defining how likely it is that a single pixel belongs to wound or skin. Otsu's thresholding is applied to generate a binary mask. Finally, everything outside the ROI is discarded (Fig. 2).

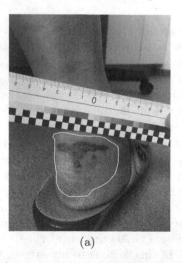 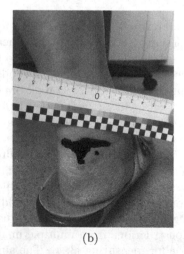

(a)   (b)

Fig. 1. (a) Paper ruler and selected region of interest shown with yellow contour. (b) The ground truth image obtained using the modified Random Walker.

To facilitate creating the ground truth masks for training the RF, the Random Walker algorithm [5], with modified edge weight function based on Quaternion Color Curvature (QCC) [6] has been used (Fig. 1(b)).

2.2 Surface area measurement

For surface area calculation, the ruler should be first detected. As shown in (Fig. 3(a)), the ruler contains a checkboard pattern with known size for easy detection. The Structure Tensor filter is used for dividing the image into uniform regions, corners, and edges according to the tensor's eigenvalues [7] for each pixel. The high eigenvalues roughly correspond to the ruler skeleton shown in (Fig. 3(b)) and the low eigenvalues to corner points (Fig. 3(c)). Identification of checkboard points is based on comparing intensities in a region around the points. Fitting a curve to the local maxima of the distance transform of the points seperates them to upper and lower points (Fig. 3(d)). Moving along this curve allows finding pairs of corresponding points by detecting intensity changes across checkerboard edges. (Fig. 3(c)).

For obtaining the local measurement parameters, a heuristical approach is used: Consider two corresponding points (p_1, p_2) as shown in (Fig. 3(c)). Along the line defined by p_1 and p_2, points $p_3, p_4, \ldots$ are placed equidistantly using $d = \|p_1 - p_2\|_2$. Extrapolating each pair of points, a grid pattern covering the wound is obtained. For measuring, each quadrilateral in the grid is unwarped from perspective distortion [8] and mapped to a square. As the "true" size of the square is known from the definition of the ruler, measuring comes down to counting the wound pixels covered by the square and using the formula

$$A_w = \frac{N_w}{N} \cdot \text{area of square} \tag{1}$$

where N is the total number of pixels and N_w is the number of wound pixels in the square. Adding these results for all squares yields the surface area of the lesion.

Evaluation We recieved 50 images of skin lesions from clinical routine. They were not taken under controlled conditions and by different persons with different commercially available (smartphone) cameras. For training the RF, this

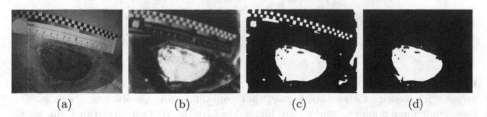

(a)   (b)   (c)   (d)

Fig. 2. (a) Original image. (b) Probability map (result of Random Forest classifier). (c) Result of Otsu's filter. (d) Segmentation result after applying the ROI.

32   Mirzaalian-Dastjerdi et al.

set of images was split into a training set of 40 images and a test set of 10 images. Splitting was done manually as the set contained multiple images for some patients. These images were all put in the training set.

As we do not know the true size of the lesions in the clinical images, evaluation of the measurements was performed using phantom images showing a geometric shape with known surface area (Fig. 3(a)). Forty phantom images with different geometric shapes of different sizes (ranging from 1.13–17.22 cm^2 were taken with an iPhone7's camera. For simulating practical use we also bent the shapes around cylindrical objects of different curvature and varied the angle of the camera slightly.

3   Results

For wound segmentation, we found a mean accuracy, sensitivity and specificity of 0.98 ± 0.02, 0.89 ± 0.13 and 0.99 ± 0.01, respectively, where accuracy is defined as the proportion of correctly classified pixels according to the ground truth. Fig. 4 shows a plot of these three values for each of the test images. Fig. 5 depicts three different results of segmented wounds.

For the measurement evaluation based on the phantom images we found an absolute error of 0.32 ± 0.27 cm^2 and a relative error of 5.2 ± 4.3 %. Tab. 1 shows the results grouped into flat images and images with lower and higher curvature.

Among these 40 images, 16 images consisted of eight pairs showing the same shape with slightly different size (differences ranging from 0.43 to 1.22 cm^2 and 7

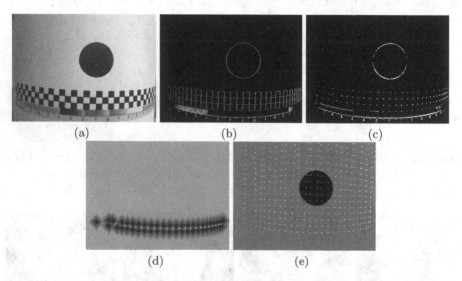

Fig. 3. (a) Phantom image. (b) Result of structure tensor filter containing high eigenvalues. (c) Result of structure tensor filter containing low eigenvalues. Two corresponding corner points p_1 and p_2 are highlighted (red). (d) Distance transform, local maxima shown with white points. (e) Obtained grid pattern and "wound segmentation" (black circle).

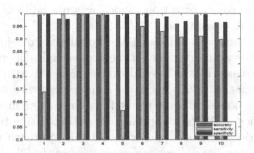

Fig. 4. The accuracy (red), sensitivity (green) and specificity (blue) parameters of wound segmentation of 10 patient wound images (bars were truncated for better visualization).

Table 1. Results for ruler-based measurements. Values for absolute and relative error are given as mean ± standard deviation.

Type of Image	absolute error (cm²)	relative error (%)	Min Area (cm²)	Max Area (cm²)
Flat (N=20)	0.23±0.21	4.54±4.86	2.80	17.22
Low Curvature (N=12)	0.42±0.34	5.03±2.98	1.13	9.73
High Curvature (N=8)	0.39±0.23	7.28±3.63	2.80	8.98
All (N=40)	0.32±0.27	5.24±4.29	1.13	17.22

to 15 %). The true mean of surface areas in the group of smaller shapes was $\mu_s = 5.57\,\mathrm{cm}^2$ compared to $\mu_l = 6.33\,\mathrm{cm}^2$ for the group of larger shapes. Even though the measurements reflect this difference ($\bar{\mu}_s = 5.73\,\mathrm{cm}^2$ and $\bar{\mu}_l = 6.52\,\mathrm{cm}^2$), a paired, one-tailed t-test did not yield a significant difference.

3.1 Discussion and conclusion

We presented first results of our method for segmenting and measuring skin lesions from a single image with acceptable error also for lesions on a bent surface. A limitation of this study is the small number of data. For segmentation we only could test our method on 10 images and a proper cross-validation was not possible due to having multiple images of the same lesion. Skin lesions are greatly varying in appearance (color and texture), so the approach must be tested using

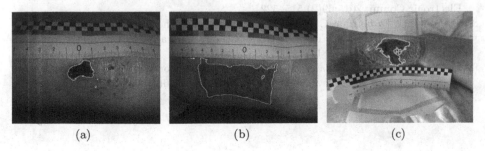

(a)	(b)	(c)

Fig. 5. (a) and (b) Examples of good segmentations. (c) A weak segmentation result (the red region is misclassified as wound).

more training and test images. Also color correction (which was not addressed in this article) may help stabilizing the results [4].

For measuring the area, our method is still lacking the possibility to reject images not taken perpendicular to the wound surface. If the angle is only slightly changed, the errors can quickly increase. It was beyond the scope of this study, addressing this problem more systematically. Also here the sample size was quite small, which also could explain the non-significant result for detecting changes in surface area. We have also studied a different approach for extrapolating the ruler points based on the cross ratio [9]; as we quickly found this approach to be less stable and to have greater error, we did not pursue it further. In [3], the announced measurement error is approximately 10% for available photographic techniques and the precision may vary with wound size. We found comparable results for our method, however, so far we have only addressed evaluation based on phantom images. Also, a systematic precision analysis was out of the scope of this work, due to the small amount of clinical images that contained the ruler.

Providing a method for rejecting images taken from great angles and tools for correcting failed segmentations could improve our approach. Further research with more data is necessary for validating this method.

References

1. Foltynski P, Ladyzynski P, Wojcicki JM. A new smartphone-based method for wound area measurement. Artific Organs. 2014;38(4):346–352.
2. Liu X, Kim W, Schmidt R, et al. Wound measurement by curvature maps: a feasibility study. Phys Measure. 2006;27(11):1107.
3. Treuillet S, Albouy B, Lucas Y. Three-dimensional assessment of skin wounds using a standard digital camera. IEEE Trans Med Imaging. 2009;28(5):752–762.
4. Wannous H, Lucas Y, Treuillet S. Enhanced assessment of the wound-healing process by accurate multiview tissue classification. IEEE Trans Med Imaging. 2011;30(2):315–326.
5. Grady L. Random walks for image segmentation. IEEE Trans Pattern Anal Machine Intell. 2006;28(11):1768–1783.
6. Shi L, Funt B, Hamarneh G. Quaternion color curvature. In: Color and Imaging Conference. vol. 2008. Society for Imaging Science and Technology; 2008. p. 338–341.
7. Baghaie A, Yu Z. Structure tensor based image interpolation method. AEU Int J Electronic Comm. 2015;69(2):515–522.
8. Jagannathan L, Jawahar C. Perspective correction methods for camera based document analysis. In: Proc. First Int. Workshop on Camera-based Document Analysis and Recognition; 2005. p. 148–154.
9. Lei G. Recognition of planar objects in 3-D space from single perspective views using cross ratio. IEEE Trans Robotic Automat. 1990;6(4):432–437.

Abstract: Deep Hashing for Large-Scale Medical Image Retrieval

Sailesh Conjeti[1,2], Magdalini Paschali[2], Abhijit Guha Roy[2,3], Nassir Navab[2,4]

[1] Deutsches Zentrum für Neurodegenerative Erkrankungen (DZNE), Bonn, Germany
[2]Computer Aided Medical Procedures, Technische Universität München, Germany.
[2]AI-med, Ludwig-Maximilian Universität München, Germany.
[4]Computer Aided Medical Procedures, Johns Hopkins University, USA.
sailesh.conjeti@dzne.de

Adoption of content-based image retrieval systems (CBIR) requires efficient indexing of the data contents in order to respond to visual queries without explicitly relying on textual keywords. Searching for similar data is closely related to the fundamental problem of nearest neighbor search. Exhaustive comparison of a query across the database is infeasible in large-scale retrieval as it is computationally expensive [1]. Towards this, we propose scalable image retrieval techniques that employing hashing to learn semantics-preserving binary codes for indexing and retrieval. We leverage deep learning for end-to-end learning of hash-codes that are tailored for retrieval in large-scale medical image databases. Developing medical image CBIR systems is particularly challenging due to variability in image acquisition (contrast agents, protocol variations), anatomical variability, high-dimensionality of the data etc. We recently introduced Deep Residual Hashing (DRH) [2] and Deep Multiple Instance Hashing (DMIH) [3] which are deep hashing methods for medical image retrieval. DRH uses residual networks that terminate in dedicated binarization layers that generate hash-codes. It was trained with a multi-class variant of neighborhood component analysis (NCA) with dedicated losses such as quantization and bit-balance to improve hash code quality. DMIH extends DRH to a scenario of multiple instance learning by introduction of the multiple-instance pooling layer that aggregates representations from across member instances within a bag of samples. The aforementioned deep hashing methods were exhaustively validated and their fidelity was demonstrated on scenarios of retrieval on highly heterogeneous databases with significant population variability such as cardiopulmonary chest X-rays, breast mammography and breast histology, with highly competitive retrieval time (< 100 ms).

References

1. Conjeti S, Katouzian A, Kazi A, et al. Metric hashing forests. Med Image Anal. 2016;34:13–29.
2. Conjeti S, Roy AG, Katouzian A, et al.; Springer. Hashing with residual networks for image retrieval. Proc MICCAI. 2017; p. 541–549.
3. Conjeti S, Paschali M, Katouzian A, et al. Deep multiple instance hashing for scalable medical image retrieval. Proc MICCAI. 2017; p. 550–558.

Abstract: Physiological Parameter Estimation from Multispectral Images Unleashed

Sebastian J. Wirkert[1], Anant S. Vemuri[1], Hannes G. Kenngott[2],
Sara Moccia[1,3,4], Michael Götz[2][5], Benjamin F. B. Mayer[2],
Klaus H. Maier-Hein[5], Daniel S. Elson[6,7], Lena Maier-Hein[1]

[1] Div. of Computer Assisted Medical Interventions, DKFZ, Heidelberg, Germany
[2] Dept. for General, Visceral and Transplantation Surgery, Heidelberg University
Hospital, Germany
[3] Dept. of Advanced Robotics, Istituto Italiano di Tecnologia, Genoa, Italy
[4] Dept. of Electronics, Information and Bioengineering, Politecnico di Milano, Italy
[5] Div. for Medical and Biological Informatics, DKFZ, Heidelberg, Germany
[6] Hamlyn Centre for Robotic Surgery, Imperial College London, UK
[7] Dept. of Surgery and Cancer, Imperial College London, UK
`s.wirkert@dkfz-heidelberg.de`

Multispectral imaging in laparoscopy can provide tissue reflectance measurements for each point in the image at multiple wavelengths of light. These reflectances encode information on important physiological parameters not visible to the naked eye. Fast decoding of the data during surgery, however, remains challenging. While model-based methods suffer from inaccurate base assumptions, a major bottleneck related to competing machine learning-based solutions is the lack of labelled training data. In this paper, we address this issue with the first transfer learning-based method to physiological parameter estimation from multispectral images. It relies on a highly generic tissue model that aims to capture the full range of optical tissue parameters that can potentially be observed in vivo. Adaptation of the model to a specific clinical application based on unlabelled in vivo data is achieved using a new concept of domain adaptation that explicitly addresses the high variance often introduced by conventional covariance-shift correction methods. According to comprehensive in silico and in vivo experiments our approach enables accurate parameter estimation for various tissue types without the need for incorporating specific prior knowledge on optical properties and could thus pave the way for many exciting applications in multispectral laparoscopy.

This work was first presented at MICCAI 2017 [1].

Literaturverzeichnis

1. Wirkert SJ, Vemuri AS, Kenngott HG, et al. Physiological parameter estimation from multispectral images unleashed. In: Medical Image Computing and Computer-Assisted Intervention - MICCAI 2017. Lect Notes Comput Sci. Springer, Cham; 2017. p. 134–141.

Abstract: Probabilistic Appearance Models for Medical Image Analysis

Julia Krüger, Jan Ehrhardt, Heinz Handels

Institute of Medical Informatics, Universitat zu Lübeck
krueger@imi.uni-luebeck.de

The identification of one-to-one point correspondences between image objects is one key aspect and at the same time the most challenging part of generating statistical shape and appearance models. Using probabilistic correspondences between samples instead of accurately placed landmarks for shape models [1] eliminated the need of extensive and time consuming landmark and correspondence determination, and furthermore, the dependency of the quality of the generated model on potentially wrong correspondences was reduced.

Recently, we represented a probabilistic approach for statistical appearance models, using probabilistic instead of one-to-one correspondences [2]. The basis of the presented approach is a sparse representation of images by a set of independent feature vectors that combine position and appearance information. The optimization problem for the generation of a model as well as the model adaption to an image is formulated using a single global optimization criterion, which is derived from a MAP-approach with respect to model parameters that directly affect shape and appearance of the considered object. The criterion is minimized by means of an expectation maximization approach that alternates between the estimation of the correspondence probabilities and the optimization of the model parameters. Thereby, analytical closed form solutions can be derived for the optimization for all the parameters.

The advantages of the proposed method include: (1) eliminated preprocessing/predefinition of landmark correspondences, (2) increased robustness for non-corresponding regions in corrupted training or test data, (3) additional information given by correspondence probabilities, (4) closed form solution for model generation and adaption. Without the need for additional measures or methods the approach can be naturally applied to a variety of problems, among other, multi-organ segmentation, image reconstruction, model generation based on partial/corrupted training data, and detection and classification of pathological image regions.

Acknowledgement. This work is supported by the DFG (HA 2355/7-2).

References

1. Hufnagel H, Pennec X, Ehrhardt J, et al. Generation of a statistical shape model with probabilistic point correspondences and the expectation maximization-iterative closest point algorithm. IJCARS. 2008;2:265 – 273.

2. Krüger J, Ehrhardt J, Handels H. Statistical appearance models based on probabilistic correspondences. Med Image Anal. 2017;37:146 – 159.

Abstract: Robust Multi-Scale Anatomical Landmark Detection in Incomplete 3D-CT Data

Florin C. Ghesu[1,2], Bogdan Georgescu[1], Sasa Grbic[1], Andreas Maier[2],
Joachim Hornegger[2], Dorin Comaniciu[1]

[1]Siemens Healthineers, Medical Imaging Technologies, Princeton, NJ, USA
[2]Pattern Recognition Lab, Friedrich-Alexander-Universität, Erlangen, Germany
`florin.c.ghesu@fau.de`

An essential prerequisite for comprehensive medical image analysis is the robust and fast detection of anatomical structures in the human body. To this point, machine learning techniques are most often applied to address this problem, exploiting large annotated image databases to estimate parametric models for anatomy appearance. However, the performance of these methods is generally limited, due to suboptimal and exhaustive search strategies applied on large volumetric image data, e.g., 3D-CT scans. Most importantly, these techniques do not effectively address cases of incomplete data, i.e., scans taken with a partial field-of-view. We address these challenges by unifying the anatomy appearance model and the search strategy in the form of a behavior-learning task. This is solved using the capabilities of deep reinforcement learning with multi-scale image analysis and robust statistical shape modeling [1]. These mechanisms enable the teaching of intelligent artificial agents to find and follow optimal navigation paths in the image scale-space, that converge to the locations of target anatomical structures. At the same time, such navigation paths can account for missing structures to ensure the robust and spatially-coherent detection of the observed anatomical landmarks. Finally, we show how the identified landmarks can be used as robust guidance in estimating the extent of the body-region, captured by the CT scan. Experiments demonstrate that our solution outperforms a state-of-the-art deep learning method in detecting different anatomical structures, without any failure, on a dataset of over 2300 3D-CT volumes. In particular, our method achieves 0% false-positive and 0% false-negative rates at detecting the landmarks or recognizing their absence from the field-of-view of the scan. Most importantly, the detection-time of the reference method is reduced by 15−20 times to under 40 ms, an unmatched real-time performance for large 3D-CT data.

References

1. Ghesu FC, Georgescu B, Grbic S, et al. Robust multi-scale anatomical landmark detection in incomplete 3D-CT data. Proc MICCAI. 2017;Part I:194–202.

Abstract: Exploring Sparsity in CNNs for Medical Image Segmentation
BRIEFnet

Mattias P. Heinrich[1], Ozan Oktay[2]

[1]Institut für Medizinische Informatik, Universität zu Lübeck
[2]Biomedical Image Analysis Group, Imperial College London
heinrich@imi.uni-luebeck.de

Deep convolutional neural networks can evidently achieve astonishing accuracies for multiple medical image analysis tasks, in particular segmentation and detection. However, the actual translation of deep learning into clinical practice is so far very limited, in part because their extensive computations rely on specialised GPU hardware that is not easily available in clinical environments.

In our recent MICCAI paper [1], we proposed a new architecture *BRIEFnet*[1] that uses very sparse, binary convolutions and thereby substantially reduces the model complexity. It can be trained from scratch in few minutes and enables inference in few seconds on a CPU. The approach separates the convolution operation into a sparse, binary sampling of few locations within an arbitrarily large receptive field followed by a nonlinearity and a channel-wise 1×1 convolution (Fig. 1). In contrast to previous fully convolutional networks, no contracting path or pooling layers are required and the number of trainable weights is reduced by orders of magnitude. We validated the BRIEFnet on a challenging dataset [2] for the segmentation of the pancreas and achieve state-of-the-art accuracy, outperforming approaches with dilated convolutions or multi-resolution architectures.

References

1. Heinrich MP, Oktay O. BRIEFnet: Deep pancreas segmentation using binary sparse convolutions. In: Proc MICCAI. Springer; 2017. p. 329–337.

---

[1] Implementation available at http://github.com/mattiaspaul/BRIEFnet

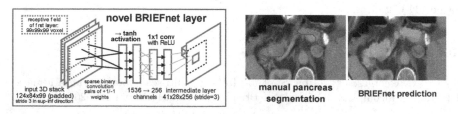

Fig. 1. Concept of sparse binary CNN block that achieves 64.5% Dice for 3D pancreas segmentation when incorporated into light-weight dual-path network.

2. Xu Z, Lee CP, et al. Evaluation of six registration methods for the human abdomen on clinically acquired CT. IEEE Trans Biomed Eng. 2016;63(8):1563–1572.

Abstract: Fast MRI Whole Brain Segmentation with Fully Convolutional Neural Networks

Abhijit Guha Roy[1,2], Sailesh Conjeti[2,3], Nassir Navab[2,4], Christian Wachinger[1]

[1]Artificial Intelligence in Medical Imaging (AI-Med), KJP, LMU München, Germany.
[2]Computer Aided Medical Procedures, Technische Universität München, Germany.
[3]German Center for Neurodegenerative Diseases (DZNE), Bonn, Germany.
[4]Computer Aided Medical Procedures, Johns Hopkins University, USA.
abhijit.guha-roy@tum.de

Whole brain segmentation from structural MRI-T1 scan is a prerequisite for most morphological analyses, but requires hours of processing time and therefore delays the availability of image markers after scan acquisition. We introduced a fully convolution neural network (F-CNN) that segments a brain scan in several seconds [1]. Training deep F-CNNs for semantic image segmentation requires access to abundant labeled data. While large datasets of unlabeled image data are available in medical applications, access to manually labeled data is very limited. To aid training of this complex network with limited data, we propose to pre-train on auxiliary labels created from existing segmentation software *FreeSurfer* [2]. The network is pre-trained on a large dataset with auxiliary labels and then fine-tuned with a small dataset with manual annotations [1]. The architecture consist of 3 encoder-decoder based 2D F-CNNs, segmenting slices along coronal, axial and sagittal axes. These predictions are aggregated to obtain the final segmentation. Dense connections are introduced within each encoder/decoder block to promote feature re-usability and ease of training. Apart from these, long skip connections and unpooling layers for upsampling in the decoder are used. The network is learnt by optimizing a joint loss function of weighted Logistic loss and Dice loss. The weights are set to tackle class imbalance and to encourage reliable contour estimation. In an extensive set of evaluations on several datasets that cover a wide age range, pathology, and different scanners, we demonstrated that our method achieves robust and superior performance to state-of-the-art atlas based methods, while being orders of magnitude faster. This drastic speed up greatly facilitates the processing of large data repositories and enables wide spread integration of imaging biomarkers in the routine clinical practice by making them almost instantaneously available.

References

1. Error corrective boosting for learning fully convolutional networks with limited data. Springer 2017.
2. Whole brain segmentation: automated labeling of neuroanatomical structures in the human brain. In Neuron; 2002.

Patient Surface Model and Internal Anatomical Landmarks Embedding

Xia Zhong[1], Norbert Strobel[2,4], Annette Birkhold[2], Markus Kowarschik[2], Rebecca Fahrig[2], Andreas Maier[1,3]

[1]Pattern Recognition Lab, FAU Erlangen-Nürnberg
[2]Siemens Healthcare GmbH, Forchheim Germany
[3]Erlangen Graduate School in Advanced Optical Technologies(SAOT)
[4]Fakultät für Elektrotechnik, Hochschule für angewandte Wissenschaften Würzburg-Schweinfurt
xia.zhong@fau.de

Abstract. The patient surface model has shown to be a useful asset to improve existing diagnostic and interventional tasks in a clinical environment. For example, in combination with RGB-D cameras, a patient surface model can be used to automate and accelerate the diagnostic imaging workflow, manage patient dose, and provide navigation assistance. A shortcoming of today's patient surface models, however, is that, internal anatomical landmarks are not present. In this paper, we introduce a method to estimate internal anatomical landmarks based on the surface model of a patient. Our method relies on two major steps. First, we fit a template surface model is to a segmented surface of a CT dataset with annotated internal landmarks using keypoint and feature descriptor based rigid alignment and atlas-based non-rigid registration. In a second step, we find for each internal landmark a neighborhood on the template surface and learn a generalized linear embedding between neighboring surface vertices in the template and the internal landmark. We trained and evaluated our method using cross-validation in 20 datasets over 50 internal landmarks. We compared the performance of four different generalized linear models. The best mean estimation error over all the landmarks was achieved using the lasso regression method with a mean error of 12.19 ± 6.98 mm.

1 Introduction

Patient modeling has shown great potential in medical applications. One reason is that RGB-D cameras have become more easily available. For example, in the diagnostic environment, Singh et al. [1] demonstrated that a patient surface model can be fitted to the patient using a RGB-D camera ahead of CT scans to automate and accelerate the workflow. In the interventional environment, a patient surface model was used to estimate the skin dose [2], monitor the breathing motion, or provide navigation assistance [3]. The patient model used in these applications is a surface model. Related activities described in the literature derive an articulated skeleton [4], model the shape of the surface model and compare different estimation methods [5]. Unfortunately, clinical relevant internal anatomical landmarks are not included in the surface model, as it only models the outer shape of a patient.

In this paper, we propose a method for finding internal landmarks of the human body e.g. vertebra, based on a surface model and evaluate its accuracy. Once internal landmarks are found, we can embed an appropriately adjusted spine model into the surface model. As organs have a fixed position relative to the spine, fitting a spine model to a surface model can, for example, be used for organ-specific positioning of a C-arm system.

2   Materials and methods

Our learning-based method embeds the internal landmarks into a patient surface model. We use CT datasets with annotated landmarks to train our method. For each CT data set, the surface is segmented and represented as a surface mesh x. We register a template surface model $\hat{x}$ to this segmented surface. Afterwards, we learn the mapping function $\mathcal{M}_i$ to establish the relation between model $\hat{x}$ and associated landmark l such that

$$\mathcal{M}_i = \arg \min_{\mathcal{M}_i} \sum_t \| l_{t,i} - \mathcal{M}_i(\hat{x}_t) \|_2^2 \qquad (1)$$

2.1   Surface model registration and fitting

We first trained an Atlas for the patient model using the Civilian American and European Surface Anthropometry Resource Project (CAESAR) data. Using an active shape model (ASM), a patient surface model can be described as $\hat{x}_t = \bar{x} + Db_t$, where the $\bar{x}$ is the mean surface model in the atlas, D describes a matrix comprising the modes of variation, and b_t is the associated weighting vector. Then, for each segmented surface model x_t, we need to find the best fitting weighting vector b_t and associated rigid transformation $\mathcal{T}_t$ by minimizing

$$b_t, \mathcal{T}_t = \arg \min_{b, \mathcal{T}} \mathcal{D} \left(x - \mathcal{T}(\bar{x} + Db) \right)^2 \qquad (2)$$

In Eq. (2), the function $\mathcal{D}$ calculates the minimal distance between two meshes. To solve this minimization problem efficiently, we rely on alternating minimization. We first estimate the transformation $\mathcal{T}$ based on a given b. This is a well-known surface mesh rigid registration problem and can be solved using feature descriptors e.g. HoG, SPIN, and LDSIFT [6] and feature matching. The challenge in our case is that the two meshes may partially overlap and the deformation between two meshes may be non-rigid. As patients usually are positioned head first, supine, i.e., are on their back, the outer shape of the patient may potentially lack distinctive key points. To establish correspondences between feature points robustly, we first sample the key points as propsed by

Surface Model with Internal Landmarks 45

Sahillioğlu et al. [7], such that the sampling is almost uniform. In this way, we avoid accumulation of feature points in high curvature regions when identifying key points. For each key point, we calculate the LDSIFT feature descriptor, which is robust to non-rigid deformations [6]. We further incorporate the prior knowledge, that the transformation $\mathcal{T}$ comprises mainly translations and that rotation is very limited. In our actual implementation, we divided the surface mesh into eight primary districts using the principal axis of the mesh, and rejected any cross-district matching. Due to the non-rigid deformation between two meshes, we may find ambiguity in rigid transformation. To counteract this effect, we consider all feasible results using RANSAC as motion cluster and use mean shift algorithm to search the cluster center of the biggest cluster. This cluster center is used as our motion estimation $\mathcal{T}_t$. Knowing the transformation $\mathcal{T}_t$, the weighting factor $\boldsymbol{b}_t$ can be estimated by minimizing

$$\boldsymbol{b}_t = \arg\min_{\boldsymbol{b}} \mathcal{D}\left(\boldsymbol{x} - \mathcal{T}_t(\bar{\boldsymbol{x}} + \boldsymbol{D}\boldsymbol{b})\right)^2 + \alpha_1 \mathcal{R}\left(\boldsymbol{x}, \hat{\boldsymbol{x}}\right) \tag{3}$$

where the scalar α is a parameter, and the function $\mathcal{R}$ calculates the overlap ratio between the segmented and the estimated surface mesh. This function regularizes the minimization problem such that the estimated surface will not be degenerated. After this step, the residual error between estimated and segmented surface is minimized using non-rigid mesh registration, as proposed by Allen et al. [8].

2.2 Surface and internal landmark embedding

After fitting the surface model $\hat{\boldsymbol{x}}$ to the segmented CT surface $\boldsymbol{x}$, we look for the mapping $\mathcal{M}_i$ between $\hat{\boldsymbol{x}}$ and the annotated internal landmarks l_i in CT data sets. For the ith landmark in the tth CT data $l_{t,i}$, we assume that the landmark position (coordinates) can be expressed as a generalized linear combination of neighboring vertices $\hat{\boldsymbol{x}}_{t,j} \in \mathcal{N}(l_i)$. The neighborhood is defined using k-nearest neighbor with Mahalanobis metric. We used the covariance matrix of the surface model $\boldsymbol{x}$ to calculate the Mahalanobis distance. We select a large neighborhood such that the residual error due to non-linearity in mapping is minimized. The number and indicies of neighborhood vertices can vary in each data set. We use the unions according to the indicies as the neighborhood for each internal landmark. To describe this more formally, we introduce matrix $\boldsymbol{X}_{\mathcal{N}(l_i)} = [X_{1,\mathcal{N}(l_i)}^T, \cdots, X_{N,\mathcal{N}(l_i)}^T]^T$ and matrix $\boldsymbol{L}_i = [l_{1,i}^T, \cdots, l_{1,i}^T]^T$ where matrix $X_{t,\mathcal{N}(l_i)} = [\boldsymbol{x}_{t,1}, \cdots, \boldsymbol{x}_{t,M}]$ comprises all vertices in an associated neighborhood for the tth data set and the landmark $l_{t,i}$. The scalar N denotes the number of dataset and the scalar M denotes the number of neighboring vertices. At this point, we can formulate a generalized linear mapping with a cost function for the linear mapping weighting vector $\boldsymbol{w}_i$ for landmarks $l_{t,i}$.

$$\boldsymbol{w}_i = \arg\min_{\boldsymbol{w}_i} \|\boldsymbol{X}_{\mathcal{N}(l_i)}\boldsymbol{w}_i - \boldsymbol{L}_i\|^2 + \lambda \mathcal{P}(\boldsymbol{w}_i) \tag{4}$$

In Eq. (1), the scalar λ is a Lagrange multiplier for the penalty function $\mathcal{P}$. The penalty function $\mathcal{P}$ is different for each generalized model. In ridge regression, the L2 norm of w is used while in lasso, the L1 norm is used respectively. The elastic net regression using a mixture of L1 and L2 norm while in linear embedding the sum of w is used. We investigated the linear embedding [9], ridge regression, lasso regression and elastic net regression method to estimate the landmark position. Noted, that in case of linear embedding regression, the minimization problem can be solved in closed form.

3   Evaluation and results

We trained our algorithm using Anatomy3 from the Visceral dataset [10]. This dataset comprises 20 full-body CT scans with 50 associated internal landmarks in each dataset. An example of the dataset can be found in Fig. 2. We evaluated our algorithm using leave-one-out cross-validation and the estimation error is given in mean ± standard deviation in mm. We compared the estimation result using linear embedding (LLE), ridge regression (Ridge), lasso regression (Lasso) and elastic net regression (Elastic). The results are shown in Fig. 1. As we can see from the results, in most of the cases, the ridge regression has the worst performance with an overall estimation error of 22.19 ± 12.36 mm. The closed-form solution of LLE method outperformed ridge regression and reduced the mean error to 13.43 ± 12.00 mm. Using elastic regression method, the standard deviation was reduced further and the mean estimation error was 12.71 ± 7.32 mm. The best performance was achieved using lasso regression. The overall landmark estimation error then was 12.19 ± 6.98 mm.

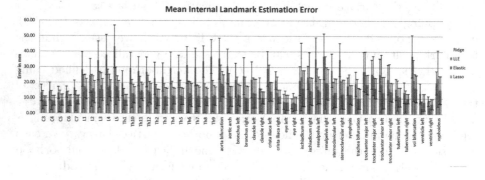

Fig. 1. Mean internal landmark estimation error using linear embedding (LLE), ridge regression (Ridge), elastic net regression (Elastic) and lasso regression (Lasso).

4   Discussion

The goal of our work has been to position anatomical landmarks inside a surface based on surface vertices close to associated landmarks. We found that our approach based on a linear mapping relative to a template surface yielded good matches between predicted landmark positions and their actual positions. The results also indicate that our template fitting method is robust as the accuracy for the template fitting is crucial for the subsequent internal landmark estimation. We can also see from the results that the ridge and LLE methods have a higher estimation error than Elastic and Lasso regression. One of the reasons can be that by introducing L1 norm as a regularizer, the Elastic and Lasso regression impose the sparsity of weighting vector w. This might be an indication that we could improve our neighborhood selection method and only include vertices which are significant for the estimation. In this work, we do not investigate the mapping using non-linear methods as the number of our datasets is limited. So far, we estimated internal landmarks independently and have not yet considered their joint estimation. As human anatomy follows certain rules there should be a potential to improve our results by exploiting any mutual relationships between them. Therefore, for certain groups of landmarks, e.g., the spine, an active shape model of the spine could potentially further improve the estimation result. We see our work of embedding the internal landmarks to the surface model as adding

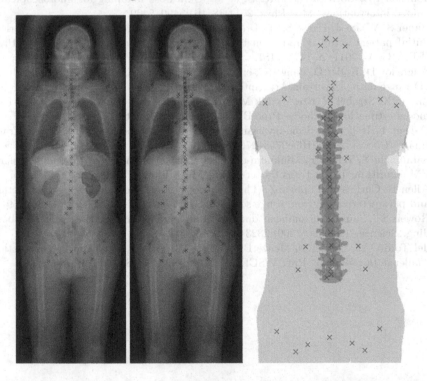

Fig. 2. A sample of the Anatomy3 training set is shown on the left. The annotated internal landmarks are indicated using red crosses and the segmented internal organs are shown in different colors. The middle figure shows the output of our algorithm, i.e., internal landmarks derived based on the surface. The result on the right demonstrates the same idea, but this time a patient surface model was used which was generated based on patient meta data such as height and weight.

prior information to our datasets. In Fig. 2, we show an example of fitting an adapted spline model using the estimated internal landmarks. In future work, we will look into the refinement method of this initial estimation when pre-operative image data is available, i.e., we will try to calculate an a posteriori estimate based on our a-priori estimate.

Acknowledgement. We gratefully acknowledge the support of Siemens Health-ineers, Forchheim, Germany. We thank Siemens Corporate Technology for pro-viding the avatar database. Note that the concepts and information presented in this paper are based on research, and they are not commercially available.

References

1. Singh V, Chang Y, Ma K, et al. Estimating a patient surface model for optimizing the medical scanning workflow. Proc MICCAI. 2014; p. 472–479.
2. Johnson PB, Borrego D, Balter S, et al. Skin dose mapping for fluoroscopically guided interventions. Med Phys. 2011;38(10):5490–5499.
3. Bauer S, Wasza J, Haase S, et al. Multi-modal surface registration for markerless initial patient setup in radiation therapy using Microsoft's kinect sensor. Proc IEEE ICCV. 2011; p. 1175–1181.
4. Anguelov D, Koller D, Pang HC, et al. Recovering articulated object models from 3D range data. Uncertain Artif Intell. 2004; p. 18–26.
5. Zhong X, Strobel N, Kowarschik M, et al. Comparison of default patient surface model estimation methods. Proc BVM. 2017; p. 281–286.
6. Darom T, Keller Y. Scale-invariant features for 3-D mesh models. IEEE Trans Image Process. 2012;21(5):2758–2769.
7. Sahillioğlu Y, Yemez Y. Minimum-distortion isometric shape correspondence using EM algorithm. IEEE Trans Pattern Anal Mach Intell. 2012;34(11):2203–2215.
8. Allen B, Curless B, Popović Z. The space of human body shapes: reconstruction and parameterization from range scans. ACM Trans Graph. 2003;22(3):587–594.
9. Roweis ST, Saul LK. Nonlinear dimensionality reduction by locally linear embed-ding. Science. 2000;290(5500):2323–2326.
10. del Toro OAJ, Goksel O, Menze B, et al. VISCERAL: visual concept extraction challenge in radiology. Proc VISCERAL Challenge at ISBI. 2014; p. 6–15.

Comparison of Self-similarity Measures for Multi-modal Non-rigid Registration of 3D-PLI Brain Images

Sharib Ali[1], Dehui Lin[1], Markus Axer[2], Karl Rohr[1]

[1]Dept. of Bioinformatics and Functional Genomics, Biomedical Computer Vision Group, BIOQUANT, IPMB, DKFZ, University of Heidelberg, Germany
[2]Institute of Neuroscience and Medicine 1, Research Centre Jülich, Jülich, Germany
s.ali@dkfz-heidelberg.de

Abstract. We introduce self-similarity measures in a spline-based non-rigid registration method. We applied our method to register multi-modal 3D polarized light imaging and blockface image data of human and rat brain sections. Quantitative evaluations demonstrate that using self-similarity measures increases the accuracy and robustness compared to a traditional mutual information measure.

1 Introduction

Multi-modal image registration is important in medical applications. Depending on the image modalities, the registration of images of different modalities is challenging due to significant differences in image intensities. In order to tackle such problems, multi-modal local measures can be used. However, the choice of such measures depends on many factors such as the statistical distribution of the intensities and local contextual information (e.g., edges, texture, and structure of an object).

In this contribution, we compare different multi-modal local measures for registration of high-resolution 3D polarized light imaging (3D-PLI, transmittance) data of both human brain (complex and asymmetric structures) and rat brain (less complex, symmetric structures) with their corresponding reference blockface images. Blockface (BF) images (Fig. 1 (a, c)) are acquired by a CCD camera using unstained brain sections before cutting while 3D-PLI images are obtained using a large area polarimeter [1] (Fig. 1 (b, d)). Tissue sectioning and mounting causes severe local tissue deformations and hence registration becomes an inevitable task [2].

In previous work, 3D-PLI images of the human brain were registered to reference blockface images using normalized mutual information (NMI) [3] and normalized cross-correlation [2]. While [3] used fluid registration, [2] employed an elastic deformation model. [4] used B-splines and mutual information (MI) for registering 3D-PLI of a rat brain. Similarity measures play a crucial role for registering multi-modal data. Even though traditionally used MI or NMI measures exploit the statistical relationship between image intensities, they do not consider contextual information and hence in case of complex and spatially dependent intensity relations (as in 3D-PLI data), they tend to be sensitive (less robust) leading to inaccurate registration results. In contrast, patch-based similarity metrics take into account local contextual information for registering multi-modal images [5, 6]. Self-similarity descriptors are the class of patch-based similarity descriptors that are invariant to monotonically increasing intensity rescalings [7]. The relation of the pixel of interest to the neighborhood pixels is encoded in a signature descriptor. These descriptors are computed within a defined search space demonstrating their self-similarity property. The descriptors capture self-similarity in terms of their color, edges, repetitive patterns, and complex textures in a unified way. Such self-similarity descriptors were used for image denoising [8], image matching in videos [9], medical image registration [5, 7], and motion estimation [7]. Correlation transform and census transform are other approaches for determining self-similarities [6].

In this contribution, we describe and compare different local measures based on self-similarity and MI for multi-modal non-rigid registration of 3D-PLI data of human and rat brain. The measures are integrated into a spline-based energy minimization scheme using an elastic deformation model.

2   Method

2.1   Self-similarity descriptors

Self-similarity descriptors are vectors computed for an n-connected neighborhood window $\mathcal{N}$ of radius r centered at pixel $\mathbf{x}$ with size $(2r+1)^2$ (*i.e.* a connectivity of $n = \{(2r+1)^2 - 1\}$ exists $\forall r \geq 1$). Thus, for a given pixel $\mathbf{x}$ of an image $g(\mathbf{x}) \in \Omega : \Omega \longrightarrow \mathbb{R}$, centered within a window $\mathcal{N}$ there exists an n-connectivity association (*i.e.* $n = 8$ for $r = 1$). The descriptors are computed for all pixels in $\mathcal{N}$ using their corresponding patch pixels centered at each pixel (Fig. 2).

MIND descriptor Self-similarity descriptors can be determined as the sum-of-squared differences between pixels in a window $\mathcal{N}$ centered at $\mathbf{x}$ of an image $g(\mathbf{x})$ and its shifted versions represented by patches $\mathcal{P}_i$ centered at each $\mathbf{x}_i$ in

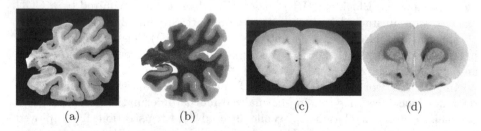

(a)   (b)   (c)   (d)

Fig. 1. Blockface images (a, c) and 3D-PLI transmittance images (b, d) of human (left) and rat (right) brain sections.

$g(\mathbf{x})$. The similarity measure can be written as a cost $C_{\mathcal{P}_i}(\mathbf{x})$

$$C_{\mathcal{P}_i}(\mathbf{x}) = \sum_{j=0}^{n} \left(g(\mathbf{x}_j) - g(\mathbf{p}_{\mathbf{x}_i}^j)\right)^2, \quad \text{with} \quad \mathbf{x}_j \in \mathcal{N} \text{ and } \mathbf{p}_{\mathbf{x}_i}^j \in \mathcal{P}_i \qquad (1)$$

where $\mathbf{x}_0$ and $\mathbf{p}_{\mathbf{x}_i}^0$ are the center pixels of the window $\mathcal{N}$ of the image $g(\mathbf{x})$ and the patch $\mathcal{P}_i$ of the shifted image $g(\mathbf{x}_i)$, respectively. The normalized self-similarity descriptors commonly known as MIND [5] in medical image analysis can be expressed in terms of a non-negative monotonically decreasing Gaussian function with the local variance of the image intensities $\sigma_{\mathbf{x}}^2$ as

$$C'_{\mathcal{P}_i}(\mathbf{x}) = \exp^{-\frac{C_{\mathcal{P}_i}(\mathbf{x})}{\sigma_{\mathbf{x}}^2}} \qquad (2)$$

CoT descriptor In [6] it was shown that correlation transforms (CoTs) for each pixel in $\mathcal{N}$ using neighborhood information can be utilized to obtain self-similarity normalized descriptors. Since CoTs compute for each pixel a value based on the mean and standard deviation of the image intensities within a local patch, CoTs are invariant to local intensity variations and hence can be used for multi-modal 3D-PLI data [2]. For each pixel in $\mathcal{N}$ we can compute CoT from a patch $\mathcal{P}_i$ surrounding that pixel as

$$CoT_{\mathcal{P}_i}(\mathbf{x}) = (g(\mathbf{x}_j) - \mu_{\mathcal{P}_i})/\sigma_{\mathcal{P}_i}, \quad \text{with} \quad \mathbf{x}_j \in \mathcal{N} \qquad (3)$$

where $\mu_{\mathcal{P}_i}$ and $\sigma_{\mathcal{P}_i}$ are the mean and standard deviation in the patch, respectively. [2] used the absolute value of CoT and a clipping technique to avoid division by small values for the standard deviation below a certain threshold T_σ in homogeneous regions. The extended correlation transform $\overline{CoT}_{\mathcal{P}_i}(\mathbf{x})$ can be formulated as

$$\overline{CoT}_{\mathcal{P}_i}(\mathbf{x}) = |g(\mathbf{x}_j) - \mu_{\mathcal{P}_i}|/\text{clip}(\sigma_{\mathcal{P}_i}, [T_\sigma, \infty]) \qquad (4)$$

2.2   Scalar conversion of descriptors

Each patch matrix centered at $\mathbf{x}$ can be represented as a *sorted* self-similarity descriptor vector $\mathbf{Sd}$. We then use the *sorted* descriptor vector for each pixel $\mathbf{x}$

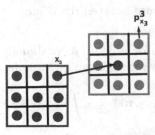

Fig. 2. $\mathbf{x}_i$ (dark grey dots, $i \in [1,8]$) are the neighbors of $\mathbf{x}$ (blue dot) in $\mathcal{N}$. A patch $\mathcal{P}_i$ is centered at the third element $\mathbf{x}_0$ of $\mathcal{N}$ and is represented by the light grey neighborhood pixels $p_{\mathbf{x}_3}^j$.

Table 1. Evaluation of multi-modal similarity metrics for non-rigid registration.

Simlarity	TRE in pixels (mean±stdDev)						
	Human brain				Rat brain		
	#637	#673	#688	Mean	#131	#161	Mean
MI	6.31±6.3	3.84±2.8	5.71±5.2	5.28±4.8	12.07±5.6	15.97±7.2	14.02±6.4
MIND	4.49±3.6	3.73±2.5	4.57±3.8	4.26±3.3	9.81±6.4	10.19±3.8	10.00±5.1
CoT	**3.50±2.7**	**3.62±2.3**	**3.57±3.0**	**3.56±2.7**	**7.13±3.8**	**6.28±2.6**	**6.70±3.2**

in an image g to compute the normalized scalar value

$$SdN(\mathbf{x}) = \left(\frac{\mathbf{Sd}[n/2] - \mathbf{Sd}[0]}{\mathbf{Sd}[0] + \mathbf{Sd}[n]} - \frac{1}{|\mathcal{N}|} \sum_i \mathbf{Sd}[i] \right) / \sqrt{\sigma_{\mathbf{Sd}}^2 + \epsilon^2} \tag{5}$$

where $\mathbf{Sd}[.]$ represents a scalar value corresponding to the index location ". ", $\sigma_{\mathbf{Sd}}$ is the standard deviation of the descriptor vector and $\epsilon > 0$ is a small value to avoid division by zero.

2.3   Energy minimization scheme

The self-similarity descriptors described above are integrated as data term for non-rigid registration based on Gaussian elastic body splines (GEBS). In addition, we used a mutual information measure [10]. GEBS are based on the Navier equation of linear elasticity. For intensity-based registration, an energy-minimizing functional E_{GEBS} has been proposed [2] to compute the deformation field $\mathbf{u}$ for registration of a source image g_1 with a target image g_2

$$E_{GEBS}(\mathbf{u}) = E_{Data,I}(g_1, g_2, \mathbf{u}^I) + \lambda_I E_I(\mathbf{u}, \mathbf{u}^I) + \lambda_E \, E_{elastic}(\mathbf{u}) \tag{6}$$

E_I and $E_{elastic}$ are two regularization terms with $\{\lambda_I, \lambda_E\}$ controlling the trade-off between regularization and the data term. (6) has been formulated in a way such that the minimization w.r.t. the searched deformation field $\mathbf{u}$ can be obtained in analytic form. Besides $\mathbf{u}$, (6) comprises a second deformation field $\mathbf{u}^I$ which is computed based on the intensity information. $E_{Data,I}$ in (6) represents an intensity similarity measure between the deformed source and target image.

Integration of mutual information A local analytic measure of mutual information (MI) as similarity measure can be formulated as [10]:

$$E_{Data,I}(g_1, g_2, \mathbf{u}^I) = - \int \log_2 \left(\epsilon + |\sin \theta| \right) d\mathbf{x}, \tag{7}$$

with $\theta = \arccos \frac{\nabla g_1(\mathbf{x}+\mathbf{u}^I) \cdot \nabla g_2(\mathbf{x})}{\|\nabla g_1(\mathbf{x}+\mathbf{u}^I)\| \|\nabla g_2(\mathbf{x})\|}$ defined in a local neighborhood of $\mathbf{x}$ and a constant $\epsilon > 0$.

Integration of self-similarity descriptors Self-similarity descriptor vectors are first converted to their corresponding normalized scalar feature map SdN. The sum of squared differences between SdN_{g_1} and SdN_{g_2} computed for a local neighborhood window $\mathcal{N}$ of g_1 and g_2, respectively, should be minimized. Thus, the data term can be formulated as

$$E_{Data,I}\left(g_1, g_2, \mathbf{u}^I\right) = \sum_{\mathbf{x} \in \Omega} \left(SdN_{g_1}(\mathbf{x} + \mathbf{u}^I) - SdN_{g_2}(\mathbf{x}) \right)^2 \qquad (8)$$

In order to handle large deformations, we use a multi-resolution scheme for the minimization of (6) and Levenberg/Marquardt optimization.

3 Experimental results

We have evaluated each self-similarity measure integrated in our spline-based non-rigid registration approach using three human brain sections and two rat brain sections ($64\mu m$ spatial resolution). Ground truth correspondences between the considered 3D-PLI data and the BF reference have been manually defined by an expert (on average 114 correspondences per section for human brain and 25 per section for rat brain). The target registration error (TRE) is used as performance measure. Image pairs were rigidly pre-registered using the method in [2]. In Table 1, it can be seen that non-rigid registration utilizing the self-similarity metric based on the correlation transform (CoT, [2]) yields the least TRE for all brain sections (3D-PLI to BF), and a mean error of 3.56 ± 2.7 pixels and 6.70 ± 3.2 pixels for human and rat brain, respectively. It can also be observed that the MIND descriptor based similarity measure performed better than MI for most of the brain sections with a mean error of 4.26 ± 3.3 pixels and 10.0 ± 5.1 pixels for human and rat brain, respectively, which is about 1 pixel and 4 pixels better than MI for human and rat brain, respectively. Visual assessment of the registration results presented in Fig. 3 show that the CoT-based self-similarity metric yields accurate results for both human (left) and rat data (right).

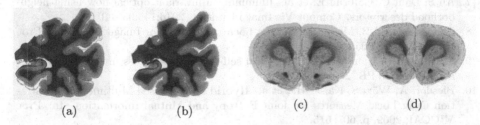

(a)   (b)   (c)   (d)

Fig. 3. Edge overlay (reference blockface image represented as red edges overlaid with source transmittance image): Rigidly registered BF and 3D-PLI images (a, c), and non-rigid registration with CoT-based self-similarity descriptor (b, d).

4   Discussion and conclusions

We have shown that self-similarity metrics improve the registration result compared to a traditional mutual information measure. For 3D-PLI images with different context information (i.e., rat and human brains), we showed that self-similarity metrics are well suited to handle intensity variability and improve the accuracy since contextual information about local structures are exploited along with their property of intensity invariance.

Acknowledgement. This project was funded by the Helmholtz Association through the Helmholtz Portfolio theme "Supercomputing and Modeling for the Human Brain" and by the European Union through the Horizon 2020 Research and Innovation Programme under Grant Agreement No. 7202070 (Human Brain Project SGA1).

References

1. Axer M, Gräßel D, Kleiner M, et al. High-resolution fiber tract reconstruction in the human brain by means of three-dimensional polarized light imaging. Front Neuroinf. 2011;5(34).
2. Ali S, Rohr K, Axer M, et al. Elastic registration of high-resolution 3D PLI data of the human brain. Proc ISBI. 2017; p. 1151–1155.
3. Palm C, Axer M, Gräßel D, et al. Towards ultra-high resolution fibre tract mapping of the human brain - registration of polarised light images and reorientation of fibre vectors. Frontiers Hum Neurosci. 2010;4(9).
4. Schubert N, Axer M, Schober M, et al. 3D Reconstructed Cyto-, Muscarinic M2 Receptor, and Fiber Architecture of the Rat Brain Registered to the Waxholm Space Atlas. Front Neuroanatom. 2016;10(51).
5. Heinrich MP, Jenkinson M, Bhushan M, et al. MIND: modality independent neighbourhood descriptor for multi-modal deformable registration. Medical Image Analysis. 2012;16(7):1423–1435.
6. Drulea M, Nedevschi S. Motion Estimation Using the Correlation Transform. IEEE Trans Image Process. 2013;22(8):3260–3270.
7. Ali S, Daul C, Galbrun E, et al. Illumination invariant optical flow using neighborhood descriptors. Comput Vis Image Underst. 2016;145:95–110.
8. Buades A, Coll B, Morel JM. A Non-Local Algorithm for Image Denoising. Proc IEEE CVPR. 2005; p. 60–65.
9. Shechtman E, Irani M. Matching local self-similarities across images and videos. Proc IEEE CVPR. 2007; p. 1–8.
10. Biesdorf A, Wörz S, Kaiser HJ, et al. Hybrid Spline-Based Multimodal Registration using Local Measures for Joint Entropy and Mutual Information. In: Proc MICCAI; 2009. p. 607–615.

Two-Step Trajectory Visualization for Robot-Assisted Spine Radiofrequency Ablations

Nico Merten[1,4], Simon Adler[2,4], Magnus Hanses[2,4], Sylvia Saalfeld[1,4],
Mathias Becker[3], Bernhard Preim[1,4]

[1]Department of Simulation and Graphics, Otto-von-Guericke-University Magdeburg
[2]Fraunhofer Institute for Factory Operation and Automation (IFF), Magdeburg
[3]Institute of Neuroradiology, University Hospital Magdeburg
[4]Research Campus STIMULATE, Magdeburg
nmerten@isg.cs.uni-magdeburg.de

Abstract. Radiofrequency Ablations (RFAs) can be employed for the treatment of spine metastases. Instruments are therefor inserted through the vertebra's pedicle into cancerous tissue within the vertebral body. This requires high precision during interventions. We present a two-step method to increase risk awareness during intervention planning and execution of manual and robot-assisted spine RFAs. Three medical experts evaluated our method and stated that it yields two advantages: First, improved visualizations for manual interventions and second, increased safety in hand-guided, robot-assisted setups.

1 Introduction

The health of bones depends on the well-balanced communication between osteoclastic and osteoblastic bone cells, which break down and synthesize bone tissue, respectively [1]. Infiltrating cancer cells can disturb this balance [2].

Many patients with vertebral metastases are in palliative care and suffer from symptoms such as pain and motor deficits. In very severe cases they may also suffer from paraplegia or spinal cord transections. Chemo- and radiation therapy, and surgery are mainly used for treatment. Radiofrequency Ablations (RFAs) can be used as an image-guided and minimally invasive alternative or additional therapy [3]. A transpedicular RFA is the most common approach, where a pathway is created by hammering a cannula and trocar through a vertebra's pedicle. Pedicles are the bony connections between the vertebra and the vertebral arch that encompass the spinal canal laterally. After pathways were created, RFA needles are inserted to perform an ablation and cancer cells within the vertebral body are coagulated. RFAs are effective [4], but must be performed with high precision, because the pedicle is between 5 to 8 mm thick. This results in physical stress for surgeons. Fig. 1 shows a Dyna-Computed Tomography (Dyna-CT) scan of a conserved vertebra and it illustrates the spatial relation between a pedicle and an inserted drill. The scan was recorded after drill insertion and the pathway's contour is highlighted in yellow for better visibility.

In this work, we focus on manually implemented and hand-guided, robot-assisted RFAs for spine metastases. A hand-guided robot augments the surgeon's abilities with tremor-free [5], scaled [6] and constrained motions [7]. Therefore, we propose to combine robot assistance with image-guided interventions, where highly accurate motions are derived from diagnostic image scans. The main benefits are increased intervention and patient safety.

Our clinical partners use CT and Magnetic Resonance Imaging (MRI) scans for diagnosis. This combination enables them to conclude about the metastasis' origin and the bone density. This knowledge is important, because the RFA needles have to be inserted deep enough into the vertebra and metastasis to be effective. Depending on the primary tumor's location, the metastasis will be very hard or soft [8]. Therefore, the physician has to be aware of the required forces beforehand: Instruments have to be inserted deep enough while avoiding pedicle fractures and injuries of the lung, the aorta, or the spinal canal.

2   Materials and methods

We propose a two-step method using diagnostic image scans to increase safety during instrument insertion. Fig. 2 shows these steps (orange boxes) with respect to the clinical workflow (blue boxes). The first step, a Map Visualization of Trajectory Risk, uses the CT scans to present the risk of multiple trajectories with respect to the instrument's size and the absolute, minimum distance to risk structures. When a trajectory is chosen, a Force Prediction is conducted to assess a single trajectory in more detail.

2.1   Step 1: map visualization of trajectory risk

Fig. 3 depicts our conceptual map visualization to present risk categories for multiple trajectories. Physicians have some spatial freedom to define a trajectory. All possible paths to a target point (TP) lie inside the red triangle and

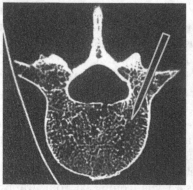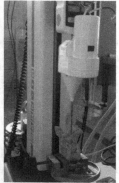

Fig. 1. Left: 10 s Dyna-CT scan with highlighted insertion path for a conserved lumbar vertebrae. Right: Experimental setup where forces are measured during automatic drill insertion with constant velocity of 2 mm/s.

the parameters that define this zone are the pedicle's width and height, and the instrument's diameter. The clinically feasible paths lie in the yellow and green triangle. The color-coding is related to Rieder et al. [9], but in contrast to their work, we convey risk awareness and do not visualize coagulation zones. Yellow color-coded trajectories are only somewhat safe. Trajectories are assigned to this category if their absolute distance to risk structures, such as the spinal canal, lies in an user-defined interval, e.g., between 2 and 5 mm.

2.2 Step 2: force prediction from diagnostic scans

Anatomical densities, thus Hounsfield Units (HUs) in Dyna-CT scans, vary for cortical, cancellous, and metastatic bone tissues. Our medical partners reported that the required drill force depends on the type of bone tissue. Therefore, we evaluated how feed rate changes correlate with HU changes in image scans. Here, feed rate describes the velocity at which the drill is advanced into the vertebra.

Experimental Setup: We built a construction to insert a hollow drill with an outer diameter of 3 mm and an inner diameter of 2 mm with a constant velocity of 2 mm/s into five series of two lumbar and one thoracic vertebrae

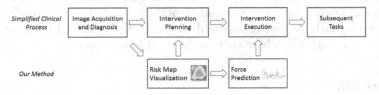

Fig. 2. Our proposed two step method to assist manual and robot-assisted RFAs. Our two-step method (orange boxes) is presented in relation to the clinical stage (blue boxes), where it should be used.

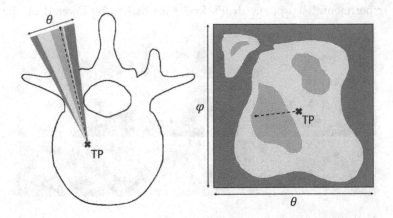

Fig. 3. Given a Target Point (TP) and the pedicle's size, trajectories get categorized and color-coded. The dashed line is the user-defined trajectory to TP. Each path can be described as a triple (TP, θ, ϕ), where θ is the horizontal and ϕ the vertical angle.

each (Fig. 1). During drilling the timestamps, covered distance, and feed rate forces were logged. First results show that forces up to 10 N are required to insert the drill into conserved lumbar vertebrae.

Image Acquisition and Processing: Dyna-CT scans were recorded before and after drilling. For all scans, all acquisition parameters were kept the same. In consultation with our medical partners, we set the acquisition time to be 10 s to get scans whose image quality is comparable to those in clinical routine.

The main difference between both scans are the low intensity values from the drill hole in the second scan, which are close to air. Therefore, to segment and assess only the intensity values from the drill hole, we use a two-step image processing chain: First, the scan with the drill hole is subtracted from the reference scan without drill hole. After subtraction an intensity threshold is applied to segment the cylindric drill path. Due to image noise and minor rigid registration inaccuracies, the result images contain many segmentation artifacts (Fig. 4(A)).

We address this problem by applying a Principal Component Analysis (PCA) on the result images, where the eigenvector with the largest eigenvalue represents the drilling direction. Knowing the drill's outer diameter, we can assume a virtual cylinder, which we use to mask the drill hole in the reference images (Fig. 4(B)). Then, the trajectory is divided into equidistant sample points and the step size equals the smallest voxel dimension. Finally, the intensity values are perpendicularly projected on the drill path. The averaged intensity values can be seen in Figure 5, where they are plotted in orange.

3   Results

To compare the measured force and averaged HU values, both value sets are normalized before plotting (Fig. 5). Steep graph curve changes indicate transitions between bone tissues with different anatomical densities. Because of restrictions in our experimental setup, the drill's feed rate had to be lowered at the corti-

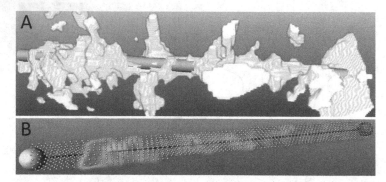

Fig. 4. (A) Remaining intensity values after image subtraction and thresholding with a high number of segmentation artifacts. (B) The drill was inserted from the yellow to the red sphere. The red area on the left is the result of high intensity values: It depicts the position of the vertebral corticalis, which is harder than the vertebral body.

calis. Therefore, the force graph curve (blue) has an offset of 2mm to the right. First results show that force changes imply changing image intensity values, but changing intensities can, but do not have to, result in force changes.

3.1 Evaluation

We evaluated our method by interviewing three clinical experts and we asked them to assess our method's feasibility. The experts stated that our method can increase intervention safety for manual, but especially for hand-guided, robot-assisted spine RFAs. The reason is the combination of map and graph visualizations to convey risk awareness. One expert also advised us not to use conserved vertebrae in the future, because fresh or dried bones have different mechanical properties than conserved bones.

Our method does not influence the current clinical workflow, as it can be used on image scans that are already recorded for diagnosis and intervention planning. The force prediction requires no additional effort from the physician. The risk map requires the physician to detect anatomical structures such as the pedicle and the spinal canal, and to define a safety interval to apply the categorization.

4 Discussion

We presented a two-step method to convey risk awareness that increases safety for manual and hand-guided, robot-assisted spine RFA. Both steps do not require much additional effort from physicians.

We think that the risk map visualization is underused and we plan to evaluate how it can be used during intervention execution, e.g., if the drill's distance to risk structures comes close or falls below a user-defined minimum threshold, the drill's feed rate is decreased or all movement is stopped, respectively.

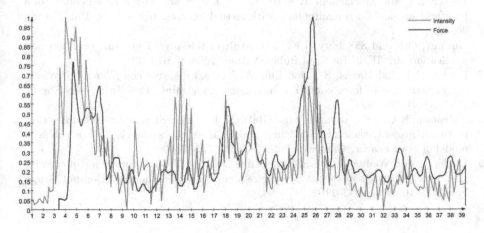

Fig. 5. Normalized forces (blue) and normalized, averaged intensities (orange) during insertion with constant velocity through a lumbar pedicle (Fig. 1).

The force prediction is highly relevant for robot-assisted setups. We argue that force changes imply changing image intensity values. Therefore, if measured force changes cannot be confirmed by changing image intensity values, the system should warn the physician during intervention. Our method predicts these changes from diagnostic image scans using an effortless image processing chain consisting of image subtraction, thresholding, and a PCA analysis.

Drilling is a complex task. The required force to move the drill depends on the drill's feed rate and rotation speed. Both can be measured during intervention execution. Because of the discussions with our medical partners, we are aware that mechanical properties of conserved and non-conserved vertebrae are different. Therefore, we plan to extend the experiments to non-conserved vertebrae, if current observations are confirmed by additional experiments.

Acknowledgement. This work is partly funded by the Federal Ministry of Education and Research within the Forschungscampus STIMULATE (13GW0095A, 13GW0095B). We thank Karin Fischer and Steffen Serowy for preparing and scanning the vertebrae we used for this work and their valuable feedback.

References

1. Ortiz, A and Lin, S. Osteolytic and osteoblastic bone metastases: two extremes of the same spectrum? In: Prevention of Bone Metastases. Springer; 2012. p. 225–233.
2. Abrams, H L and Spiro, R and Goldstein, N . Metastases in carcinoma: analysis of 1000 autopsied cases. Cancer. 1950;3(1):74–85.
3. Gazis, A N and Beuing, O and Franke, J et al . Bipolar radiofrequency ablation of spinal tumors: predictability, safety and outcome. Spine J. 2014;14(4):604–608.
4. Callstrom, M R and Charboneau, J W and Goetz, M P et al . Image-guided ablation of painful metastatic bone tumors: a new and effective approach to a difficult problem. Skeletal Radiol. 2006;35(1):1–15.
5. Becker, B C and Maclachlan, R A and Lobes, L A et al . Vision-based control of a handheld surgical micromanipulator with virtual fixtures. IEEE Trans Rob Autom. 2013;29(3):674–683.
6. Guthart, G S and Salisbury, J K. The intuitive telesurgery system: overview and application. In: IEEE Int Conf Robot Autom; 2000. p. 618–621.
7. Davies, B L and Harris, S J and Lin, W J et al . Active compliance in robotic surgery: the use of force control as a dynamic constraint. Proc Inst Mech Eng H. 1997;211(4):285–292.
8. Halvorson, K G and Sevcik, M A and Ghilardi, J R et al . Similarities and differences in tumor growth, skeletal remodeling and pain in an osteolytic and osteoblastic model of bone cancer. Clinical J Pain. 2006;22(7):587–600.
9. Rieder, C and Weihusen, A and Schumann, C et al . Visual support for interactive post-interventional assessment of radiofrequency ablation therapy. Comput Graph Forum. 2010;29(3):1093–1102.

Unsupervised Pathology Detection in Medical Images using Learning-based Methods

Hristina Uzunova, Heinz Handels, Jan Ehrhardt

Institut für Medizinische Informatik, Universität zu Lübeck
uzunova@imi.uni-luebeck.de

Abstract. Detecting pathologies automatically is challenging because of their big variability. As the usual supervised machine learning approaches would only be able to detect one type of pathologies, in this work we pursue an unsupervised approach: learn the entire variability of healthy data and detect pathologies by their differences to the learned norm. Two methods have been developed based on this principle: A modified PatchMatch algorithm shows plausible results on contrasting brain tumors, but bad generalization ability for other types of data. A CVAE-based method on the other hand performs significantly better and ca. 17 times faster on the brain data and can be generalized to other pathologies, e.g. lung tumors. Not only is the achieved Dice coefficient of 0.55 comparable to other supervised methods on this data, moreover this method reliably detects different pathology types and needs no ground-truth.

1 Introduction

Pathology detection in medical images is an important task of medical image computing and analysis. Pathologies would often cause missing correspondences for processes like image registration and therefore should be marked ahead as such, e.g. by using probability masking. However, the big variability of possible pathologies is a challenge to automatic detection methods. Supervised machine-learning algorithms for segmentation like [1] would usually use big training sets of ground-truth data to learn the appearance of a single pathological structure. However, to make it possible to detect a range of pathology types in this work we pursue another unsupervised approach: learn the entire variability of normal healthy tissue and detect pathologies based on their differences to what has been learned. This idea has been used in [2] for the detection of brain lesions, by modeling the healthy data with a probabilistic appearance model and in [3] for the segmentation of anomalies in OCT images by using GANs. Such approaches are usually less accurate, but suitable for all possible anomalies and do not need any ground-truth data.

In this work we present two different unsupervised detection approaches. (1) A modified PatchMatch algorithm to establish comparison between a set of healthy patients images and a pathological test image. (2) A conditional variational autoencoder (CVAE) – a neural network which models healthy data by mapping it to a less dimensional latent space with a given prior distribution.

2   Materials and methods

2.1   Multi-scale PatchMatch

Assuming pathologies are structures strongly differing from the normal tissue variability, we hypothesize that they can be detected by finding the biggest differences between a test image and multiple healthy example images. An efficient approach to compare image regions is the PatchMatch [4] algorithm, which finds the approximate nearest matches between image patches by stochastic neighborhood search, as suggested in [5].

To adapt PatchMatch to our approach, where we aim to compare one test image I_{test} to n healthy patients example images, we first calculate feature vectors $\mathbf{d_j}$ on small patches around the position j. For every feature $\mathbf{d}_j \in I_{test}$ a closest matching feature in every example image $\mathbf{f}_j^i, i = 1, \ldots, n$ can be found using PatchMatch. Now we assume that pathologies have big distances even to their nearest neighbors, thus a distance image I_{dist} is computed $I_{dist}(j) = \min_i \Delta(\mathbf{d}_j, \mathbf{f}_j^i)$ where high values correspond to pathologies.

In our work we tested HOG [6], SSC [7] and Needle features [8], where the last were chosen as they lead to best differentiation. The Needle features consider multiple scales of an image and consist of the concatenated vectorized patches on the same relative position of every scale, thus they contain both fine and coarse information of the image.

In order to increase the discrimination ability, we propose two extensions of PatchMatch related to locality and multi-resolution. The original PatchMatch algorithm does not necessarily result in big distances for pathological patches. By usually starting off with a random initialization of correspondences and finally randomly searching through the whole image for better matches, the algorithm is able to match patches on very distant relative positions. In the case of medical images this is not a desired effect, as those are (or can easily get) roughly aligned and hence same structures have similar positions. To avoid problems such as matching a tumor border patch to a distant head border patch, locality information needs to be integrated into PatchMatch. For this purpose we limit the radius in the random selection steps to 20 and also introduce a multi-scale PatchMatch approach using the Needle features.

Assume Needle features with l scales $s_0, \ldots, s_l$ are given, where s_l is the coarsest one. The multi-scale PatchMatch first considers s_l and performs as usual by starting randomly (with a limited radius) and finding the best match position $p_{l_{best}}$. Now the next scale s_{l-1} is concatenated to s_l and PatchMatch is performed on the longer features starting at $p_{l_{best}}$. This process is iteratively repeated until s_0 is reached. This way the coarse information on the last levels ensures that the rough location of the match is found in the first few iterations and then refined by using the local information of the first levels in the further process.

2.2   Conditional variational autoencoder

An autoencoder aims to reconstruct input data, by using a low-dimensional latent space representation. In particular a variational autoencoder (VAE) is a neural network that assumes a prior distribution of the latent space (typically normal distribution) and learns to map data to its latent vectors z (encoding), then pursue a best possible reconstruction of the input data by only using latent vectors (decoding). Furthermore, VAEs can be conditioned (CVAE) [9], by adding an extra prior semantic information about the data, e.g. a label. This way the z-space distribution is learned per condition and more control over the learned space and reconstruction of images is possible.

Our CVAE architecture is shown in Fig. 1. Inspired by the previous patch-based locality approach, we train the CVAE on patches (32×32). Furthermore, we integrate locality information, by using relative to the size continuous positions $c \in [0,1] \times [0,1]$ of the patches as condition. Note that an assumption about the rough alignment of the images is made. We chose a simple fully-connected architecture containing 3 hidden layers in the encoder and decoder each. Also different dimensions of z are possible, here 20 and 5 showed best performance.

Our CVAE is designed to map the variability of healthy tissue per position to a normal distribution, thus pathological patches should automatically be mapped far from the center of the distribution and can be detected by their high (e.g. euclidean) distances to the mean of the learned z-space. Another possibility is however that by only learning healthy tissue, the autoencoder is not able to adequately encode and reconstruct pathological patches, hence big distances between the original and reconstructed images appear in pathological areas. Those two assumptions are not strictly disjoint and, as experiments would show, should be used together, combined to a third assumption: pathologies have both large reconstruction and z-space distances, which corresponds to multiplying both distances.

3   Experiments and results

Two data sets of 2D images with different pathologies and anomalies have been used to test our approach. (1) BRATS: 220 Brain MRI T1c images with ground-

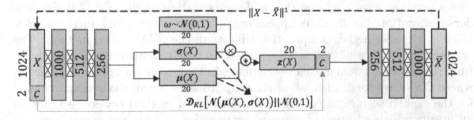

Fig. 1. CVAE architecture. Vectorized patch X and reconstruction $\bar{X}$; fully-connected encoder (blue) and decoder (red) layers; condition (green); z-space (purple) where $z = \mu + \sigma \times \omega$, with random $\omega \sim \mathcal{N}(0,1)$. Dashed lines correspond to loss functions $\mathcal{D}_{KL}$ – Kullback-Leibler divergence and $|| \cdot || - l^1$ norm. Numbers denote size of layers.

truth segmentations of high-grade glioblastomas from the BRATS challenge data set. The segmentations allow a selection of non-pathological patches for training. All images are extracted from the same slice of the original 3D volumes. (2) Lungs: 46 Lung CT slices containing different pathologies with no suitable ground-truth available. As it is important for the images to be roughly aligned to each other, they all have been cut using a bounding box around the structures (brain or lungs). For this reason the sizes of the images vary, but the relative positions of the structures approximately match.

Both PatchMatch and the CVAE-based approaches (with the three detection assumptions) have been compared to each other in our experiments. For the BRATS data set we used a 4-fold cross-validation. For the CVAE training we chose 150000 patches not containing pathologies on random positions to avoid learning only discrete positions and used $dim(\mathbf{z}) = 20$. In the test data set for both methods we only included data that contains visible pathologies. As the skull-stripping of the BRATS images leaves very uneven borders, causing high distances, all distance images have been multiplied with the Gaussian smoothed masks of the brains. To evaluate the differentiation ability a ROC analysis is executed and the area under curve (AUC) calculated. Sensitivity and specificity values are calculated on the Youden index of the ROC, and regrading those a lower threshold is chosen as a percentage of the maximum distance. The resulting segmentations are then evaluated with Dice coefficient. Only labels corresponding to the tumor core are evaluated.

For the Lungs data set no suitable ground-truth was available, therefore picking patches not containing pathologies for training was impossible. For this reason 35 images without obvious pathologies were picked for training and the remaining ones for testing. For the CVAE training 5000 patches on random positions were extracted and $dim(\mathbf{z}) = 5$ was chosen. Because of the missing ground-truth no adequate quantitative evaluation of the results is possible. However, having this small amount of testing images enables a visual evaluation.

The results of all methods on the BRATS data are shown in Tab. 1. Clearly, the ROC analysis shows that all methods are able to establish differentiation between healthy and pathological tissue (AUC $\gg 0.5$), however best results in terms of all evaluation metrics are achieved when using the combination of reconstruction and z-space distances resulting off the CVAE method. PatchMatch shows very low sensitivity and thus bad segmentation results (Fig. 2 typical undersegmentation, big distances appear only at contrasting areas), furthermore it has a ~ 17 times higher computation time than the CVAE-based method. The achieved mean Dice of 0.55 is a segmentation result comparable to the results from [10] where it would make the 6th place, but not to newer approaches like [1], where CNNs are used. Still, all of those approaches are supervised and trained for the explicit segmentation of glioblastomas. Our method however establishes an unsupervised detection of different pathologies that are not necessarily considered by the used ground-truth, but would still cause missing correspondences. Furthermore, 2D layers with no visible pathologies would often contain parts of overflowing 3D segmentations. Thus right detection by our method would result

Table 1. BRATS results. Shown are CVAE reconstruction, z-space and combined distances and PatchMatch distances. Evaluation metrics are mean over all images and folds: Area under curve (AUC) from ROC analysis, sensitivity and specificity at Youden index and Dice coefficient of segmentation with ROC picked threshold. Subscripts correspond to statistical significance (p<0.001) in a one-sided t-test ($\diamond$ – compared to PatchMatch, $\star$ – compared to CVAE-combined).

	CVAE-reconstr	CVAE-z-space	CVAE-combined	PatchMatch
Dice	$0.49 \pm 0.26^{\diamond\star}$	$0.51 \pm 0.26^{\diamond\star}$	$0.55 \pm 0.27^{\diamond}$	$0.44 \pm 0.25^{\star}$
Sensitivity	0.89	0.88	0.91	0.55
Specificity	0.81	0.85	0.86	0.83
AUC	0.94	0.92	0.95	0.81

in bad Dice coefficients. Even though the Lungs data set is fundamentally different, the visual evaluation showed that the CVAE method still has the ability to detect present pathologies (Fig. 3 big distances correspond to pathological structures). Interestingly, z-space distances here seem to rather correspond to edges than pathological structures, as pathologies typically have the same intensity values as healthy tissue. Still, combining them with the reconstruction distances performs well. On the other hand, the PatchMatch algorithm turned out to be fully unsuitable for the pathology detection on this data set, proving its poor generalization ability.

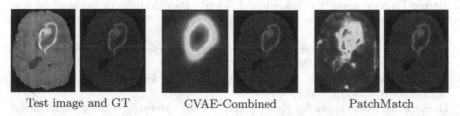

Test image and GT   CVAE-Combined   PatchMatch

Fig. 2. BRATS segmentation results. Shown are the resulting distance images (growing values: blue → red) and segmentations of the CVAE-combined and PatchMatch method. Successful detection by the CVAE combined method (middle) and typical undersegmentation of the PatchMatch method.

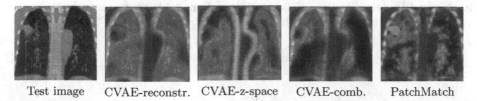

Test image   CVAE-reconstr.   CVAE-z-space   CVAE-comb.   PatchMatch

Fig. 3. Lungs detection results with the CVAE and PatchMatch methods. Left to right: Test image, reconstruction, z-space and combined distance images, PatchMatch distance image.

4   Discussion

We presented two methods for unsupervised pathology detection. A multi-scale PatchMatch approach proves to be suitable for the detection of contrasting tumors in brain MRIs, however fails at homogenous pathologies in lung CT scans. On the other hand, the proposed CVAE detection method performs significantly better and faster on both data sets and tends to establish good detection. Even though this method does not achieve perfect accuracy in terms of pathology segmentation, it is unsupervised and hence no ground-truth data is needed for training. Furthermore different structures causing missing correspondences are detected, and thus this method could be of a significant advantage combined with a registration method.

References

1. Kamnitsas K, Ferrante E, Parisot S, et al. DeepMedic for brain tumor segmentation. Proc MICCAI. 2016; p. 138–149.
2. Krüger J, Ehrhardt J, Handels H. Probabilistic appearance models for segmentation and classification. Proc ICCV. 2015; p. 1698–1706.
3. Schlegl T, Seeböck P, Waldstein SM, et al. Unsupervised anomaly detection with generative adversarial networks to guide marker discovery. Inf Process Med Imaging. 2017; p. 146–157.
4. Barnes C, Shechtman E, Finkelstein A, et al. PatchMatch: A randomized correspondence algorithm for structural image editing. Proc ACM SIGGRAPH. 2009;28(3).
5. Faktor A, Irani M. Clustering by composition: unsupervised discovery of image categories. Proc ECCV. 2012; p. 474–487.
6. Dalal N, Triggs B. Histograms of oriented gradients for human detection. Proc IEEE CVPR. 2005; p. 886–893.
7. Heinrich MP, Jenkinson M, Papie z BW, et al. Towards realtime multimodal fusion for image-guided interventions using self-similarities. Proc MICCAI. 2013; p. 187–194.
8. Lotan O, Irani M. Needle-Match: reliable patch matching under high uncertainty. Proc IEEE CVPR. 2016 June; p. 439–448.
9. Kingma DP, Mohamed S, Jimenez Rezende D, et al. Semi-supervised learning with deep generative models. Adv Neural Inf Process Syst. 2014;27:3581–3589.
10. Menze BH, Jakab A, Bauer S, et al. The multimodal brain tumor image segmentation benchmark (BRATS). IEEE Trans Med Imaging. 2015;34(10):1993–2024.

Classification of Lobular and Ductal Breast Carcinomas by Texture Analysis in DCE-MRI Data

Kai Nie, Gabriel Mistelbauer, Bernhard Preim

Department of Simulation and Graphics, OvG University Magdeburg
kai@isg.cs.uni-magdeburg.de

Abstract. Breast cancer can be distinguished into several subtypes, where invasive ductal carcinomas (IDC) and invasive lobular carcinomas (ILC) are the two most common subtypes. These two types of tumor grow at a different speed and exhibit different metastatic patterns. Although both types are malignant, they show different treatment results for the same therapy. Accurate distinction between these two subtypes is helpful for determining therapy strategies. In this paper, we classify IDC and ILC based on their characteristic texture features, which are extracted from a three-dimensional co-occurrence matrix. The texture features at different time points are used instead of the features from a single time point. We employ a non-linear support vector machine (SVM) algorithm and a random forests method as classifiers to separate IDC and ILC via their texture features and achieve a high accuracy of the classification result.

1 Introduction

Invasive lobular carcinoma (ILC) and invasive ductal carcinoma (IDC) are the most common subtypes of breast cancer, which accounts for 80% and 15% of all invasive breast tumors, respectively [1]. The characteristic differences between ILC and IDC are commonly shown in their distinct clinical presentations, morphologic and molecular features, and genomic profiles. The ILC is more likely to occur in older patients, to be larger in size, and to be estrogen receptor-positive. It also has a higher incidence of contralateral breast cancer [2]. Meanwhile, the treatment effect of chemotherapy for patients with ILC is lower than with IDC, while patients with ILC derive greater benefit from hormonal therapy [3]. Thus, to distinguish these two subtypes plays a great role. The common classification scheme of IDC and ILC is based on their histological analysis or genomic testing [4], while morphologically the texture differences between these two cancer subtypes are promising to discriminate them [5].

A variety of texture extraction schemes for breast MRI data was tested in [5]. The result shows that the gray level co-occurrence matrix (GLCM) based parameters are superior to other texture parameters in breast tumor classification. Aiming at the various features extracted from GLCM, Nie et al. [6] introduced a fuzzy c-means (FCM) based method to eliminate interference elements from texture features to simplify the calculation and improve the classification accuracy. Compared with standard MRI, dynamic contrast-enhanced (DCE) MRI captures the contrast agent (CA) accumulation over time, providing temporal dynamic features which enrich the characteristics of MRI data. Preim et al. [7] developed a new tool to quantify the heterogeneity of a tumor by combining dynamic temporal information to predict malignancy. Similar to the work in [7], Chang et al. [8] combined the texture features with kinetic curves, which reflect the temporal information of breast tumors, to recognize the molecular markers of a tumor. We use the characteristics of breast tumor structure change over time in DCE-MRI data extracting texture features at different time points to identify the breast cancer subtypes.

2   Material and methods

2.1   Image data

Our data set comprises 54 malignant tumor lesions (18 ILC and 36 IDC) from 49 patients. All tumors are large lesions, where the smallest volume of the lesion is 212.39 μl. A 1T scanner (Philips Medical Systems) was used to acquire these data sets with the following parameters: in-plane resolution $\approx 0.67 \times 0.67$ mm^2, matrix $\approx 500 \times 500$ pixels, slice thickness = 3 mm, slice gap = 1.5 mm, echo time = 6 ms, number of acquisitions = 5–6, total acquisition time = 300–400 s. Since the first time point is acquired before the contrast agent (CA) injection, the tumor is hard to be observed (Fig. 2 (a)). Hence, the images are collected from the second time point to the fifth time point, whereas the fourth time point is the peak time point. An elastic registration method [9] is employed to overcome motion artifacts due to thorax expansion through breathing. All these images have already been segmented by our collaborating radiologist, who is an expert in breast cancer diagnosis.

2.2   Methods

The pipeline of our approach is shown in Fig. 1. We use mask files provided by a radiologist to segment tumors from the DCE-MRI data. The three-dimensional (3D) texture features are extracted from each lesion to construct a training set and a test set for the classifiers.

The intensity change is the intuitive representation of temporal information of DCE-MRI data, where the characteristics of malignant tumors are manifested as the intensity increases with time until the peak time point and then decreases rapidly. Fig. 2 shows the intensity of a malignant tumor at different time points. The intensity of a tumor shows a great change after the contrast agent (CA) arrival (Fig. 2 (b) to Fig. 2 (d)), which are accompanied by texture feature changes. The peak time point appears in Fig. 2 (d), where the average intensity of the tumor reaches the maximum value. Although the texture shows its largest intensity and most details at the peak time point, it appears that over-smoothing and contrast within texture is lacking, compared with other time points (the value differences are shown in Tab. 1). After introducing the texture information at other time points, we get more elements for the texture analysis of the same tumor. The number of black voxels on the background would change the texture feature values and affect the classification accuracy [9]. In order to reduce the influence, we select the smallest region manually, which can contain the whole tumor. The 3D GLCM is employed to extract the texture features and generate 12 Haralick features (Tab. 1).

Tab. 1 shows the temporally changed texture feature mean values of a malignant tumor. The feature values at the first time point are not included, since its low intensity makes the texture features hard to be extracted. Where TP means time point, F1 to F12 represent different characteristics, which are energy, entropy, correlation, contrast, variance, sum mean value, inertia, cluster shade, cluster tendency, homogeneity, maximum probability and inverse variance.

There are two tumor subtypes, which are segmented at the peak time point shown in Fig. 3. Although they have a different morphology, it is difficult to

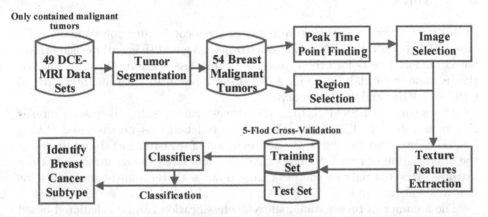

Fig. 1. The workflow of the presented approach.

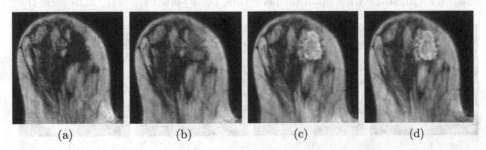

Fig. 2. A series of breast images that reflect the intensity of a malignant tumor changes over time. (a) shows the first point in time before the contrast agent injection. (b) shows the second time point 79s after the first time point. (c) and (d) are obtained at the same time interval of 79s after (b).

Table 1. Texture feature values of a malignant tumor at different time points.

TP	F1	F2	F3	F4	F5	F6	F7	F8	F9	F10	F11	F12
2	0.506	0.78	0.077	1.89	0.874	11.91	2.94	1.89	448.03	7534	0.71	0.124
3	0.506	0.77	0.057	2.02	0.873	16.32	3.31	2.02	690.55	13050	0.71	0.125
4	0.506	0.74	0.048	2.53	0.879	19.47	3.57	2.52	838.45	16613	0.71	0.122
5	0.507	0.73	0.049	2.64	0.885	19.13	3.55	2.64	799.65	15532	0.71	0.118

determine the subtypes of these malignant tumors by observing the image directly. In order to extract 3D texture features of each lesion, 13 directions and 3 distances ($d = 1, 2, 4$) are used to generate a co-occurrence matrix, which shows that the tumor has 468 features at each time point describing its texture.

In order to deal with such large number of data, we employ nonlinear SVM and random forests [10] classifying texture features to distinguish breast cancer subtypes. The classification accuracy is evaluated via 5-fold cross-validation.

3   Results

In this section, we study the performance of the second-order polynomial kernel-based SVM (quadratic SVM) and Bootstrap-aggregated (bagged) decision trees-based random forests for breast cancer subtype classification. Our implementation is done in Matlab 2016a on a Windows 7 platform with an Intel Core i5 CPU at 3.3GHz and 8GB memory.

The accuracy of SVM classifiers for breast cancer subtype classification is shown in Tab. 2 and Tab. 3. Where IDC is labeled as positive and ILC is labeled as negative, inv.duc is the abbreviation of invasive ductal and inv.lob is the abbreviation of invasive lobular. We also compared the accuracy of texture features extracted only at the peak time point with the multi-time points (at four different time points).

The accuracy of breast tumor subtype classification can be calculated based on Tab. 2 and Tab. 3, where the accuracy of SVM classifier and random forests classifier with single time point (at peak time point) is 70.4% and 72.2%, and the

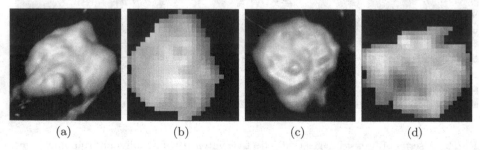

(a)   (b)   (c)   (d)

Fig. 3. Two subtypes of breast cancer, which have similar size, and whose types are hard to distinguish. (a) a volume rendering image of an ILC; (b) an axial view of (a); (c) a volume rendering image of an IDC; (d) an axial view of (c).

	Peak time point		Multi-time points	
inv.duc	26	10	138	6
inv.lob	6	12	8	64
Sensitivity	72.2%		95.8%	
Specificity	66.7%		88.9%	

Table 2. Confusion matrix of breast cancer subtype identified with single time point and different time points by SVM classifier.

	Peak time point		Multi-time points	
inv.duc	31	5	138	6
inv.lob	10	8	15	57
Sensitivity	86.1%		95.8%	
Specificity	44.4%		79.2%	

Table 3. Confusion matrix of breast cancer subtype identified with single time point and different time points by random forests.

accuracy of SVM classifier and random forests classifier with multi-time points is 93.5% and 90.3%.

4 Discussion

Compared to the common method, which is based on histology and genetic testing, the texture feature-based classification method simplifies the diagnostic process. The accuracy of more than 90% from our results shows that this method has a high potential in clinical diagnosis.

The SVM classifier shows a higher performance than the random forests classifier. Although the random forests keep a higher performance for IDC classification, the low accuracy for ILC reduced the overall performance. Besides, we partly tested the correlation between texture features and classification results. If any of these three features, energy, variance or maximum probability, has been removed from the texture features set, the SVM classification result would increase to 77.8% at the peak time point while the random forests classification result decreases to 64.8%. Otherwise, the classification result which extracted texture features from multi-time points show a slight decline ($-1\% \sim -2\%$) for both classifiers when any texture feature is removed.

We employed the SVM classifier and the random forests classifier with different time point texture features to identify the subtype of breast cancer. Compared with the method that only extracts texture features at the peak time point, the classification accuracy is significantly improved when the texture features at different time points are taken into account. The texture extraction at different time points makes full use of the temporal dynamics in DCE-MRI data. Despite of getting a high accuracy for breast cancer subtype classification, there are some limitations of our approach. We only consider the two most common subtypes of breast cancer and ignore the mixed ductal/lobular carcinoma and other rare subtypes, such as inflammatory breast cancer and phyllodes tumors of the breast. In the future, we want to develop a hybrid classifier to improve the accuracy that makes the rare subtype classification possible. Meanwhile, we want to analyze the effect of each texture feature on the classification accuracy and remove the features which have a minimum correlation or negative effect to improve the stability of the classification performance.

Acknowledgement. We would like to thank U. Preim, Klinikum Magdeburg, Germany for providing the breast DCE-MRI data and diagnostic report.

References

1. Li CI, Anderson BO, Daling JR, et al. Trends in incidence rates of invasive lobular and ductal breast carcinoma. JAMA. 2003;289(11):1421–1424.
2. Chen Z, Yang J, Li S, et al. Invasive lobular carcinoma of the breast: a special histological type compared with invasive ductal carcinoma. PLoS One. 2017;12(9).
3. Barroso-Sousa R, Metzger-Filho O. Differences between invasive lobular and invasive ductal carcinoma of the breast: results and therapeutic implications. Ther Adv Med Oncol. 2016;8(4):261–266.
4. Korkola JE, DeVries S, Fridlyand J, et al. Differentiation of lobular versus ductal breast carcinomas by expression microarray analysis. Cancer Res. 2003;63(21):7167–7175.
5. Holli K, Lääperi AL, Harrison L, et al. Characterization of breast cancer types by texture analysis of magnetic resonance images. Acad Radiol. 2010;17(2):135–141.
6. Nie K, Glaßer S, Niemann U, et al. Classification of DCE-MRI data for breast cancer diagnosis combining contrast agent dynamics and texture features. Procs BVM. 2017; p. 325–330.
7. Preim U, Glaßer S, Preim B, et al. Computer-aided diagnosis in breast DCE-MRI-quantification of the heterogeneity of breast lesions. Eur J Radiol. 2012;81(7):1532–1538.
8. Chang RF, Chen HH, Chang YC, et al. Quantification of breast tumor heterogeneity for ER status, HER2 status, and TN molecular subtype evaluation on DCE-MRI. Magn Reson Imaging. 2016;34(6):809–819.
9. Rueckert D, Sonoda LI, Hayes C, et al. Nonrigid registration using free-form deformations: application to breast MR images. IEEE Trans Med Imaging. 1999;18(8):712–721.
10. Breiman L. Random forests. Mach Learn. 2001;45(1):5–32.

Abstract: Revealing Hidden Potentials of the q-Space Signal in Breast Cancer

Paul Jaeger[1], Sebastian Bickelhaupt[2], Frederik Bernd Laun[2,3],
Wolfgang Lederer[4], Daniel Heidi[5], Tristan Anselm Kuder[6], Daniel Paech[2],
David Bonekamp[2], Alexander Radbruch[2], Stefan Delorme[2],
Heinz-Peter Schlemmer[2], Franziska Steudle[2], Klaus H. Maier-Hein[1]

[1]Medical Image Computing, German Cancer Research Center (DKFZ),
Heidelberg, Germany
[2]Department of Raiology, DKFZ, Heidelberg, Germany
[3]Institute of Radiology, University Hospital Erlangen, Germany
[4]Radiological Practice at the ATOS Clinic, Heidelberg, Germany
[5]Radiology Center Mannheim (RZM), Germany
[6]Medical Physics in Radiology, DKFZ, Heidelberg, Germany
`p.jaeger@dkfz.de`

Mammography screening for early detection of breast lesions currently suffers from high amounts of false positive findings, which result in unnecessary invasive biopsies. Diffusion-weighted MR images (DWI) can help to reduce many of these false-positive findings prior to biopsy. Current approaches estimate tissue properties by means of quantitative parameters taken from generative, biophysical models fit to the q-space signal under certain assumptions regarding noise and spatial homogeneity. This process is prone to fitting instability and partial information loss due to model simplicity. We reveal unexplored potentials of the signal by integrating all data processing components into a convolutional neural network (CNN) architecture that is designed to propagate clinical target information down to the raw input images. This approach enables simultaneous and target-specific optimization of image normalization, signal exploitation, global representation learning and classification. On a multicentric data set of 222 patients we demonstrate that our approach significantly improves clinical decision making with respect to the current state of the art, preventing 63 out of 100 unnecessary biopsies. Notably, this work has previously been published at MICCAI 2017 [1]. Subsequent experiments including automated lesion detection and a comprehensive comparison to conventional radiomics approaches will be part of an extended presentation.

References

1. Jäger PF, Bickelhaupt S, Laun FB, et al.; Springer. Revealing hidden potentials of the q-space signal in breast cancer. Proc MICCAI. 2017; p. 664–671.

Elastic Mitral Valve Silicone Replica Made from 3D-Printable Molds Offer Advanced Surgical Training

Sandy Engelhardt[1,2,3], Simon Sauerzapf[1], Sameer Al-Maisary[3],
Matthias Karck[3], Bernhard Preim[2], Ivo Wolf[1], Raffaele De Simone[3]

[1]Faculty for Computer Science, Mannheim University of Applied Sciences, Germany
[2]Dep. of Simulation and Graphics, Magdeburg University, Germany
[3]Departement of Cardiac Surgery, Heidelberg University Hospital, Germany
sandy.engelhardt@isg.cs.uni-magdeburg.de

Abstract. Reconstructive mitral valve surgeries are demanding cardiac surgeries that are conducted in the mid-age of a surgical career at the earliest. Receiving years of training in patients is required to gain the experiences and skills necessary for surgical success. On top of that, the number of such surgeries is limited per hospital, therefore other means of training should be offered to facilitate a steep learning curve. Within the scope of this work, we equipped an existing physical simulator with patient-specific flexible replica of the mitral valve. We developed software to automatically produce a 3D-printable casting mold for silicone material, as this mimics properties of the valve tissue in terms of stitching and cutting. We show the feasibility of the approach and the usefulness of these models is evaluated by an experienced cardiac surgeon, successfully conducting reconstructive surgery on pathological silicone valves.

1 Introduction

Mitral valve reconstruction is one of the most challenging procedures in cardiac surgery due to the pathomorphological complexity of the valve. This kind of procedure requires a lot of personal experience, skill and dexterity. During surgery, spontaneous decisions have to be made resulting in a potential change of the surgical techniques and strategy, which is especially challenging for trainee cardiac surgeons. Performing this surgery using minimally invasive approaches, endoscopically or through direct vision, is even more demanding for the surgeon when working with long-shafted instruments to stitch sutures in different angles than usual. Though it has been shown to be effective and beneficial for patients [1], the application of minimally invasive approaches remains concentrated in high-volume centers and it is therefore not conducted by the majority of the surgeons on a regular basis.

The current situation forces surgeons to develop most of their skills mainly in patients, which is truly unacceptable. To overcome this, physical surgical simulators became commercially available in the last years. The Mitral valve holder (LifeLike BioTissue Inc., Ontario, Canada) or the MA-TRAC High Fidelity Minimally invasive Mitral Valve Repair simulator (Maastricht Trading Company, Inc., Maastricht, The Netherlands) are equipped with mitral valves made of silicone. Others offer valves made of felt, e.g. for the MICS MVR Simulator (Fehling Inc., Acworth, Georgia, USA), Fig. 3. However, these valves are generic, lack patient-individual features and are therefore not suitable to address strategies for specific pathologies. Providing patient-specific replica reflecting the realistic anatomy and tissue before the actual operation takes place would be beneficial in terms of accurately planning and training critical steps of the reconstructive method applied in real surgery.

Existing works already addressed direct 3D-printing of the mitral valve using acrylonitrile butadiene styrene (ABS) plastic material [2]. It goes without saying that stiff material hinders adequate surgical training. Vukicevic et al. [3] also used direct printing, but employed multi-material elastomeric TangoPlus materials (Stratasys, Eden Prairie, Minnesota, USA) that were compared to freshly harvested porcine leaflet tissue. All TangoPlus varieties were less stiff than the maximum tensile elastic modulus of mitral valve tissue. Regardless of the tissue stiffness, surgical eligibility of the material in terms of realistic stitching properties also needs to be evaluated. Furthermore, this approach requires expensive printer and materials. Ilina et al. [4] produced silicone heart valve models from a patient-specific 3D-printable mold. Surgeons reported good tissue properties (realistic flexibility, cuts and holds sutures well without tearing) from their personal experiences and considered the silicone models to be useful for surgical planning. The main focus of their work were pediatric congenital heart valves.

The aim of this work is to produce elastic patient-individual 3D-models of the mitral valve for adult surgery, that can be fixated into the existing MICS MVR surgical simulator to consider crucial techniques of reconstructive surgery.

2 Materials and methods

Together with the involved surgeons, we identified the following requirements for physical replica of patient-specific valves:

- R1: the leaflets should reflect end-systolic shape of patient-specific valve, such that the morphology of potential prolapsing segments are visible,
- R2: stitching properties of the material should be realistic such that rounded needles can be inserted and sutures pass through with similar tissue resistance as in real surgery,
- R3: the model must be fixable into the MICS MVR simulator to provide a realistic port-to-valve relation,
- R4: low-cost materials for 3D-printing and no specific printer should be used to facilitate reproducibility of the approach by other groups,
- R5: total production time should be ≤ 2 days and the process as automated as possible to facilitate integration into the patient workflow management.

We decided to produce silicone valves, as they were positively evaluated by surgeons for congenital heart valves [4] (R2). A potential casting mold for the silicone must consist of different pieces, including a valve holder (R3), that can be sticked together and easily opened up.

2.1   Generation of generic mold parts

The generic parts of the mold were once created in a CAD program to fit into the MICS MVR surgical simulator (Fehling Inc., Acworth, Georgia, USA), Fig. 1. The mold is comprised of an upper and lower part forming the outer shell. A valve holder (Fig. 2) is placed inside the mold such that silicone connects to the ring of the holder during silicone casting (R3). The outer parts are equipped with a chute to ease casting of silicone into the mold. The valve holder has two additional holes with a double function: They are used as air ducts that enables air to flow out when displaced by the silicone, otherwise larger air bubbles would remain inside the mold (R2). Secondly, their walls have threads in order to anchor the holder in the simulator (R3).

2.2   Automatic augmentation with patient-specific parts

Mitral valve models are interactively segmented from 3D echocardiography by an expert using the MITK-Plugin Mitralyzer [5], which is based on the open source framework Medical Imaging Interaction Toolkit. The resulting systolic surface model is then used to add patient-specificity to the mold (R1). The

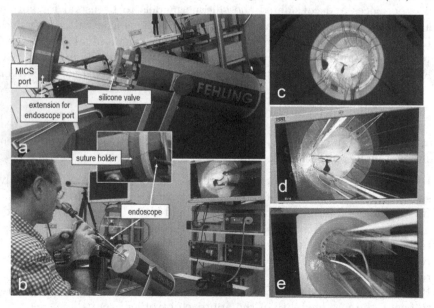

Fig. 1. a) Minimally invasive cardiac surgery (MICS) mitral valve repair (MVR) simulator with novel endoscopic port component, suture holder and a patient-individual valve b) Surgeon performs leaflet resection and annuloplasty c) Direct view onto the valve through the port d) Endoscopic view e) Implantation of a printed prosthetic ring.

model is rotated and transformed to the center of the generic parts. A collar
around the annulus is created in the size of the inner hole of the generic parts
(Fig. 2). Then, the free leaflet ends are connected to each other to close the
gap between the leaflets tips. After Laplacian smoothing with 20 iterations, the
negative form of the patient-specific part is created as follows: The extended
valve surface is used as an implicit function in the Visualization Toolkit (VTK)
to clip two 3D grid cubes: the first time with a defined offset in the direction
of the surface normals and the second time without offset. The offset describes
the later valve thickness. The resulting counterparts of the mold are shown in
Fig. 2, top row right. This geometry is clipped with a cylinder, connected to
the generic parts of the mold and finally exported to stl.

2.3   Slicing, printing and silicone casting

The stl-file is loaded into the open-source and widely used slicing software Ultimaker Cura 3.0. The generated gcode-file is then sent to the Ultimaker 2+
printer (Ultimaker B.V., Geldermalsen, The Netherlands) to print the mold
pieces in polylactide (PLA). PLA is a cheap, biodegradable and bioactive ther-
moplastic aliphatic polyester derived from renewable resources (R4). Of course,
other software, printers and stiff materials could be used for mold production.
After printing, support material must be removed.

For simulating mitral valve tissue, we created a silicone mixture using Dragon
Skin® silicone 10 Fast (Smooth On, Inc., Macungie, PA, USA). The silicone
rubbers were mixed 1A:1B by volume. Per valve, roughly 100 ml is needed. A
slacker component is added to the silicone mixture in a ratio of 1:10 to improve
flowability. Slacker changes the "feel" of the silicone rubber to a softer material.
It also alters the rebound properties of the silicone, making it feel more like
human tissue (R2). Pot life of the silicone is around 8 min. Leukoplast tights
the mold parts together during casting through the chute. Afterwards, the parts
are put into a vacuum pump for vacuum degassing. Cure time is around 75 min
for this specific silicone mixture. Then, the mold parts can be easily detached and
the free leaflet ends need to be manually separated into anterior and posterior
leaflet by a scalpel. Finally, the valve can be inserted into the simulator. The
full process of silicone valve production is shown in Fig. 2.

3   Results

3.1   Feasibility

A set of three different valves with leaflet thickness of 1.5 mm were created
according to the proposed pipeline and fixed subsequently in the simulator: a
normal, a prolapsed and an ischemic valve (Fig. 3). This set includes the two
main categories of valve pathologies. Creating a mold, and placing the pour
hole for silicone with a chute close to the posterior part of the leaflets enables
easy filling without wasting material. Furthermore, we observed that all bubbles

are reduced in comparison to other filling strategies, such as filling one side of the mold and placing the other side on top of that (R2). We used the low-cost Ultimaker 2+ for printing the molds (R4) with a layer thickness of 0.2 mm. The printer has only little tolerances when printing PLA, such that individual mold parts could be sticked together. Staircase artifacts from the layers were hardly visible on the final silicone models. The estimated total producing time for one silicone valve, including 3D printing, is more than 12 hours, which means that one has to start 1-2 days before surgery. To further save time, the generic valve holder can be printed in advance to have it on stock (R5).

3.2   Usefulness

Evaluation is carried out by an experienced surgeon, who conducted a valve repair by leaflet plasty and annuloplasty on the silicone valves (Fig. 1). Afterwards, he filled out a questionnaire assessing the models. In the following, we sum up the answers: He found the silicone material to have a realistic flexibility. It cuts and holds sutures well without tearing when employing different reconstructive techniques (R2). However, a human valve tissue would probably tear more rapidly according to his experiences. Position in the simulator, shape, size and thickness of the valve was assessed as realistic (R3). Visual comparison of the silicone model to the virtual model revealed, that the silicone leaflets remain in their end systolic shape as acquired by echocardiography (Fig. 2 and 3; R1).

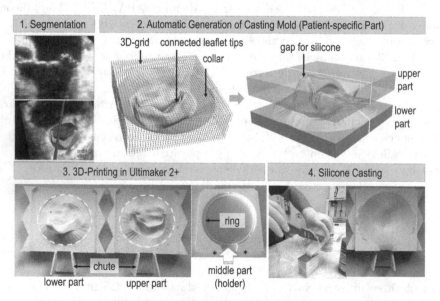

Fig. 2. Process of silicone valve production. Generic CAD-parts become algorithmically extended with the patient-specific geometry indicated by the yellow dashed circles. The yellow solid line has the purpose to visualize the gap between the counterparts. Large arrow shows direction of silicone flow. Asterisks mark position of air ducts.

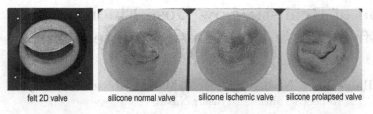

Fig. 3. Valves
in holder.

felt 2D valve   silicone normal valve   silicone ischemic valve   silicone prolapsed valve

One point of criticism was that the correct course of the annulus was not easily recognizable. The difference in tissue between valve and surrounding is better distinguishable in real patients. All in all, the silicone models were considered to be extremely useful for surgical planning and for training of difficult cases, as they also improve visual 3D perception of the individual pathology.

4   Discussion

Within the scope of this work, we propose a novel pipeline for creation of patient-specific mitral valve replica that satisfy the given requirements. As can be seen in Fig. 2, some steps of the full pipeline are conducted automatically, while others require manual work to be conducted. To speed up the process, a robust automatic approach for valve segmentation [5] should be used (R5). All in all, we could produce similar results and feedback from end user as by Ilina et al. [4]. In contrast to their work, our silicone leaflets appear thinner and better stay in their systolic shape. We furthermore propose a different mold creation process and a stable valve anchor that directly connects to the silicone during casting.

Future work will include integration of individual regional leaflet thicknesses, the structures of chordae tendinae, papillary muscles and surrounding anatomy. This would also offer cardiologists to gain experiences and procedural training in novel catheter-based structural interventions [3]. Furthermore, the simulator enables training of recent optical tracking measurement procedures [6].

References

1. Mick SL, Keshavamurthy S, Gillinov AM. Mitral valve repair versus replacement. Ann Cardiothorac Surg. 2015;4(3):230–7.
2. Witschey RTW, Pouch AM, McGarvey JR, et al. Three-dimensional ultrasound-derived Physical Mitral Valve Modeling. Ann Thorac Surg. 2014;98:691–4.
3. Vukicevic M, Puperi DS, Grande-Allen JK, et al. 3D printed modeling of the mitral valve for catheter-based structural interventions. Ann Biomed Eng. 2017;45(2):508–519.
4. Ilina A, Lasso A, Jolley MA, et al. Patient-specific pediatric silicone heart valve models based on 3D ultrasound. In: Proc SPIE 10135; 2017. p. 1013516.
5. Engelhardt S, Lichtenberg N, Al-Maisary S, et al. Towards automatic assessment of the mitral valve coaptation zone from 4D ultrasound. In: Functional Imaging and Modelling of the Heart. 9126; 2015. p. 137–145.
6. Engelhardt S, Wolf I, Al-Maisary S, et al. Intraoperative quantitative mitral valve analysis using optical tracking technology. Ann Thorac Surg. 2016;101(5):1950–6.

Simulation of Realistic Low Dose Fluoroscopic Images from their High Dose Counterparts

Sai Gokul Hariharan[1,2], Norbert Strobel[2,4], Markus Kowarschik[1,2], Rebecca Fahrig[2,5], Nassir Navab[1,3]

[1]Computer Aided Medical Procedures (CAMP), Technische Universität München, Munich, Germany
[2]Siemens Healthineers, Advanced Therapies, Forchheim, Germany
[3]Whiting School of Engineering, Johns Hopkins University, Baltimore, USA
[4]Fakultät für Elektrotechnik, Hochschule für angewandte Wissenschaften Würzburg-Schweinfurt, Schweinfurt, Germany
[5] Pattern Recognition Lab, Friedrich-Alexander-Universität Erlangen-Nürnberg (FAU), Erlangen, Germany
saigokul.hariharan@tum.de

Abstract. Learning based denoising methods have attracted increasing interest in the recent past. These methods rely on data pairs. In the case of denoising, the data pairs are usually noise corrupted images and their noise-free counterparts, if available. Otherwise an associated high-dose X-ray image can be used instead as a practical alternative. As the current image processing techniques are not yet able to provide the necessary image quality at very low dose levels, it is usually not possible to acquire clinical sequences. As variation in the data is extremely important for learning based methods, phantom data alone cannot be used to train a network and achieve optimal performance. A possibility to overcome this issue is to simulate low dose images from the related high dose images. However, to make sure that the simulated low dose images are realistic (replicate the properties of real low dose images), image noise attributes associated with low dose image acquisition need to be taken into account. In their paper we introduce a novel method to simulate low dose images from high dose images based on modelling the X-ray image formation process. This way, we can better account for imaging parameters such as system gain and electronic noise. We have evaluated our method by comparing several corresponding regions of the simulated lower dose images with that of real lower dose images using a two sample Kolmogorov-Smirnov Test at 5% significance. Out of 40 pairs, in 85% of the cases the hypothesis that the corresponding regions (from the low and simulated low dose images) belong to the same distribution has been accepted.

1 Introduction

Exposure to high X-ray radiation has always been an important issue for patients as well as the clinicians. For instance, there are procedures based on fluoroscopic guidance, such as the treatment of chronic total occlusion (CTO) that can last for several hours. In addition, procedures may be repeated, for example, due to failed initial attempts. As a consequence, patients as well as staff (in due course) may be exposed to non-negligible amount of radiation. The potential consequences of high radiation exposures fall under two categories namely stochastic (cancer) and deterministic risks (skin injury, hair loss). According to the ALARA principle, radiation doses can be lowered only if it is possible to maintain the necessary image quality needed to carry out a clinical task safely. This has provided an opportunity to reduce X-ray exposure using sophisticated image processing techniques, if one can manage to keep the image quality up to the required standard.

Learning based methods on the other hand have been shown to solve complicated problems if sufficient training data is available. Zhang et al. [1] have developed a deep learning based blind denoising algorithm for optical still images corrupted by additive white noise. Wolternik et al. [2] have employed a generative adversarial network for denoising low dose CT volumes to transform them into regular dose images. Although there are several methods proposed for optical images and CT volumes, there is limited literature for denoising of X-ray images/sequences that involves deep learning. Matviychuk et al. [3] have published a learning based method for X-ray image denoising. The results published in this paper are, however, computed using DICOM images, i.e., the images (ground truth or the expected output) have already been processed by an imaging system before it has been stored in DICOM format. As a consequence, the data has most likely undergone some gray level point transform as well as image quality enhancement. In order to generate noisy data they have added additive Gaussian noise to their ground truth images. Since actual X-ray images involve Poisson as well as Gaussian noise, simply adding Gaussian noise to a final result may yield results that differ from what one may encounter in a more realistic environment.

In fact, researchers have tried adding noise to high dose images to simulate low dose images making the assumption that the sequences are corrupted by Poisson (and) or Gaussian noise in the past. Unfortunately, they have usually relied on image formation models that do not fully account for how X-ray images are acquired in practice, i.e., when different gain factors are used and when noise levels depend on particular X-ray examination protocols. Often the assumption is made that the detector gain is one. This may not always be true as a higher gain is usually applied when the dose is low to make better utilization of the available dynamic range of the D/A converter. Moreover, at ultra-low dose levels and high gain, even small amounts of electronic noise start to matter, and the noise itself may also depend on the detector gain used. Finally, researchers have used sequences stored in DICOM format for generating noise corrupted images. In general, these sequences are tone mapped versions of the Poisson-Gaussian corrupted sequences and no longer represent actual pixel values whose brightness is proportional to the amount of X-ray quanta received. Unless system dependent parameters are taken into account, it may not be possible to simulate realistic noisy low dose sequences from high dose. And if pairs of associated noisy (low dose) and noise free (high dose) clinical sequences are not available, it is difficult to develop learning based methods. As a solution, we propose a novel method to generate low dose images from high dose images such that the simulated low dose images have the same image characteristics as if they have actually been taken at a lower dose.

2   Materials and methods

Many noise simulation approaches have been developed assuming that the noise is either signal independent homogeneous additive white Gaussian noise with a known variance or signal dependent Poisson noise with a system gain of 1. However, in real X-ray applications the situation is more complicated. For example, the noise has various sources (e.g., Poisson noise, electronic noise, quantization noise) and, depending on the imaging situation, different gains are applied. To take this into account, we introduce an image formation model first. We then describe the low dose simulation method that depends on this model.

2.1   Image formation and noise model

The formation of images from X-ray quanta can be assumed to follow a linear model [4]. The mean gray value $\bar{y}[i,j]$ at a particular location $[i,j]$ has a linear relationship with respect to the incident mean X-ray air kerma $\bar{x}$ at that location. That is, the measured mean quanta, $\bar{x}[i,j]$, is scaled by the detector gain, α, and shifted by the overall system offset p.

$$\bar{y}[i,j] = \alpha \cdot \bar{x}[i,j] + p \tag{1}$$

The quantum nature of X-ray photons can be modelled using a Poisson distribution. The presence of electronic noise, e.g., due to read out noise and dark noise, can be modelled using a Gaussian distribution with zero mean. The formation of an image (assuming flat field correction) can thus be represented as

$$y[i,j] = \alpha \cdot (x[i,j] + \eta_a[i,j]) + p + \eta_q[i,j] = \alpha \cdot x[i,j] + p + \eta[i,j] \tag{2}$$

Here x, η_a, η_q and y represent the quanta, electronic noise due to analog sensor read out, electronic noise due to quantization (analog to digital conversion) and the noise-corrupted detector pixel value, respectively. The overall additive noise can be represented as η. The gain is typically chosen such that the resulting pixel values occupy as much of the available dynamic range as possible before quantization takes place. The choice of the detector gain determines the amount of Poisson noise present in the images.

2.2   Generation of low dose images from high dose images

Let us assume that we acquire a high dose image $y_h[i,j]$ as well as a low dose image $y_l[i,j]$ of the same object using the same tube voltage.

$$y_h[i,j] = \alpha_h \cdot x_h[i,j] + p_h + \eta_h[i,j] \tag{3}$$

$$y_l[i,j] = \alpha_l \cdot x_l[i,j] + p_l + \eta_l[i,j] \qquad (4)$$

The mean dose at a particular pixel in the high dose image should be a scaled version (by a factor c) of the mean dose of the corresponding pixel in the low dose image, i.e.

$$\bar{x}_l[i,j] = [\bar{x}_h[i,j] \cdot c] \qquad (5)$$

From equations 3, 4 and 5, the mean gray values of the low dose and high dose can be related a follows

$$\bar{y}_{h \to l}[i,j] = \left[\frac{\alpha_l}{\alpha_h} \cdot c \cdot \bar{y}_h[i,j] + p_l - c \cdot \frac{\alpha_l}{\alpha_h} \cdot p_h \right] \qquad (6)$$

From Eq. 6, it can be observed that the noise-free low dose image $\bar{y}_{h \to l}$ can be derived from the noise-free high dose image by scaling and adding an offset. Using these transform parameters helps in retaining the mean of low dose images. i.e, the mean gray values of $y_{h \to l}$ are the same as found in y_l. This transformation can also be performed by analysing several corresponding regions of the low and high dose images and obtaining the scaling factor as well as the offset. The transformation also scales the electronic noise due to analog sensor read out (η_a) to match that of low dose images.

The next step is to add noise to the linearly transformed high dose image, $\bar{y}_{h \to l}$, such that its noise level matches the one found in the original low dose images. We perform this in the generalized Anscombe domain by adding an appropriate amount of white Gaussian noise. The generalized Anscombe transform (GAT) has been designed to stabilize signal-dependent noise to a known constant (usually unit variance) [5]. We use the system parameters of the low dose image, α_l, p_l and σ_{η_l}, and apply the transform on $\bar{y}_{h \to l}$ to obtain $\bar{y}'_{h \to l}$.

Since the signal to noise ratio is much higher in high dose images, the noise present in $\bar{y}'_{h \to l}$, will, in general, be very low (variance much less than 1). We measure the amount of noise present in the image by analysing flat patches. Taking into account the amount of noise present, we add Gaussian noise with standard deviation σ'_n to make the standard deviation of noise in $\bar{y}'_{h \to l}$ equal to one. The corrupted image in the GAT domain is represented as $y'_{h \to l}$. We then apply inverse generalized Anscombe transform on $y'_{h \to l}$ using the parameters of the low dose image, α_l, σ_{η_l} and p_l, to get back to the image domain $y_{h \to l}$.

3   Results

As only a limited selection of phantoms has been available to us, we have chosen coronary angiogram images and cerebral angiogram images to validate our procedure. Sequences using the thorax phantom have been acquired at different dose levels (100%, 81%, 50%, 28% and 15% and 7.5%) without moving the phantom. Similarly, sequences using the brain phantom have been acquired at dose levels 100%, 66%, 33% and 20%. These images have been acquired with Artis zee systems (Siemens Healthineers, Erlangen, Germany). We have made use of the sequence acquired at 100% dose, which is the clinical standard, to simulate the lower dose sequences. We have also verified that the images have been acquired at the same tube voltage. System parameters used during acquisition have been used for transforming the high dose images y_h to low dose $y_{h \to l}$.

We have validated the method by analysing the standard deviation and the mean of several corresponding flat regions in the low dose and the simulated low dose images for all fractions of the dose mentioned above. The values of the simulated images match that of the low dose images (Tab. 1 for a selection of values). In addition, in Fig. 1(a) we show an ROI of the simulated 7.5% dose images from 100% dose image of the thorax phantom. It can be observed that the simulated image (Fig. 1(c)) resembles the low dose image (Fig. 1(b)) in terms of visual appearance. Similarly, the simulated 22% dose image (Fig. 1(g)) from the 100% dose image (Fig. 1(e)) of the brain phantom matches the low dose image (Fig. 1(f)) visually. Moreover, the difference images appear to be free from structures (Fig. 1(d) and Fig. 1(h)). We have also compared the corresponding regions of the simulated low dose images generated from 100% dose images and actual low dose images using a two-sample Kolmogorov-Smirnov Test [6] at 5% significance level. The two-sample Kolmogorov-Smirnov test is a non-parametric hypothesis test that evaluates the difference between the cumulative distribution functions of the distributions of the two sample data vectors. In 85% of the cases, the hypothesis that the regions come from the same distribution has been accepted. In the cases where the hypothesis have been rejected, there

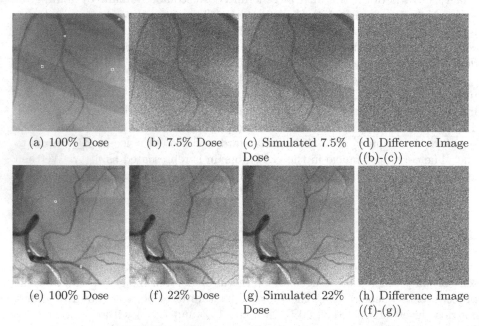

(a) 100% Dose   (b) 7.5% Dose   (c) Simulated 7.5% Dose   (d) Difference Image ((b)-(c))

(e) 100% Dose   (f) 22% Dose   (g) Simulated 22% Dose   (h) Difference Image ((f)-(g))

Fig. 1. Results (selected ROI) for the simulation of low dose images from 100% dose images of thorax (top row) and brain phantom (bottom row). Some of the regions used for comparison in Tab. 1 have been highlighted in (a) and (e).

Table 1. Comparison of Low Dose (LD) and Simulated Low Dose (SLD) Images with respect to mean (μ) and standard deviation (σ) across several regions.

| Region | Thorax Phantom | | | | Brain Phantom | | | |
| | LD (7.5%) | | SLD (7.5%) | | LD (22%) | | SLD (22%) | |
	μ	σ	μ	σ	μ	σ	μ	σ
1	67.63	12.03	68.44	12.02	22.12	1.61	21.98	1.40
2	17.87	7.49	17.84	7.82	10.67	1.26	10.63	1.09
3	38.81	8.88	39.11	8.92	13.20	1.68	13.05	1.49
4	26.24	8.47	26.79	7.89	11.77	1.23	11.49	1.16
5	68.40	12.46	69.16	12.92	15.37	1.40	15.42	1.35

is a difference in the mean and standard deviation by a factor of around 2% and 10%, respectively. These results can be explained by recalling that our input images are taken after pixel defect and flat field correction and remembering that these corrections depend on the dose level as well as on the spatial position in the image. In other words, these correction mechanisms differ for high dose and low dose images.

4 Discussion

In this paper we have proposed an effective method to simulate low dose X-ray images from higher dose X-ray images taking into consideration the system parameters. The simulation results have been found to be acceptably accurate based on both visual comparison and statistical analysis. Our future work will address the impact of scattered radiaition and will also involve data from several X-ray detectors. Furthermore, the method will be extended to flat panel C-arm CT applications, e.g., extending the approach outlined in [4].

References

1. Zhang K, Zuo W, Chen Y, et al. Beyond a gaussian denoiser: residual learning of deep CNN for image denoising. IEEE Trans Image Process. 2017.
2. Wolterink JM, Leiner T, Viergever MA, et al. Generative adversarial networks for noise reduction in low-dose CT. IEEE Trans Med Imaging. 2017.
3. Matviychuk Y, Mailhé B, Chen X, et al.; IEEE. Learning a multiscale patch-based representation for image denoising in x-ray fluoroscopy. Proc Int Conf Image Proc. 2016; p. 2330–2334.
4. Yang K, Huang SY, Packard NJ, et al. Noise variance analysis using a flat panel x-ray detector: a method for additive noise assessment with application to breast CT applications. Med Phys. 2010;37(7):3527–3537.
5. Makitalo M, Foi A. Optimal inversion of the generalized Anscombe transformation for poisson-gaussian noise. IEEE Trans Image Process. 2013;22(1):91–103.
6. Massey Jr FJ. The kolmogorov-smirnov test for goodness of fit. J Am Stat Assoc. 1951;46(253):68–78.

Towards Full-body X-ray Images

Christoph Luckner[1,2], Thomas Mertelmeier[2], Andreas Maier[1], Ludwig Ritschl[2]

[1]Pattern Recognition Lab, FAU Erlangen-Nuernberg
[2]Siemens Healthcare GmbH, Forchheim
christoph.luckner@fau.de

Abstract. Digital tomosynthesis is a tomographic imaging technique whose upsurge is mainly caused by breast imaging. However, it might also be useful in orthopedics due to its high in-plane resolution as well as the fact that tomosynthetic slices do not suffer from magnification or distortion, making measurements possible, for example, even without the need of any calibration object. Since the reading time of such a reconstruction is higher compared to conventional 2-D radiographs, a simple parallel projection of the volume can be computed to get an overview of the volume. However, this leads to a rather blurred image impression since all artifacts and inhomogeneities in the reconstructed volume as well as certain anatomical structures which are not necessary for the diagnosis, will end up in the projection. We propose a method which selects the slices to be projected into a smart synthetic X-ray image in a way which is optimal w.r.t to the sharpness of predefined ROIs (e. g. knee, spine or hip). Therefore, two Laplacian-based auto-focus measures are combined with a thin-plate spline yielding a sharp and homogenous image impression within the smart radiograph. It was shown that the auto-focus method is able to select the same slice as have been selected during an expert annotation. Upon visual inspection, it could be determined that the proposed method achieves higher contrast and clearly better visibility of complex bone structures like spine or hip.

1 Introduction

Digital tomosynthesis (DT) is a tomographic imaging technique using flat panel detectors, which allows creating multiple tomographic images in a specified plane. Its upsurge is mainly caused by breast imaging, however, it might also be useful in orthopedics. Even though DT is characterized by an incomplete data acquisition, meaning that it fails to provide a complete and isotropic 3-D imaging of the scanned object, especially its high in-plane resolution as well as the fact that reconstructed slices do not suffer from magnification or distortion compensate its drawbacks. The former yields that DT provides excellent visibility of fine structures, necessary for the assessment of high contrast structures like bone and joint structures, which can be difficult to assess in conventional 2-D radiographs. The latter may allow the usage of tomosynthetic datasets for surgical planning or the assessment of pathologies since measurements are easily possible even without the need of a dedicated calibration object [1, 2]. Since the reading time of a tomosynthetic volume is increased compared to plain 2-D X-rays, a synthetic radiograph can be created based on the 3-D reconstruction by performing a simple parallel projection of all slices. However, this leads to a rather blurred image impression since all artifacts and inhomogeneities in the reconstructed tomo-volume, as well as certain anatomical structures which are not necessary for the diagnosis, will end up in the synthetic radiograph. We, instead, propose a method which selects the slices to be projected into the smart synthetic X-ray image (sSR) in a way which is optimal in terms of sharpness of predefined regions of interest (ROIs).

2   Materials and methods

In the following, the image acquisition and reconstruction process using filtered backprojection will be outlined. Then, the proposed algorithm to generate sSR using auto-focus measures and thin-plate splines is presented. The results were compared to an average intensity projection and the current state-of-the-art acquisition technique for full-body imaging - the source-tilting technique.

2.1   Image acquisition and reconstruction

The acquisition geometry as well as the parallel-shift line trajectory (indicated as blue arrows) is shown in Fig. 1. The chosen trajectory allows lying as well as standing acquisitions and thus is also capable of weight-bearing acquisitions. The distance between source and detector is denoted as SID. N_u and N_v is the number of pixels in u- and v direction and the corresponding isotropic pixel pitch is denoted as d_u and d_v, respectively. The acquired projections form the basis for the reconstruction, which uses the cone-angle to obtain depth information. To cope with aliasing artifacts due to the scanning geometry a slice thickness filter as introduced in [3] is used as preprocessing step before the reconstruction, which is performed using the widely-used filtered backprojection. The reconstruction will be denoted as $V(\boldsymbol{x}, z)$, with $\boldsymbol{x} = (x, y)$, consisting of N_x and N_y isotropic pixels in x- and y-direction and N_z slices with slice thickness d_z in z-direction.

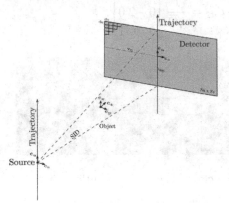

Fig. 1. Acquisition geometry and parallel-shift trajectory (indicated as blue arrows) [3].

88   Luckner et al.

2.2 Smart x-ray image generation

The generation of a smart synthetic radiograph consists of four subsequent steps:

1. Define one (or multiple) ROI $\mathcal{R}$ in a tomosynthesis slice. A set of ROIs (knees, hip, lumbar spine, thoracic sp. and cervical sp.) is illustrated in Fig. 2.
$$\mathcal{R}(z) \equiv V(\boldsymbol{x}, z), \text{ with } x, y \in \mathcal{R}$$
2. Compute focus measures α for each ROI $\mathcal{R}$ within each slice.
3. Use best, i.e. sharpest, slice as seed point for a thin-plate spline (TPS).
4. Project the optimal slices (according to the TPS) into the sSR.

Auto-focus measure To determine the degree of focus for a slice z inside an ROI $\mathcal{R}$, we compute two Laplacian-based auto-focus measures α.

The first measure, the Energy of Laplacian (LAPE) [4], is defined as

$$\alpha_{\text{LAPE}}(\mathcal{R}(z)) = \sum_{x,y} \Delta\mathcal{R}(\boldsymbol{x}, z)^2 \qquad (1)$$

where $\Delta\mathcal{R}$ is the image Laplacian obtained by a convolution of a slice z of the ROI $\mathcal{R}$ with the Laplacian masks

$$\mathcal{L}_x = [1 \quad -2 \quad 1] \text{ and } \mathcal{L}_y = \mathcal{L}_x^T$$

The second measure, the diagonal Laplacian (LAPD) [4], is defined as

$$\alpha_{\text{LAPD}}(\mathcal{R}(z)) = |\mathcal{R}(z) * \hat{\mathcal{L}}_x| + |\mathcal{R}(z) * \hat{\mathcal{L}}_y| + |\mathcal{R}(z) * \mathcal{L}_{d1}| + |\mathcal{R}(z) * \mathcal{L}_{d2}| \qquad (2)$$

with $\hat{\mathcal{L}}_x = -\mathcal{L}_x = [-1\, 2\, -1]$ and $\hat{\mathcal{L}}_y = \hat{\mathcal{L}}_x^T$ as modified convolution masks to detect vertical and horizontal structures, and $\mathcal{L}_{d1}$ and $\mathcal{L}_{d2}$ to detect diagonal structures, which are given by

$$\mathcal{L}_{d1} = \frac{1}{\sqrt{2}} \begin{bmatrix} 0 & 0 & 1 \\ 0 & -2 & 0 \\ 1 & 0 & 0 \end{bmatrix} \text{ and } \mathcal{L}_{d2} = \frac{1}{\sqrt{2}} \begin{bmatrix} 1 & 0 & 0 \\ 0 & -2 & 0 \\ 0 & 0 & 1 \end{bmatrix}$$

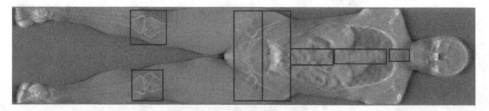

Fig. 2. Central slice of a tomosynthetic reconstruction. The ROIs are outlined in blue.

Since auto-focus measures are prone to noise and artifacts, we apply a moving average filter as a post-processing step to the computed auto-focues measures, to cope with outliers.

Finally, the mean value over the two smoothed auto-focus measures $\widehat{\alpha}$ is computed to obtain a combined and slice-dependent measure for the amount of focus within an ROI. Thus, selecting the best, i.e. sharpest, slice $z_{\mathcal{R}}^*$ for an ROI $\mathcal{R}$ is a simple maximum operation over all slices z

$$z_{\mathcal{R}}^* = \max_z \{0.5 \cdot (\widehat{\alpha}_{\mathrm{LAPE}}(\mathcal{R}(z)) + \widehat{\alpha}_{\mathrm{LAPD}}(\mathcal{R}(z)))\} \tag{3}$$

Thin-plate spline In order to obtain a smooth and homogeneous image impression, we propose to use a thin-plate smoothing spline (TPS). The TPS fits a mapping function $f(\boldsymbol{x})$ matching the set of coordinate inputs for each ROI $\{\boldsymbol{x}_1 \cdots \boldsymbol{x}_R\}$ with the set of optimal slices $\{z_{\mathcal{R}_1}^* \cdots z_{\mathcal{R}_R}^*\}$, by minimizing the following energy function E

$$E(f(\boldsymbol{x})) = \lambda \cdot \sum_{r=1}^{R} \|z_r^* - f(\bar{\boldsymbol{x}}_r)\|^2 + (1-\lambda) \iint \left[\left(\tfrac{\partial^2 f}{\partial x^2}\right)^2 + 2\left(\tfrac{\partial^2 f}{\partial x \partial y}\right)^2 + \left(\tfrac{\partial^2 f}{\partial y^2}\right)^2 \right] \mathrm{d}x\,\mathrm{d}y \tag{4}$$

with $\bar{\boldsymbol{x}}_r$ as central point of the r-th ROI, and λ as smoothing parameter controlling the amount of how much non-ridged transformation is allowed [5].

The determined function f maps each image pixel to a certain slice which is optimal according to the auto-focus measures and the smoothness criterion. Since the resulting value is not necessarily an integer, we apply linear interpolation between the two neighboring slices to obtain the actual projection value.

2.3   Experiment

For proof of concept, we simulated a scan with a female XCAT full-body phantom [6]. In total 380 anterior-posterior noise-free projections (1440x1440 pixel á 0.296 mm with SID = 180 cm and a parallel-shift of 5 mm) were acquired using the presented trajectory and reconstructed using filtered backprojection with $N_z = 100$, a slice thickness $d_z = 3$ mm and an isotropic pixel size $d_x = d_y = 1$ mm.

For evaluation an average intensity projection, i.e. a parallel projection over all slices as well as a conventional full-body radiograph acquired with the Siemens Healthineers SmartOrtho^{TM}-technique was generated.

3   Results

Fig. 3 shows a plot of the auto-focus measures for the right knee, the upper part of the hip, as well as the cervical spine. The dotted red line indicates the expert-annotated ground truth (GT), regarding which slices are optimal w.r.t. sharpness. From this data, we computed the TPS which is presented in Fig. 4. The black dots indicate the sampling points, i.e. the central points of the ROIs $\bar{x}$ and the corresponding slice $z_{\mathcal{R}}^*$. For illustration, the 3-D view, as well as the y-z plane, is shown. Fig. 5 shows a comparison of the full-body smart synthetic radiograph (sSR), an average intensity projection (AIP) as well as a conventional 2-D full-body acquisition (CR). The computation time of the complete algorithm was about 2 seconds.

4   Discussion

We proposed an algorithm which automatically generates a smart synthetic radiograph from a tomosynthetic reconstruction. It was shown that it is possible to use auto-focus measures to select the slices within a reconstruction which were also considered to be optimal during an expert annotation. Yet, in Fig. 3(c) the method did not work as expected which might be due to low image contrast. The obtained thin-plate spline ensures that predefined ROIs are clearly visible and guarantees an overall homogeneous image impression. Furthermore, the double S-shape of the spine is clearly visible in Fig. 4(b). While on the one hand, the smart radiograph has an overall sharp impression especially of the spine as can be seen in Fig. 5, the standard synthetic radiograph suffers from overlapping structures and the state-of-the-art full-body radiograph approach from overlapping structures and distortion and magnification. As a topic for future research,

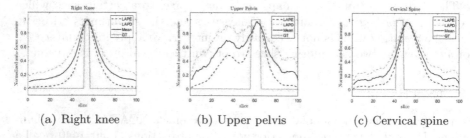

(a) Right knee   (b) Upper pelvis   (c) Cervical spine

Fig. 3. Auto-focus measures for the right knee (a), the upper pelvis (b) and the cervical spine (c). LAPE is plotted in blue, LAPD in green and the combined mean focus measure in black. The dotted red line indicates the expert-annotated ground truth (GT).

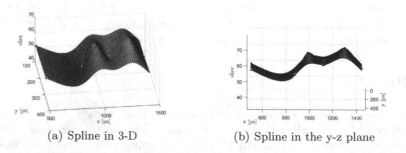

(a) Spline in 3-D   (b) Spline in the y-z plane

Fig. 4. Exemplary thin-plate spline in 3-D and the corresponding y-z plane view.

Fig. 5. Comparison of an average intesity projection [AIP] (a,d), the smart synthetic radiograph [sSR] (b,e) and a conventional 2-D full-body acquistion [CR] (c,f) for the full body (a,b,c) and a detail view of the spine (d,e,f).

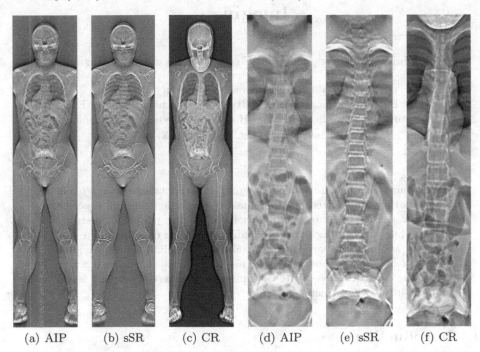

(a) AIP   (b) sSR   (c) CR   (d) AIP   (e) sSR   (f) CR

the selection of the ROIs, which is currently done manually, could be replaced by an automated detection using, for instance, deep neural networks.

Disclaimer. The concepts and information presented in this paper are based on research and are not commercially available.

References

1. Dobbins JT. Tomosynthesis imaging: at a translational crossroads. Med Phys. 2009;36(6):1956–1967.
2. Lauritsch G, Härer WH. A theoretical framework for filtered backprojection in tomosynthesis. Proc SPIE. 1998;3338(2):1127–1137.
3. Luckner C, et al. Parallel-shift tomosynthesis for orthopedic applications. Proc SPIE. 2018.
4. Sun Y, Duthaler S, Nelson BJ. Autofocusing in computer microscopy: selecting the optimal focus algorithm. Microscope Res Tech. 2004;65(3):139–149.
5. Bookstein FL. Principal warps: thin-plate splines and the decomposition of deformations. IEEE Trans Pattern Anal Mach Intell. 1989;11(6):567–585.
6. Segars WP, et al. Realistic CT simulation using the 4D XCAT phantom. Med Phys. 2008;35(8):3800–3808.

Influence of Excitation Signal Coupling on Reconstructed Images in Magnetic Particle Imaging

Anselm von Gladiss[1], Matthias Graeser[2,3], Thorsten M. Buzug[1]

[1] Institute of Medical Engineering, University of Lübeck
[2] Section for Biomedical Imaging, University Medical Center Hamburg-Eppendorf
[3] Institute for Biomedical Imaging, Hamburg University of Technology
{gladiss,buzug}@imt.uni-luebeck.de

Abstract. In Magnetic Particle Imaging, superparamagnetic iron oxide nanoparticles are excited by an oscillating magnetic field that is generated by sending coils. In multidimensional set-ups, perfect geometrical decoupling cannot be achieved. Remaining coupling can distort the trajectory and introduce artefacts, thus active decoupling is introduced at costs of high power consumption. This work uses a device with active coupling control to investigate the influence of different coupling levels on the image reconstruction.

1 Introduction

Magnetic Particle Imaging (MPI) is an emerging medical imaging technology that visualises superparamagnetic iron oxide nanoparticles in a field of view (FOV). MPI features a very high temporal resolution in the range of milliseconds and has potential of submillimeter spatial resolution. It does not rely on ionising radiation as other tracer based imaging modalities (e. g. PET or SPECT) and is therefore tailored to be applied in medical imaging [1, 2, 3, 4].

In MPI, the nanoparticles are excited by oscillating sinusoidal magnetic fields

$$\mathrm{H}_{\mathrm{D}_i} = A_i \sin(2\pi f_i t) \cdot \mathbf{e}_i \tag{1}$$

in different spatial directions $i \in \{\text{x,y,z}\}$ forming a trajectory as in Fig. 1. For spatial encoding a static magnetic gradient field is introduced featuring a field free point (FFP). Now, only the particles nearby the FFP contribute to the receive signal. The excitation signal $\mathrm{H}_{\mathrm{D}_i}$ moves the FFP over the FOV which encodes the temporal receive signal spatially. Due to the non-linear magnetisation behaviour of the nanoparticles, a receive signal can be detected whose spectrum contains the excitation frequency f_i and higher harmonics [1]. The total harmonic spectrum is a fingerprint of the particles and can be used for identifying them inside the FOV.

A system matrix can be used to reconstruct the receive signal into an image that shows the spatial distribution of the particles inside the FOV. The system matrix $\mathbf{S}$ is obtained by placing a particle sample on priorly defined positions in the FOV subsequentially and performing a measurement at each position. The spectrum of the receive signal $\mathbf{u}$ is stored in the system matrix. This collection of measurements encodes the particle signal to the spatial concentration of nanoparticles $\mathbf{c}$ in the FOV. Later, arbitrary particle distributions can be reconstructed by solving a linear system of equations using the spectrum of the receive signal and the system matrix

$$\mathbf{S} \cdot \mathbf{c} = \mathbf{u} \tag{2}$$

System matrix reconstruction relies on the stability and consistency of a system. This means, that e. g. the driven trajectory must be the same for both system matrix acquisition and measurements.

Recently, it has been proposed to reconstruct MPI measurements with a hybrid system matrix, that has not been acquired in the scanning device but in a magnetic particle spectrometer (MPS). Although this is an important step towards reducing the calibration time in MPI and therefore increasing the efficiency of MPI scanning devices, new requirements have to be met, as the driven trajectory in both the MPS and the MPI scanning device must be the same.

1.1   Excitation signal coupling

According to Faraday's law of induction the time-variant excitation signal from one sending coil may couple into another sending coil causing a twisted trajectory as displayed in Fig. 1. Conventional multidimensional MPI scanner set-ups feature orthogonal sending coils that should prevent signal coupling. In practice, coupling may occur due to accuracy limitations in hardware assembly. Then, the magnetic drive field H_{D_i} features not only one frequency as in Eq. 1, but is superposed by the coupled signals $H_{D\kappa_{ij}}$ of other spatial directions j

$$H_{D_i} + \sum_{j,j \neq i} H_{D\kappa_{ij}} = A_i \sin(2\pi f_i t) \cdot \mathbf{e}_i + \sum_{j,j \neq i} A_{\kappa_{ij}} \sin(2\pi f_{\kappa_{ij}} t) \cdot \mathbf{e}_i \tag{3}$$

Here, the effective field coupling ratio κ_{ij} defines the coupling ratio from sending coil j into i:

$$\kappa_{ij} = H_{D\kappa_{ij}}/H_{D_j} \tag{4}$$

In order to cope for the signal coupling, a software decoupling can be implemented that monitors the current on the sending coils and identifies the coupled signals. The cancellation signal $H_{canc\kappa_{ij}}$ is generated with a phase shift of $\Delta\phi = 180°$ and fed back into the signal path in order to cancel out the coupling signal $H_{D\kappa_{ij}} \to 0$.

This contribution discusses the influence of signal excitation coupling for system matrix reconstruction. The software decoupling is used to manipulate the trajectory by introducing an additional signal that corresponds to signal coupling.

Fig. 1. Excitation signal in MPI for (a) 1D and (b) 2D excitation. In 1D, the nanoparticles are excited along a line. The superposition of excitation signals in 2D forms a Lissajous trajectory. The trajectory without signal coupling is visualised in blue. Introducing a field coupling of $\kappa_{yx} = 10\,\%$ in y-direction, the trajectory is twisted (red).

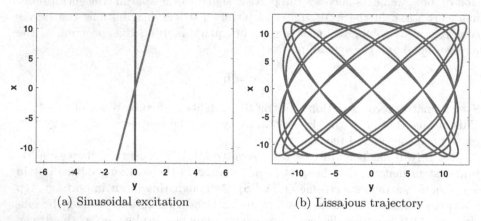

(a) Sinusoidal excitation   (b) Lissajous trajectory

2 Material and methods

The measurements have been carried out using an MPS featuring excitation and receive coils in different orthogonal spatial directions and switchable magnetic offset fields [5]. Furthermore, the currents on the sending coils are monitored by a software decoupling unit that ensures a maximum effective field coupling of $\kappa_{ij} \leq 0.1\,\%$. Also, an accuracy of $99.9\,\%$ for the amplitudes of the excitation signals with a maximal phase error of $0.2°$ is guaranteed.

It has been shown, that an MPS can be used to acquire a hybrid system matrix [6]. The spatial positions inside the gradient field of an MPI scanning device are emulated subsequentially by applying different magnetic offset fields. Furthermore, phantoms can be emulated with an MPS [7]. The phantom is discretised into distinct spatial positions that are emulated by the MPS using the magnetic offset fields. The addition of the receive signals at those positions corresponds to a phantom measurement in an MPI scanning device.

2.1 Hybrid system matrices

Hybrid system matrices have been acquired in the xy-plane using 29×29 emulated spatial positions. First, two hybrid system matrices with 1D excitation in x-direction have been acquired with a magnetic field strength of $A_x = 12\,\mathrm{mT}$ and an excitation frequency of $f_x \approx 24.51\,\mathrm{kHz}$. One of them will serve as a system matrix in the reconstruction, the other one will be used to emulate the phantom 2.2. Then, the same excitation frequency has been introduced in y-direction $f_{\kappa_{yx}} = f_x$ with a magnetic field strength of $A_{\kappa_{yx}} = 0.12\,\mathrm{mT}$ and $A_{\kappa_{yx}} = 1.2\,\mathrm{mT}$ representing an excitation signal coupling from sending coil x into y of $\kappa_{yx} = 1\,\%$ and $\kappa_{yx} = 10\,\%$.

In order to acquire hybrid system matrices with 2D excitation, another excitation signal has been introduced in y-direction with a frequency of $f_y \approx 26.04\,\mathrm{kHz}$

and a magnetic field strength of $A_y = 12\,\text{mT}$. The same signal coupling as in the 1D case has been introduced ($\kappa_{yx} = 1\,\%$, $\kappa_{yx} = 10\,\%$). The influence of signal coupling on the FFP trajectory can be seen in Fig. 1.

2.2 Phantom and reconstruction

The phantoms are emulated by choosing single spatial positions out of the system matrices that feature a defined field coupling. As a reference, the same phantom is emulated using one system matrix that has been acquired without field coupling. Out of the 1D excitation measurements, a 2 dot phantom in the centre of the FOV is emulated. A 9 dot grid has been emulated using the 2D excitation measurements. The reconstructed reference phantoms can be seen in Fig. 3 (a) and (f). The images are reconstructed by solving the underdetermined linear system of equations (Eq. 2) as described in [8] using a regularised Kaczmarz algorithm. The normalised root mean square error (NRMSE) σ between the reconstruction of the reference and field coupling measurements is calculated.

3 Results

3.1 System functions

Fig. 2 shows frequency components of the hybrid system matrices, i. e. system functions. Fig. 2 (a) and (c) display the reference system function for 1D and 2D excitation without field coupling. In contrast, Fig. 2 (b) and (d) show the same system functions after introducing a field coupling of $\kappa_{yx} = 10\,\%$. These system functions with coupling are twisted in comparison to their reference. Furthermore, wave peaks that are clearly separated smear when introducing coupling in 2D excitation.

3.2 Reconstructed images

Fig. 3 shows reconstruction results of the emulated phantoms. The reconstructed reference images (a) and (d) show the 2 dot phantom for 1D excitation and the

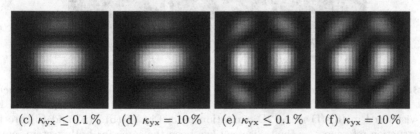

(c) $\kappa_{yx} \leq 0.1\,\%$ (d) $\kappa_{yx} = 10\,\%$ (e) $\kappa_{yx} \leq 0.1\,\%$ (f) $\kappa_{yx} = 10\,\%$

Fig. 2. Frequency components of hybrid system matrices corresponding to (a)-(b) the 3rd harmonic and (c)-(d) a mixing frequency around the 6th harmonic of the excitation frequencies. (a) and (b) were obtained using 1D excitation as in Fig. 1 (a). (c) and (d) have been acquired using 2D excitation as in Fig. 1 (b). For (b) and (d) a field coupling of $\kappa_{yx} = 10\,\%$ has been introduced from sending coil x to y.

9 dot grid for 2D excitation. The 2 dot phantom is not reconstructed as 2 dots but as two lines which indicates a strong spatial resolution in the direction of excitation but a poor one orthogonal to it. After twisting the excitation trajectory background noise increases. Furthermore, the centre of the reconstructed lines begins to blur. This effect increases with increasing emulated coupling. Though, the 2 dots of the phantom are still represented mainly by two lines as in the reference image (a). The NRMSE of Fig. 3 (b) and (c) in comparison to its reference is $\sigma = 3.81\,\%$ and $\sigma = 5.34\,\%$.

The single dots of the 9 dot grid are reconstructed into a point cloud consisting of one bright pixel, the centre, and neighbouring pixels (Fig. 3 (d)). As for 1D excitation, the background noise increases when introducing field coupling. Furthermore, the reconstruction of the dots blurs out. The NRMSE increases to $\sigma = 4.58\,\%$ and $\sigma = 6.19\,\%$. For a high coupling factor of $\kappa_{yx} = 10\,\%$, the centres of different point clouds move by one pixel (e. g. lower left corner).

4   Discussion

It has been shown, that a small coupling of $\kappa_{yx} = 1\,\%$ has a large effect on the reconstructed images in terms of image quality and NRMSE. After introducing coupling signals, background noise appears in the reconstructed images. Furthermore, the reconstructed dots are starting to blur out.

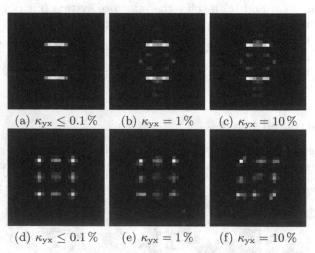

(a) $\kappa_{yx} \leq 0.1\,\%$ (b) $\kappa_{yx} = 1\,\%$ (c) $\kappa_{yx} = 10\,\%$

(d) $\kappa_{yx} \leq 0.1\,\%$ (e) $\kappa_{yx} = 1\,\%$ (f) $\kappa_{yx} = 10\,\%$

Fig. 3. Reconstructed images of emulated phantoms. (a)-(c) show a reconstructed 2 dot phantom using 1D excitation as in Fig. 1 (a). A 9 dot grid phantom has been visualised in (d)-(f) using 2D excitation as in Fig. 1 (b). (a) and (d) are the reconstruction references as the trajectory has been the same for both system matrix acquisition and phantom measurement. After introducing a field coupling of $\kappa_{yx} = 1\,\%$ and $\kappa_{yx} = 10\,\%$, background noise appears in the reconstructed images. Furthermore, the NRMSE σ increases. With increasing field coupling the reconstructed image is twisted in comparison to its reference for 2D excitation.

Although a twist in the system function can be identified (Fig. 2 (b)), this twist is not visible in the reconstructed images (Fig. 3 (c)). As the spatial resolution in y direction is poor when exciting only in the direction of x, this twist in the y direction cannot be observed in the reconstructed images. The twist of the system function in Fig. 2 (d) can also be seen in Fig. 3 (f). In this work, the field coupling has only been emulated from sending coil x into y. In a real scenario, signal coupling may also occur from sending coil y into x which will increase the mismatch between the driven trajectories and therefore, deteriorate the reconstructed images.

Image reconstruction has been performed using a system matrix. If the system matrix has been acquired in the same scanning device as the measurement, signal coupling is no issue if it is supposed to be stable inside the same device. In order to reduce the calibration time in MPI, it is important to be able to measure the system matrix in a dedicated device [6]. Then, the driven trajectory including the coupled signals must be the same as in the imaging device in order to avoid artefacts in the reconstructed images.

In this work, the influence of excitation signal coupling on the reconstructed images has been examined using system matrix reconstruction. The signal coupling has been emulated by superposing corresponding signals to the excitation signal. It has been shown, that a small change in the driven trajectory has a large impact on the reconstructed images.

Acknowledgement. The authors thankfully acknowledge the financial support by the German Research Foundation (DFG, grant number BU 1436/10-1) and the Federal Ministry of Education and Research (BMBF, grant number 13GW0069A).

References

1. Gleich B, Weizenecker J. Tomographic imaging using the nonlinear response of magnetic particles. Nature. 2005;435(7046):1214–7.
2. Panagiotopoulos N, Vogt F, Barkhausen J, et al. Magnetic particle imaging: current developments and future directions. Int J Nanomed. 2015; p. 3097.
3. Ferguson RM, Khandhar AP, Kemp SJ, et al. Magnetic particle imaging with tailored iron oxide nanoparticle tracers. IEEE Trans Med Imaging. 2015;34(5):1077–1084.
4. Borgert J, Schmidt JD, Schmale I, et al. Perspectives on clinical magnetic particle imaging. Biomed Technik. 2013;58(6).
5. Graeser M, von Gladiss A, Weber M, et al. Two dimensional magnetic particle spectrometry. Phys Med Biol. 2017;62(9):3378–3391.
6. von Gladiss A, Graeser M, Szwargulski P, et al. Hybrid system calibration for multidimensional magnetic particle imaging. Phys Med Biol. 2017;62(9):3392–3406.
7. Schmidt D, Graeser M, von Gladiss A, et al. Imaging characterization of MPI tracers employing offset measurements in a two dimensional magnetic particle spectrometer. Int J Mag Part Imaging. 2016;1(2).
8. Knopp T, Rahmer J, Sattel TF, et al. Weighted iterative reconstruction for magnetic particle imaging. Phys Med Biol. 2010;55(6):1577–1589

A Joint Probabilistic Model for Speckle Variance, Amplitude Decorrelation and Interframe Variance (IFV) Optical Coherence Tomography Angiography

Stefan B. Ploner[1], Christian Riess[1], Julia Schottenhamml[1,2], Eric M. Moult[2], Nadia K. Waheed[3], James G. Fujimoto[2], Andreas Maier[1]

[1]Pattern Recognition Lab, FAU Erlangen-Nürnberg, Germany
[2]Department of Electrical Engineering and Computer Science, Research Laboratory for Electronics, Massachusetts Institute of Technology, Cambridge, MA, USA
[3]Ophthalmology, New England Eye Center, Tufts Medical Center, Boston, MA, USA
stefan.ploner@fau.de

Abstract. Optical Coherence Tomography Angiography (OCTA) is a general method to visualize blood flow in biological tissue. Despite its good results in practice, the commonly used Amplitude Decorrelation OCTA (AD-OCTA) measure suffers from a well-understood objective function, which makes it challenging to mathematically model post processing tasks like, e.g., denoising. In this paper, a probabilistic model is developed for the three OCTA measures Speckle Variance OCTA, AD-OCTA and the newly proposed Interframe Variance OCTA (IFV-OCTA) to enable further tasks like regularization-based denoising. From a theoretical point of view, IFV-OCTA is shown to be in-between the other two methods and can act as a link between them. A small sized observer study suggests that the image quality of IFV-OCTA is comparable to the other methods. IFV-OCTA is a promising OCTA measure for algorithms that require a dependency on the interscan time.

1 Introduction

Optical Coherence Tomography (OCT) is a 3D imaging modality based on low coherence interferometry that achieves micron-scale resolution in biological tissue [1]. Its fast acquisition speed, up to real time imaging, and the non-invasiveness led to its adaption in many clinical fields, in particular in ophthalmology. By analyzing the differences of repeated scans, an angiographic signal can be formed, which is called OCT angiography (OCTA). In contrast to doppler techniques, which are based on the signal's phase information, the herein compared OCTA measures are only dependent on the signal intensity.

In this work, a common probabilistic model is developed for three different OCTA measures, which are Speckle Variance OCTA (SV-OCTA) [2], Amplitude Decorrelation OCTA (AD-OCTA) [3] and a newly proposed method. Whereas SV-OCTA has, as the name tells, a clear probabilistic interpretation, namely the variance of the signal, such an interpretation was missing for AD-OCTA. We derived a probabilistic model, whose solution is equivalent to the AD-OCTA method. We further introduce the Interframe Variance OCTA (IFV-OCTA) method, which acts as a link between SV-OCTA and AD-OCTA.

Finally, we compared the image quality of the three methods in an observer study, which was performed on the full 3D volume. Five different cases were analyzed by five expert graders.

2   Materials and methods

First, the probabilistic model for the three OCTA measures is introduced. Then, the details of the observer study are described.

2.1   Probabilistic models

For each OCTA measure, an objective function L is formulated based on the voxel intensities $a_i, i \in 1, \ldots, N$, where N is the number of repeated B-scans per location in the OCT scan protocol and $\mu = \frac{1}{N} \sum_{i=1}^{N} a_i$ is the mean of the intensities.

Speckle variance OCTA (SV-OCTA) The SV-OCTA method has a probabilistic interpretation, which is the variance of the repeatedly acquired samples. This can easily be shown by formulating a maximum likelihood estimation of the parameters μ and σ_{SV}^2 for the given a_i, assuming a normal distribution $\mathcal{N}$ in the objective function L_{SV}.

$$L_{SV} = \prod_{i=1}^{N} \mathcal{N}\left(a_i; \mu, \sigma_{SV}^2\right) = \prod_{i=1}^{N} \frac{1}{\sqrt{2\pi\sigma_{SV}^2}} \exp\left(-\frac{(a_i - \mu)^2}{2\sigma_{SV}^2}\right) \tag{1}$$

$$\max_{\mu,\sigma_{SV}^2}\left\{L_{SV}\right\} = \max_{\mu,\sigma_{SV}^2}\left\{\log L_{SV}\right\} = \max_{\mu,\sigma_{SV}^2}\left\{N \cdot \log \frac{1}{\sqrt{2\pi\sigma_{SV}^2}} - \sum_{i=1}^{N} \frac{(a_i - \mu)^2}{2\sigma_{SV}^2}\right\} \tag{2}$$

We then locate the σ_{SV}^2 that produces the measured data with highest probability by setting the respective derivative to zero.

$$\frac{d \log L_{SV}}{d\sigma_{SV}^2} = \frac{-N \cdot \sigma_{SV}^2 + \sum_{i=1}^{N}(a_i - \mu)^2}{2\sigma_{SV}^4} \stackrel{!}{=} 0 \tag{3}$$

$$\sigma_{SV}^2 = \frac{1}{N} \sum_{i=1}^{N}(a_i - \mu)^2 \tag{4}$$

Interframe variance (IFV-OCTA) The newly proposed Interframe Variance measure is the variance of the differences of the voxel intensities. Note that the mean value of these differences is zero due to the identical distribution of the values. Again, by setting the derivative of the new objective function L_{IFV} to zero, a direct computation formula can be derived, which is denoted in Eq. (8).

$$L_{\mathrm{IFV}} = \prod_{i=1}^{N-1} \mathcal{N}\left(a_i - a_{i+1}; 0, \sigma_{\mathrm{IFV}}^2\right) = \prod_{i=1}^{N-1} \frac{1}{\sqrt{2\pi\sigma_{\mathrm{IFV}}^2}} \exp\left(-\frac{(a_i - a_{i+1})^2}{2\sigma_{\mathrm{IFV}}^2}\right) \quad (5)$$

$$\log L_{\mathrm{IFV}} = (N-1)\cdot\log\frac{1}{\sqrt{2\pi\sigma_{\mathrm{IFV}}^2}} - \sum_{i=1}^{N-1}\frac{(a_i - a_{i+1})^2}{2\sigma_{\mathrm{IFV}}^2} \quad (6)$$

$$\frac{d\log L_{\mathrm{IFV}}}{d\sigma_{\mathrm{IFV}}^2} = \frac{-(N-1)\cdot\sigma_{\mathrm{IFV}}^2 + \sum_{i=1}^{N-1}(a_i - a_{i+1})^2}{2\sigma_{\mathrm{IFV}}^4} \overset{!}{=} 0 \quad (7)$$

$$\sigma_{\mathrm{IFV}}^2 = \frac{1}{N-1}\sum_{i=1}^{N-1}(a_i - a_{i+1})^2 \quad (8)$$

Amplitude decorrelation (AD-OCTA) The AD-OCTA method is defined by its direct computation formula [3]. Thus, this time we set up an objective function L_{AD} which yields a σ_{AD}^2 that matches the AD-OCTA computation formula. Similar to IFV-OCTA, the objective function is based on the difference between consecutive voxel intensities. However, for AD-OCTA, the difference is normalized by its amplitude through a multiplication with the factor $\frac{1}{\sqrt{a_i^2 + a_{i+1}^2}}$.

$$L_{\mathrm{AD}} = \prod_{i=1}^{N-1} \mathcal{N}\left(\frac{a_i}{\sqrt{a_i^2 + a_{i+1}^2}} - \frac{a_{i+1}}{\sqrt{a_i^2 + a_{i+1}^2}}; 0, \sigma_{\mathrm{AD}}^2\right) \quad (9)$$

$$= \prod_{i=1}^{N-1}\frac{1}{\sqrt{2\pi\sigma_{\mathrm{AD}}^2}}\exp\left(-\frac{\frac{(a_i - a_{i+1})^2}{a_i^2 + a_{i+1}^2}}{2\sigma_{\mathrm{AD}}^2}\right) \quad (10)$$

$$\log L_{\mathrm{AD}} = (N-1)\cdot\log\frac{1}{\sqrt{2\pi\sigma_{\mathrm{AD}}^2}} - \sum_{i=1}^{N-1}\frac{\frac{(a_i - a_{i+1})^2}{a_i^2 + a_{i+1}^2}}{2\sigma_{\mathrm{AD}}^2} \quad (11)$$

$$\frac{d\log L_{\mathrm{AD}}}{d\sigma_{\mathrm{AD}}^2} = \frac{-(N-1)\cdot\sigma_{\mathrm{AD}}^2 + \sum_{i=1}^{N-1}\frac{(a_i - a_{i+1})^2}{a_i^2 + a_{i+1}^2}}{2\sigma_{\mathrm{AD}}^4} \overset{!}{=} 0 \quad (12)$$

$$\sigma_{\mathrm{AD}}^2 = \frac{1}{N-1}\sum_{i=1}^{N-1}\frac{(a_i - a_{i+1})^2}{a_i^2 + a_{i+1}^2} \quad (13)$$

2.2   Swept source optical coherence tomography

Optical coherence tomography angiography was performed using an ultrahigh speed Swept Source-OCT (SS-OCT) research prototype developed at the Mas-

Table 1. Results of the observer study. The grading ranges from 1 (very good) to 5 (very bad).

	SV-OCTA	IFV-OCTA	AD-OCTA
Grade ($\mu \pm \sigma$)	2.2 ± 1.22	2.24 ± 1.13	3.16 ± 1.07

sachusetts Institute of Technology and in use at the New England Eye Center. A similar OCT system was described previously and therefore only key characteristics are summarized herein [4]. The prototype OCT instrument uses a vertical cavity surface emitting laser (VCSEL) swept light source with a 400 kHz A-scan rate. The light source is centered at $1,050$ nm wavelengths. Optical coherence tomography interferometric signals were acquired with an analog-to-digital acquisition card externally clocked at a maximum frequency of ~ 1.1 GHz using an external Mach-Zehnder interferometer. Optical coherence tomography angiography imaging was performed with 6 mm · 6 mm and 3 mm · 3 mm fields of view. For both field sizes, 5 repeated B-scans from 500 uniformly spaced locations were sequentially acquired. Each B-scan consisted of 500 A-scans, which yields an isotropic transverse sampling. The fundamental interscan time between repeated B-scans was ~ 1.5 ms, accounting for the mirror scanning duty cycle. The acquisition time for repeated B-scans was ~ 7.5 ms ($5 \cdot 1.5$ ms) per position. A total of $5 \cdot 500 \cdot 500$ A-scans were acquired per OCTA volume for a total acquisition time of ~ 3.9 s.

2.3   Observer study

Retrospective data of 5 subjects was used for this study, which were scanned at the New England Eye Center. The OCTA signal was computed with the SV-OCTA, IFV-OCTA and AD-OCTA formulas. The volumes were post processed with a volumetric median filter with radius 1. For the SV-OCTA and IFV-OCTA methods, the volumes were additionally logarithmized to optimize the intensity distribution. This step was not necessary for the AD-OCTA volume due to the intrinsic normalization. The observers were allowed to adjust the displayed intensity window. The volumetric data was viewed directly, no projection along depth was performed. 5 experts graded the vessel visibility of each volume on a scale from 1 (very good) to 5 (very bad).

3   Results

Fig. 1 shows the three OCTA measures computed at the same depth through a dataset of a healthy subject. The results of the observer study suggest that the IFV-OCTA measure is on par with the established measures (Table 1).

4   Discussion

This work's contribution is twofold. First, a probabilistic model for AD-OCTA was formulated, which was found to be a normal distribution based on the

Fig. 1. Representative slices at the same depth in the SV-OCTA, IFV-OCTA and AD-OCTA volumes. All volumes were post processed with a median filter with radius 1. The SV-OCTA and IFV-OCTA volumes were additionally logarithmized.

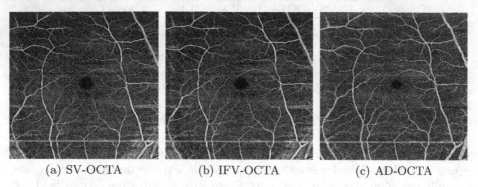

(a) SV-OCTA   (b) IFV-OCTA   (c) AD-OCTA

amplitude-normalized intensity differences. This aids in the interpretation of AD-OCTA data because the inherent model assumptions are now apparent and can be compared to underlying physical principles. Furthermore, the model can be extended with denoising priors like, e.g., total variation, to incorporate denoising in the signal reconstruction step.

Second, the newly introduced IVF-OCTA computation formula can be seen as the missing link between SV-OCTA and AD-OCTA, which is especially apparent when comparing the objective functions. In a small sized study, the image quality of IFV-OCTA was comparable to the commonly used SV-OCTA and AD-OCTA methods. In the future, the IVF-OCTA method could be used in algorithms that require a dependency on the interscan time. An example for such a method is the VISTA algorithm [5, 6], which was currently only applied to AD-OCTA data.

References

1. Huang D, Swanson EA, Lin CP, et al. Optical coherence tomography. Science. 1991 11;254(5035):1178–1181.
2. Mariampillai A, Standish BA, Moriyama EH, et al. Speckle variance detection of microvasculature using swept-source optical coherence tomography. Opt Lett. 2008;33(13):1530.
3. Jia Y, Tan O, Tokayer J, et al. Split-spectrum amplitude-decorrelation angiography with optical coherence tomography. Opt Express. 2012;20(4):4710–4725.
4. Choi W, Potsaid B, Jayaraman V, et al. Phase-sensitive swept-source optical coherence tomography imaging of the human retina with a vertical cavity surface-emitting laser light source. Opt Lett. 2013;38(3):338–340.
5. Choi W, Moult EM, Waheed NK, et al. Ultrahigh-speed, swept-source optical coherence tomography angiography in nonexudative age-related macular degeneration with geographic atrophy. Ophthalmology. 2015;122(12):2532–2544.
6. Ploner SB, Moult EM, Choi W, et al. Toward quantitative optical coherence tomography angiography: visualizing blood flow speeds in ocular pathology using variable interscan time analysis. Retina. 2016;36 Suppl 1:S118–S126.

A Simulation Study and Experimental Verification of Hand-Eye-Calibration using Monocular X-Ray

Petra Dorn[1], Peter Fischer[1,2], Holger Mönnich[2], Philip Mewes[2],
Muhammad Asim Khalil[3], Abhinav Gulhar[2], Andreas Maier[1]

[1]Lehrstuhl für Mustererkennung, FAU Erlangen-Nürnberg
[2]Siemens Healthcare GmbH, Forchheim, Germany
[3]K-tronik GmbH, Garching
petra.dorn@fau.de

Abstract. In this paper, the simultaneous hand-eye/robot-world problem $AX = ZB$ is performed using a single X-ray image instead of a stereo camera in order to avoid the additional tracking device. Our setup consists of a special X-ray marker, several image preprocessing steps, and a monocular pose estimation algorithm, for extracting the 6-D pose of the marker with respect to the X-ray source. Simulations are performed to investigate the behavior of the proposed hand-eye method when including inaccuracies of the robot and the non-isotropic errors of monocular pose estimation. The simulations were evaluated in an experimental setup, reaching an accuracy of 0.06° and 0.77 mm.

1 Introduction

In surgical interventions robots are on the advance because of their high precision and repeatability. A common topic in robotics is known as hand-eye calibration and covers the procedure of finding the rigid transformation between the camera or marker mounted onto the robot's end-effector and the robot flange, denoted as X. The state-of-the-art procedure to solve this problem is performed with optical tracking. However, additional equipment is needed. In this paper, the hand-eye calibration is performed using a C-arm system which is typically available in many operating rooms that require imaging. The theory behind the calibration can be solved with many mathematical approaches, which can differ, for example, in their parametrization for the rotation and their choice of solving rotation and translation either simultaneously or separately. Zhuang et al. and Dornaika et al. solve the problem $AX = ZB$ with the help of quaternions and compute the orientation before translation [1, 2]. Shah rewrites the rotational part in terms of a Kronecker product [3]. Li et al. present two methods where they solve rotation and translation simultaneously. Besides the Kronecker product they use dual quaternions for the second method [4]. Iterative methods, which often use the Levenberg-Marquardt algorithm for finding the minimum of the optimization problem, are presented e.g. in [5]. Each paper is based on the classical setup where either a camera is mounted on the end-effector of the robot and acquires a calibration pattern or an optical tracking system acquires a marker attached on the robot. In this paper, the tracker is replaced by a static C-arm system which acquires 2-D images of the marker. Problems arising from monocular instead of stereo view are the inaccuracies in estimation of the depth and out-of-plane rotations [6]. In simulations, the effect of the expected inaccuracies from the robot and from pose estimation of the marker with respect to the X-ray source is investigated. These results are compared with real measurements.

2   Methods

The simultaneous hand-eye and robot-world problem $AX = ZB$ is visualized in Figure 2(a). The problem describes a closed loop with the two unknown matrices X and Z which is the transformation between marker and robot flange or X-ray source and robot base, respectively. During the calibration procedure the robot flange moves to different poses, resulting in several measurements A_i – transformations from the C-arm source to the marker – and B_i – transformations from the robot base to the flange. While B is known due to the forward kinematic of the robot, A has to be estimated from the X-ray image. Each matrix of the equation $A_iX = ZB_i$ is a rigid transformation matrix which includes a 3×3 rotation matrix R and a 3×1 translation vector t. $AX = ZB$ can be split into a rotational and a translational equation

$$R_A R_X = R_Z R_B \tag{1}$$
$$R_A t_X + t_A = R_Z t_B + t_Z \tag{2}$$

For finding the pose of the marker A, the 3-D geometric model of the marker is required. Our marker has a cylindrical shape and consists of five metal beads embedded in plastic. Metal has a much higher density than plastic and can be seen easily on X-ray images (Fig. 2(b)). In order to estimate the 6-D pose from a 2-D image, which is also known as Perspective-n-point (PnP) problem, at least four metal beads have to be visible on the 2-D acquisition. The fifth bead of the

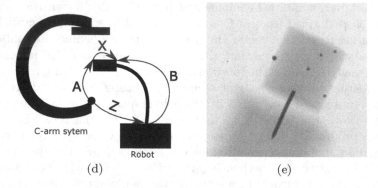

(d)   (e)

Fig. 1. a) Model for the problem $AX = ZB$, and b) 2-D acquisition of the marker.

marker is redundant, but might be necessary when two dots overlap each other. The pose estimation algorithm provided by the Visual Servoing Platform (ViSP), a modular cross platform library written in C++, is used [7]. The included dot tracker algorithm finds dots on an image automatically, and checks their shape and size. The further pose estimation algorithm, which is based on the ideas of DeMenthon and Lowe, matches a 3-D model with the projection, finds the best combination, and calculates the transformation matrix [8, 9]. Since there might be some disturbances on the X-ray image, which impair the success of the algorithm, different preprocessing steps are necessary. First, a black top-hat filter is used in order to remove large objects in the image. Second, an intensity normalization is performed. Third, this filtered image is binarized with an adaptive threshold. These implementations make use of the OpenCV library. All steps are done in order to highlight the dots and remove other disturbing objects in the image. The challenge of pose estimation is that the dimensions which mean a change in depth of the beads are more difficult to estimate. These are the z-coordinate which describes the point on the axis between X-ray source and detector, α and β which are the rotations around the x- and y-axis of the X-ray source frame.

3   Experiments

The hand-eye calibration was performed with Octave using the open source implementation from Shah [3]. The experiments are conducted both on simulated and real data.

3.1   Hand-eye simulation

The assumed geometrical distances in the synthetic setup are based on a realistic arrangement of robot, marker, and C-arm system. The movements of the robot flange were set to a range of ± 50 mm and $\pm 50°$ that was randomly sampled. After the ideal loops $A_i^* X^* = Z^* B_i^*$ with 15 measurement poses are created, Gaussian noise was added on the robot and C-arm data. The inaccuracies of the robot were simulated with a standard deviation $\sigma_{trans} = 0.2$ mm for each component of the translation and $\sigma_{rot} = 0.05°$ for each Euler angle α, β and γ. Since no valid information regarding the inaccuracies of the transformations between C-arm source and marker are given, the noise of them was varied. In the first experiment σ_{trans} and σ_{rot} were slightly increased from 0 to 1 mm and 0 to 0.5°, respectively. This was done in order to generally examine the effects of increasing noise on the accuracy of hand-eye calibration. The second experiment takes the expected inaccuracies of the monocular pose estimation into account. That means that α, β and z are assumed to be worse compared to the other components. It was of interest, whether only the overall noise or the increasing noise on single components is of importance as well. The noise level of the C-arm data was set constant to overall standard deviations $\sigma_{trans,all} = 1$ mm and

$\sigma_{rot,all} = 0.5°$. With the factor f, α, β and z are weighted with values from 0 to 10. Thus, the standard deviations of the C-arm data were set to

$$\sigma_{trans} = \frac{1}{\sqrt{f^2 + 2}} \cdot (1, 1, f)\, mm \tag{3}$$

$$\sigma_{rot} = \frac{\sqrt{0.5}}{\sqrt{2f^2 + 1}} \cdot (f, f, 1)° \tag{4}$$

In case of synthetic data the ground truth is known. Thus, the estimated transformation matrix $\widehat{X}$ can be compared directly with the correct matrix X^*. The rotational error is computed as

$$\Delta\theta = \theta(R_{X^*}^{-1} R_{\widehat{X}}) \tag{5}$$

where θ is the rotation angle given in degrees from its angle-axis representation. The translational error $\|\Delta t\|$ in mm is the norm of the difference translation vector of ground truth and noisy matrix

$$\|\Delta t\| = \|t_{X^*} - t_{\widehat{X}}\| \tag{6}$$

3.2   Verification measurements

For real measurements an industrial robot (KR 10 R1100 sixx, KUKA) and a C-arm system (ARTIS pheno, Siemens Healthineers) were used. The images have a spatial resolution of 0.16 mm per pixel. The results were compared with the simulated data, in order to figure out the inaccuracies of A and the resulting deviations of X and Z. The errors of real data can be determined as the offset

$$E_i = (ZB_i)^{-1}(A_iX) \tag{7}$$

when following each i-th closed loop of n test data. From this error matrix E_i the rotational error in degrees is computed with

$$\text{RMSE}_{rot} = \sqrt{\frac{1}{n}\sum_{i=1}^{n}(\theta(R_{E_i}))^2} \tag{8}$$

while the translational error in mm is

$$\text{RMSE}_{trans} = \sqrt{\frac{1}{n}\sum_{i=1}^{n} t_{E_i}^T t_{E_i}} \tag{9}$$

4   Results

4.1   Hand-eye simulation

With increasing rotational and translational noise on the X-ray data, the errors both of each matrix (Fig. 4.1(a)) and the closed loop errors (Fig. 4.1(b)) increase steadily.

Although the rotational error of X and Z is equal, the translational error of Z is higher. Due to the larger distance between C-arm and robot of $\|t_Z\|$ = 1007.8 mm, compared to the distance between robot flange and marker of $\|t_X\|$ = 86.6 mm, the same rotation error leads to higher deviations from the correct position. In the second experiment, the noise level was constant while the distribution between the single coordinates and angles was changed. The results in Figure 4.1 show an almost constant error level, what indicates that the overall noise level is much more important than the distribution on the components.

4.2   Verification measurements

The 24 measurements were evaluated with 6-fold cross validation, whereby five subsets were used as training data for the hand-eye calibration and one subset as test data for calculating the errors. The averaged errors of the closed loop are: $\text{RMSE}_{rot} = 0.06°$ and $\text{RMSE}_{trans} = 0.77$ mm. In order to reach the same results with synthetic data, the overall noise level of the C-arm data had to be set approximately to $\sigma_{trans,all} = 0.45$ mm and $\sigma_{rot,all} = 0.001°$. Applying these

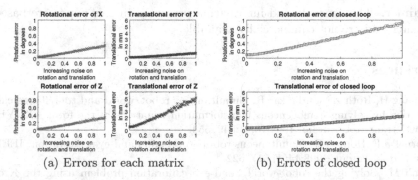

(a) Errors for each matrix   (b) Errors of closed loop

Fig. 2. Behavior of the rotational and translational errors with increasing amount of noise on A, which is the transform between C-arm and marker.

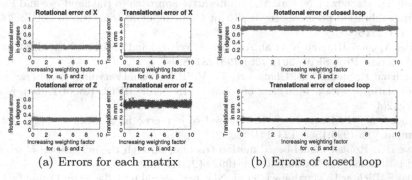

(a) Errors for each matrix   (b) Errors of closed loop

Fig. 3. Behavior of the rotational and translational errors with increasing weighting factor on α, β and z of A, which is the transform between C-arm and marker.

standard deviations on simulated data and computing the errors of each matrix results in the following values: The rotational error of X and Z is $\Delta\theta = 0.04°$, the translational error of X is $\|\Delta t\| = 0.24\,\text{mm}$, and the one of Z is $\|\Delta t\| = 0.63\,\text{mm}$. The translational error of Z is still small because the rotational error is very low.

5   Discussion and conclusion

In this paper, it could be shown that hand-eye calibration with X-ray is feasible. Moreover, the accuracy of the setup used in this paper seems to be similar to the optical tracking system [10]. The translational errors depend on a large extend on the overall rotational noise and the geometrical distance. To reach good results the estimated rotation has to be quite accurate. The inaccuracies of the depth estimation are tolerable as long as the other components can be computed accurately enough. In future work, the knowledge of the more inaccurate components could be used in order to further improve the pose estimation algorithm, e.g., by residual weighting.

Disclaimer. The concepts and information presented in this paper are based on research and are not commercially available.

References

1. Zhuang H, Roth ZS, Sudhakar R. Simultaneous robot/world and tool/flange calibration by solving homogeneous transformation equations of the form AX=YB. IEEE Trans Rob Autom. 1994;10(4):549–554.
2. Dornaika F, Horaud R. Simultaneous robot-world and hand-eye calibration. IEEE Trans Rob Autom. 1998;14(4):617–622.
3. Shah M. Solving the robot-world/hand-eye calibration problem using the Kronecker product. J Mech Robot. 2013;5(3):031007-1–031007-7.
4. Li A, Wang L, Wu D. Simultaneous robot-world and hand-eye calibration using dual-quaternions and Kronecker product. Int J Phys Sci. 2010;5(10):1530–1536.
5. Hirsh RL, DeSouza GN, Kak AC. An iterative approach to the hand-eye and base-world calibration problem. In: IEEE Int Conf Robot Autom. vol. 3. IEEE; 2001. p. 2171–2176.
6. Maier A, Choi JH, Keil A, et al. Analysis of vertical and horizontal circular C-arm trajectories. Proc SPIE. 2011;7961:7961231–8.
7. Marchand É, Spindler F, Chaumette F. ViSP for visual servoing: a generic software platform with a wide class of robot control skills. IEEE Robot Autom Mag. 2005;12(4):40–52.
8. Dementhon DF, Davis LS. Model-based object pose in 25 lines of code. Int J Comput Vis. 1995;15(1):123–141.
9. Lowe DG. Robust model-based motion tracking through the integration of search and estimation. Int J Comput Vis. 1992;8(2):113–122.
10. Ernst F, Richter L, Matthäus L, et al. Non-orthogonal tool/flange and robot/world calibration. Int J Med Robot. 2012;8(4):407–420.

Background Correction and Stitching of Histological Plaque Images

Lilli Kaufhold[1], Heike Goebel[2], Hanieh Mirzaee[1], Christoph Strecker[3],
Andreas Harloff[3], Anja Hennemuth[1,4]

[1]Fraunhofer MEVIS
[2]Universitätsklinik Köln
[3]Universitätsklinik Freiburg
[4]Charité–Universitätsmedizin Berlin
lilli.kaufhold@mevis.fraunhofer.de

Abstract. Histological examination of atherosclerotic plaques is the gold standard for the analysis of vessel plaque composition. The digitalization of the microscopic histology images results in a set of image tiles with overlapping regions of the same histological 2D slice. To allow comparison with other imaging modalities the tiles must be stitched together to a complete image of the plaque. The purpose of this work is to develop custom processing methods for the intensity correction and stitching problems. The developed methods are applied to 19 plaque images from an ongoing study. Results are compared with manual as well as automatic photo stitching.

1 Introduction

While the treatment of illnesses like acute coronary syndromes and stroke has improved, early detection of vulnerable lesions before the onset of symptoms is still subject to research [1]. In a histological analysis, ex-vivo plaque specimen are sliced into thin layers and subsequently inspected with a microscope. The digitalization of the microscopic images yields a collection of separate, but overlapping, image tiles covering different parts of the plaque. These tiles are affected by so-called vignetting, a peripheral darkening at the edge of the image tile, which is a reproduction of the optical edge of the microscopes light path (Fig. 1). It is commonplace to model the vignetting effect as a multiplication of the original image with a bias field function [2]. This function may be asymmetrical if the camera unit is not positioned perfectly over the optical axis of the microscope. The purpose of this work is to develop custom processing methods for devignetting and stitching of overlapping image tiles of histological plaque images.

Most previous publications address the problems of image fusion and intensity correction separately. The process of registering and fusing image tiles into a larger image is called stitching [3, 4, 5]. Vignetting is a common problem in conventional photography, and has therefore been addressed in this context in the literature. When possible, a straightforward way of obtaining the vignetting function is to derive it from a calibration image [6]. Other approaches derive vignetting functions from overlapping image regions [7]. For microscopic applications, Babaloukas et al. [8] have compared several common methods for intensity inhomogeneity correction and stitching. The vignetting problem is similar to intensity inhomogeneity problems that appear in other medical imaging modalities [9].

2 Materials and methods

The histological images are acquired of plaque specimen that have been surgically resected from human carotid arteries. For histological analysis, the atherosclerotic plaque is fixed in formalin, decalcified with EDTA and embedded in paraffin after a dehydration process, leading to a slight shrinkage of the tissue. The plaque is then sectioned in 1-3 μm slices, placed on a glass slide and is ready for microscopical examination after staining. The histological images in this work were acquired with a JVC KY-F75 CCD camera (lens 1.6 flat, aperture 0.05). The image size is 1240×1000 pixels and the resolution is $1.825 \mu m^2/px$.

Assuming that the intensity values of each image tile $I_i(x, y)$ result from an intensity offset $o_i \in \mathbb{R}$ and the vignetting function $v_i(x, y)$, the stitched image can be described by

$$\forall (x,y) \in \bigcup_i D_i^t : I_s(x,y) = \frac{\sum_{i,(x,y) \in D_i^t} w_i^t(x,y) \cdot \frac{I_i^t(x,y) - o_i}{v_i^t(x,y)}}{\sum_{i,(x,y) \in D_i^t} w_i^t(x,y)}$$

where the superscript t indicates that the images and functions have been translated to their correct stitching positions. D_i^t denotes the domain covered by the transformed tile i, and $w_i^t(x, y)$ is a weight function that blends the transformed images to achieve smooth transitions at the borders. The weight functions $w_i^t(x, y)$ are in this work defined as a function of the squared distances from the image tile centers. Thus, $I_s(x, y)$ equals a weighted sum of the transformed input images $I_i^t(x, y)$ where their new domains D_i^t overlap, and 0 otherwise.

2.1 Vignetting correction

As depicted in Fig. 1, one can neither assume a centered vignetting function, nor can it be obtained through heavy low-pass filtering. The number of tiles that contribute to an image varies between 1 and 4. Hence, using overlapping

Fig. 1. Histological images showing parts of a plaque specimen from the carotid artery. The vignetting, which results in a darkening towards the image edges, is clearly visible.

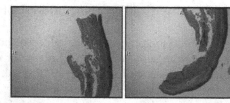

image regions for the determination of the vignetting function, as in [7], is not feasible. Prior knowledge, that can be used, is that the image background is homogeneous and that the plaque tissue has a strong texture. Moreover, the vignetting function has a smooth character. Thus, to estimate the vignetting function, a standard deviation filter is first applied in order to estimate the amount of variation in local pixel intensities. From this a background mask is obtained by thresholding as shown in Fig. 2(a). As some camera manufacturers report that the vignetting might differ for each RGB-channel, the correction is performed separately on each color channel. The vignetting function is modelled by a smooth multiplicative field, which is determined with the N3-method [9] applied to the pixels included in the background mask. The N3 method works with the logarithm of the input image to obtain an additive log-bias field. This log-bias field is modelled spatially as a linear combination of cubic B-spline functions and statistically as Gaussian probability density function. This method does not require any prior knowledge about the expected vignetting function but allows to influence the smoothness of the result through parametrization. An important parameter in the method is the distance d in voxels between the B-spline functions, which controls the frequency content and smoothness of the vignetting function. Tomazevic et al. [2] reported difficulties with N3 for images with large objects. However, by increasing d from 200 as in [2] to 500, good results were obtained as illustrated in Fig. 2(b).

2.2 Stitching

After vignetting correction, the image tiles I_i are stitched together to form a complete image I_s of the plaque. To this end, an intensity-based registration using the sum of squared differences of the gradient images is employed [10]. By

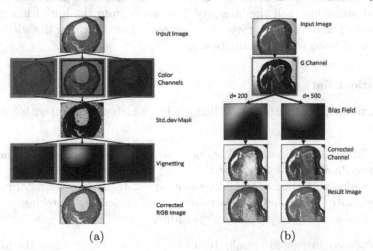

(a)   (b)

Fig. 2. Devignetting of the histological tiles. a) a joint standard deviation mask is derived from the RGB-channels; b) effect of the basis function distance d of the N3 algorithm on the devignetting result of an image with sparse background information.

using the gradient images, the structural information in the images is emphasized and after the application of the vignetting correction the gradient strengths should correspond well in overlapping regions of different image tiles. Because the camera movement between the acquisition of two image tiles is restricted to movement parallel to the histological slices, the transformation is restricted to a translation. The following cost function is minimized over the translation parameters (x_i^t, y_i^t) for each image tile I_i

$$\sum_{\substack{\cup_k D_k^t \\ (x,y) \in D_j^t}} \sum_{(x,y) \in D_j^t} \left[||\nabla I_i(x - x_i^t, y - y_i^t)||_2 - ||\nabla I_j(x - x_j^t, y - y_j^t)||_2 \right]^2$$

The user interactively defines starting positions relative to a reference tile. Subsequently the tiles are matched and merged in an iterative process.

3 Results

The described methods were implemented within a prototypical software and applied to generated test data as well as 19 histological images of carotid artery plaques from 6 patients who underwent endarterectomy.

3.1 Simulated tiling and vignetting

A plaque image, which showed a complete cross-section of a carotid artery plaque was filtered and the background was masked to ensure that it was homogeneous. Subsequently, overlapping image tiles were extracted and multiplied with a vignetting function as shown in Figure 3. The tiles were processed with the developed algorithm, and the intensity differences from the initial images were determined. The devignetting was most successful in the image tile with biggest proportion of background information.

3.2 Patient data

The patient images consisted of 2-4 image tiles, which were fused with 3 different methods:

- M1: Manual fusion with a commercially available image processing tool (Adobe Photoshop) by an expert.
- M2: Fusion with the free and fully automatic autostitch software for panorama images with a deformable registration based on feature matching [3].
- M3: Fusion with the proposed algorithms.

The results were inspected visually by a histology expert regarding the following criteria: plausibility of tile positioning and deformation, intensity differences at tile borders and blurring. Figure 3 shows an example of the achieved fusion. Figure 1 reports the assessment of all fusion results. The interactive fusion with simple blending resulted in plausible results in most cases, but intensity differences at the tile borders were visible. The proposed algorithms delivered good results for all cases and visible blurring occurred in 3 cases. In the result images from the fully automatic autostitch-algorithm, tile borders were not visible, but blurring was introduced by the image deformation, which was assumed to be implausible in 6 cases.

4   Discussion

We have presented an algorithmic approach for the fusion of image tiles of histological images for the further analysis and comparison with images from other modalities. First, the vignetting effects are corrected by applying the N3 algorithm to the background regions in all three color channels. Then, the corrected image tiles are fused by applying intensity-based registration after rough manual initialization. The results achieved on 19 plaque images, which are composed from 44 image tiles, show good results. Further work will address the automatic initialization of the fusion procedure and the registration with MR images for further analysis of the histological data.

References

1. Sanz J, Fayad ZA. Imaging of atherosclerotic cardiovascular disease. Nature. 2008;451(7181):953–957.
2. Tomaževič D, Likar B, Pernuš F. Comparative evaluation of retrospective shading correction methods. J Microsc. 2002;208(3):212–223.

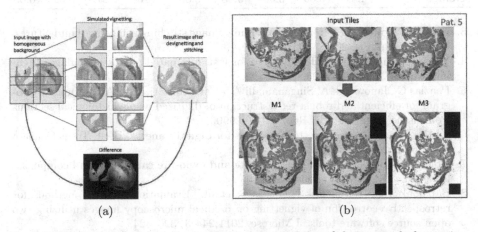

(a)   (b)

Fig. 3. Sample results. a) example of the devignetting and fusion result for an image with simulated vignetting applied to sub-image tiles; b) The manual fusion (M1) shows slight image differences at the stitching edges. The images fused with the fully automatic panorama software (M2) show implausible deformations and inhomogeneous brightness levels. The results achieved with the proposed method (M3) are shown in the rightmost image.

Table 1. Assessment of results achieved with methods M1-M3 regarding the blending of tile borders, blurring through blending and deformation, and the plausibility of the applied transformations. 0 means a good result, 1 is acceptable and 2 is bad.

Patient	Tiles	Borders			Blurring			Plausibility		
1	2	2	0	0	0	1	0	0	2	0
	2	1	0	0	0	1	0	0	2	0
	2	2	0	0	1	1	1	0	1	0
2	2	0	0	0	0	1	0	0	1	0
	2	2	0	0	0	0	0	0	0	0
3	2	1	0	0	0	0	0	0	0	0
	2	1	0	0	1	1	0	0	2	0
	3	2	1	0	2	1	0	1	1	0
4	2	1	0	0	1	1	0	0	1	0
	2	2	0	0	0	1	0	0	2	0
	2	2	0	0	0	2	0	0	2	0
5	2	2	0	0	1	1	0	0	1	0
	2	1	0	0	1	1	0	1	1	0
	3	2	0	0	1	1	0	0	1	0
	2	1	0	0	2	1	0	1	0	0
6	2	1	0	0	0	0	0	0	0	0
	4	2	0	0	1	1	1	1	1	0
	2	1	0	0	0	1	0	0	2	0
	4	2	0	0	0	1	1	0	1	0
Average		1.47	0.05	0.00	0.58	0.89	0.16	0.21	1.11	0.00

3. Brown M, Lowe DG. Automatic panoramic image stitching using invariant features. Int J Comput Vis. 2007;74(1):59–73.
4. Yang F, Deng ZS, Fan QH. A method for fast automated microscope image stitching. Micron. 2013;48:17–25.
5. Penzias G, Janowczyk A, Singanamalli A, et al. AutoStitcher: An automated program for efficient and robust reconstruction of digitized whole histological sections from tissue fragments. Sci Rep. 2016;6:29906.
6. Yu W. Practical anti-vignetting methods for digital cameras. IEEE Trans Consum Electronic. 2004;50(4):975–983.
7. Goldman DB, Chen JH; IEEE. Vignette and exposure calibration and compensation. Proc IEEE ICCV. 2005;1:899–906.
8. Babaloukas G, Tentolouris N, Liatis S, et al. Evaluation of three methods for retrospective correction of vignetting on medical microscopy images utilizing two open source software tools. J Microsc. 2011;244(3):320–324.
9. Sled JG, Zijdenbos AP, Evans AC. A nonparametric method for automatic correction of intensity nonuniformity in MRI data. IEEE Trans Med Imaging. 1998;17(1):87–97.
10. Modersitzki J. Numerical methods for Image Registration. Oxford University Press on Demand; 2004.

Towards In-Vivo X-Ray Nanoscopy
The Effect of Motion on Image Quality

Leonid Mill[1], Bastian Bier[1], Christopher Syben[1], Lasse Kling[2],
Anika Klingberg[3], Silke Christiansen[4,5], Georg Schett[3], Andreas Maier[1]

[1]Pattern Recognition Lab, Friedrich-Alexander-University Erlangen-Nuremberg
[2]Max Planck Institute for the Science of Light, Erlangen
[3]Institute of clinical Immunology, University Hospital Erlangen
[4]Freie Universität Berlin, Berlin
[5]Helmholtz Zentrum Berlin für Materialien und Energie, Berlin
`leonid.mill@fau.de`

Abstract. Novel X-Ray Microscopy (XRM) systems allow to study the internal structure of a specimen on nanoscale. A possible use of this non-destructive technology is motivated in the medical research area. *In-Vivo* investigation of medication over a period of time and its effects on perfusion and bony structure might lead to a better understanding of drug mechanisms and diseases like Osteoporosis and could lead to new approaches to their treatment. The first step towards *in-vivo* XRM imaging is to investigate the suitability of recent XRM systems for this task and subsequently to determine the system parameters. In this context, the impact of mice motion on the image quality is studied in this work. This paper aims to simulate the effects of breathing motion and muscle relaxation of the mice on the reconstructed images, which already effects the projection images. We therefore assume a mouse's respiration motion pattern, which happens four time during a single projection acquisitions, and the muscle relaxation movement due to anesthesia and simulate its impacts on image quality. Additionally, we show that a frame rate of at least 16 fps is needed to capture *in-vivo* movements in order to apply state-of-the-art motion correction methods.

1 Introduction

X-Ray Microscopy (XRM) systems are used in a variety of research areas including material sciences, medicine, and biology. One of the benefits of this technology in comparison to recent medical computed tomography (CT) applications is the high resolution of the reconstructed images with a voxelsize of up to 700 nm. This permits the investigation of structures in nano-scale in a non-destructive manner. One of these applications is the acquisition of mice bones in order to investigate the inner bony structures. We aim at the investigation in-vivo in order to detect effects of medication on the bone structure. In theory, the resolution that can be achieved with such system is sufficient. However, XRM systems are not designed to scan live moving objects such as mice. Despite of anesthesia, motion due to breathing and the relaxation of their muscles occurs during the scan. In general, motion in CT or CBCT has been investigated in various different applications [1, 2, 3]. However, combined with current exposure times in XRM of 1 s, motion blur appears in each single projection image since mice can breath up to four times during the acquisition of a single image. Furthermore, a whole acquisitions takes more than one hour resulting in motion artifacts in the reconstructions. This decreases the image quality remarkably and makes the evaluation of the medication hardly measurable.

In this work, we investigate the expected effect of this specific mouse movement on the image quality of the projections and the follow up reconstructions. Therefore, we evaluate on the one hand the effect of the exposure time on the projection images. On the other hand, we study the influence of different motion assumptions of the mouse and their influence on the reconstructions. We conduct experiments with different exposure times and discuss, what kind of motion would be observed. We evaluate the results using the Structural Similarity (SSIM) to measure the image quality.

2   Materials and methods

2.1   Experimental Setup

The simulation study is based on a scan of a high quality reconstruction of a mouse's tibia, acquired without any influence of motion. These scans have been acquired on a Xradia Versa 520 XRM system using 2000 projection images with an angular increment of $0.18°$. The mouse is placed on a rotating plate. The detector size of the system is 2024×2024 pixels with a pixel size of 1.34 μm. The resulting reconstructed volume had a size of $1980 \times 2024 \times 1999$ voxel with an isotropic resolution of 1.35 μm. Note, that this system has currently an exposure time of 1 s per projection, which is very long compared to current medical CT or CBCT systems. The same settings are used to create projection images using CONRAD [4]. For reconstruction, we used a standard FDK backprojection algorithm that consists of a cosine weighting [5], Parker redundancy weighting [6], Ram-Lak ramp filtering [5], and a backprojection step [7]. The voxel size of the reconstructions are set to 1.34 μm.

2.2   Occurring mouse motion

To model the mouse motion we consider two different kinds of motion. On the one hand we assume a breathing motion with 240 breathing cycles per minute. During one breathing cycle, an overall motion of 5 μm in the plane horizontal to the ground is assumed, which is defined in the x-y plane in the following. On the other hand, a second motion is considered as a result of muscle relaxation that appears horizontal to the x-y-plane with a total motion of 10 μm per hour. This motion is modeled as a linear movement in the z-direction. These motion assumptions are based on long term experiences of mice under anesthesia. If

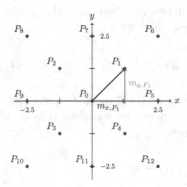

Fig. 1. Simulation of the respiration movement by shifting the volume to several points P_k in the x-y plane. For each point at a time t_j a projection is performed and the average over k projections is computed.

we combine this motion pattern with the current system's exposure time of $1\,\mathrm{s}$, we observe four breathing cycles and a relaxation motion of $\frac{1}{360}$ μm per acquired projection image. Thus, the breathing motion results in a motion blur effect in the acquired projections, which is an intra-scan motion, while the relaxation motion, which as inter-scan motion, leads to motion artifacts in the reconstruction. The model for breathing and the relaxation motion are described separately in the next sections.

2.3 Inter-scan motion

The relaxation motion is modeled as rigid object transformation in z-direction that can be incorporated into the projection matrices. For this we multiply to the j-th projection matrix $\mathbf{P}_J \in \mathbb{R}^{3\times4}$, with $j \in \{1,\dots,n\}$, the respective motion matrix $\mathbf{M}_j \in \mathbb{R}^{4\times4}$ from the right side, yielding a motion corrupted projection matrix $\mathbf{P}'_j$

$$\mathbf{P}'_j = \mathbf{P}_j \cdot \mathbf{M}_j = \mathbf{P}_j \cdot \begin{pmatrix} 1 & 0 & 0 & 0 \\ 0 & 1 & 0 & 0 \\ 0 & 0 & 1 & m_z^j \\ 0 & 0 & 0 & 1 \end{pmatrix}$$

where m_z^j indicates the movement based on muscle relaxation.

2.4 Intra-scan motion

Based on the assumptions stated above, reconstructions are created from motion blurred projections. The effect of the long exposure time can be seen as the average of several projections with variable translations. For the simulation we assume a movement of a maximum of 5 μm in a single breathing cycle and four breathing cycles per second. Thus, the different respiration motion states during the acquisition of one single projection image can be modeled with k projections for each point P_k at a time t_j (Fig. 1). Followed by an averaging over all k projections. Instead of simulating the intra-scan motion in the projection domain, we propose an alternative approach by convolving the reconstruction with a respective motion kernel that depends on the systems exposure time. The projection $p(s, \theta)$ for 2D parallel-beam can be described with

$$p(s, \theta) = \int_{-\infty}^{\infty} \int_{-\infty}^{\infty} f(x, y)\delta(x \cos \theta + y \sin \theta - s) \, dx \, dy \qquad (1)$$

which is also called the Radon transform and is denoted by $\mathbf{R}$ in the following [8]. The object density function $f(x, y)$ can be reconstructed by a convolution with the filter kernel $h(s)$ and a subsequent backprojection

$$f(x, y) = \int_{0}^{\pi} \int_{-\infty}^{\infty} p(s - t, \theta)h(t) \, dt \, d\theta \qquad (2)$$

which is in the following denoted by $\mathbf{R}^{-1}$ as the inverse Radon transform. As stated, the motion corrupted projection $\hat{p}(s, \theta)$, with the offsets $s_{i,x}$ and $s_{i,y}$ in x and y-direction, can be modeled as a weighted sum over l projections

$$\hat{p}(s, \theta) = \sum_{i=1}^{l} \omega_i \mathbf{R}\{f(x - s_{i,x}, y - s_{i,y})\} \qquad (3)$$

Thus, the motion corrupted reconstruction $\hat{f}(x, y)$ is

$$\hat{f}(x, y) = \mathbf{R}^{-1} \left\{ \sum_{i=1}^{l} \omega_i \mathbf{R}\{f(x - s_{i,x}, y - s_{i,y})\} \right\} \qquad (4)$$

using the linearity of the inverse Radon transform, the weighted sum can be pulled out

$$\hat{p}(s, \theta) = \sum_{i=1}^{l} \omega_i \mathbf{R}^{-1} \left\{ \mathbf{R}\{f(x - s_{i,x}, y - s_{i,y})\} \right\} \qquad (5)$$

Using the property that Randon transform followed by its inverse cancel out, we obtain

$$\hat{p}(s, \theta) = \sum_{i=1}^{l} \omega_i f(x - s_{i,x}, y - s_{i,y}) \qquad (6)$$

which is just the discrete formulation of a convolution of $f(x, y)$ with some filter kernel ω. Therefore by varying the number of projections l, we can simulate the strength of the motion during the acquisition of one projection. The filter kernels are created based on the concept shown in Fig. 1. For the currently used exposure time we consider all points, while for the higher frame rates we decrease the number of points.

Fig. 2. Reconstruction images of a mouse tibia. GT (left) and motion corrupted reconstruction due to respiration and muscle relaxation (right).

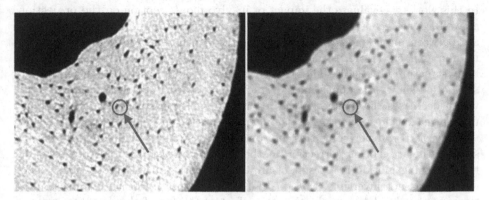

3   Results

Fig. 2 shows zoomed regions of the ground truth (GT) and the motion corrupted reconstruction, which includes breathing as well as motion due to the muscle relaxation. Motion blur is introduced in the motion corrupted image. Further, the shape and the position of the tiny bone structures changes, which is indicated with the arrow in both images. Additionally, ghost points appear in the marked area. Besides the qualitative evaluation, we obtain an SSIM of 0.732 for the motion corrupted image compared to the GT. The results of the exposure time variation experiment are shown in Fig. 3. All results are compared to the GT (a) using the SSIM. As can be seen, the SSIM values improve from 0.963 for a frame rate of 1 fps to an SSIM of 1.0 if frame rate of 32 fps is used.

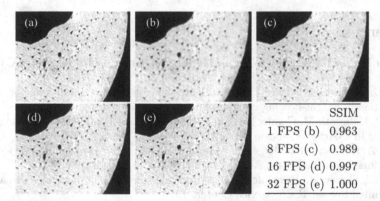

	SSIM
1 FPS (b)	0.963
8 FPS (c)	0.989
16 FPS (d)	0.997
32 FPS (e)	1.000

Fig. 3. The effect of respiration motion on reconstructed images simulated for different frame rates. Ground truth (a), 1 fps (b), 8 fps (c), 16 fps (d) and 32 fps (e) are compared in the table by means of the SSIM.

4   Discussion

In this work, we evaluate the impact of in-vivo mouse motion on the projection as well as the reconstructed image quality. We simulate motion and differentiate between inter- and intra-projection motion, which introduces blurring and motion artifacts in the reconstructions. These artifacts make diagnostics of the bony structure unfeasible. The result of the inter-scan muscle relaxation motion simulation shows the appearance of ghost points in the reconstruction images, which decreases the quality of the reconstructed bony structure. However, as muscle relaxation motion occurs as intra-projection movement, due to its slow velocity of 10 μm per hour, this motion can be estimated and compensated by state-of-the-art motion correction methods. In contrast, the blurring effect of the breathing motion is a result of an average over multiple projections. This averaging is not invertible, thus we cannot compensate for the intra-scan motion. In the simulation evaluating the effect of the fps of the detector, we can observe that the reconstruction quality increases with the fps. This can be explained by looking at the strength of the breathing motion and the system setup. The assumed breathing motion with 5 μm for a single breathing cycle and 4 cycles in a second lead to a movement of 0.625 μm for a single projection using a detector with 32 fps. Since our detector has a spacing of 1.34 μm the motion is not detectable in one projection. However, using a detector with 32 fps the breathing motion occurs between the acquisition and is therefore shifted towards an inter-scan motion, which is also compensatable with state-of-the-art motion correction methods. With the proposed simulation we have shown that in-vivo x-ray nanoscopy is feasible given that the frame rate of the detector is high enough such that all motion occurs as inter-scan motion and thus can be corrected. Motion correction itself is subject of our future work.

References

1. Berger M, Xia Y, Aichinger W, et al. Motion compensation for cone-beam CT using fourier consistency conditions. Phys Med Biol. 2017;62(17):7181.
2. Bier B, Aichert A, Felsner L, et al.. Epipolar consistency conditions for motion correction in weight-bearing imaging. Springer; 2017.
3. Bier B, Unberath M, Geimer T, et al.; Springer. Motion compensation using range imaging in C-Arm cone-beam CT. Proc MIUA. 2017; p. 561–570.
4. Maier A, Hofmann HG, Berger M, et al. CONRAD: a software framework for cone-beam imaging in radiology. Med Phys. 2013;40(11):111914–1–8.
5. Kak AC, Slaney M. Principles of computerized tomographic imaging. Piscataway, NJ, United States: IEEE Service Center; 1988.
6. Parker DL. Optimal short scan convolution reconstruction for fanbeam CT. Med Phys. 1982;9(2):254–257.
7. Rohkohl C, Lauritsch G, Nöttling A, et al. C-Arm CT: Reconstruction of dynamic high contrast objects applied to the coronary sinus. Proc IEEE NSS/MICR. 2008; p. no pagination.
8. Zeng GL. Medical image reconstruction: a conceptual tutorial. Springer; 2010.

Towards Fully Automated Determination of Laryngeal Adductor Reflex Latencies through High-Speed Laryngoscopy Image Processing

Jacob F. Fast[1], Martin Ptok[2], Michael Jungheim[2], Robin Szymanski[1], Tobias Ortmaier[1], Lüder A. Kahrs[1]

[1]Leibniz Universität Hannover, Institute of Mechatronic Systems
[2]Hannover Medical School, Department of Phoniatrics and Pediatric Audiology
jacob.fast@imes.uni-hannover.de

Abstract. Protective reflexes of the larynx help to avoid intrusion of foreign particles into the lower airways, which can lead to aspiration pneumonia. These protective mechanisms include the Laryngeal Adductor Reflex (LAR), a rapid adduction of the vocal folds. Up to now, the LAR latency could only be determined manually by visually assessing laryngoscopic high-speed video sequences obtained during and after stimulation of the larynx by water droplet impact. Here, we present a novel image processing algorithm based on difference image calculation and optical flow analysis for a more objective LAR latency determination. To evaluate our prototype algorithm, we compared the results obtained for a set of example sequences with the values given by two expert phoniatricians. The results show a very good LAR stimulation detection performance. LAR onset detection remains challenging for our algorithmic approach as well as for the human perceptive system, as demonstrated by a low inter-rater reliability.

1 Introduction

In the year 2014, respiratory diseases were responsible for 8.5 % of all deaths in the elderly population (age > 65 years) in the European Union [1]. Aspiration is an important etiologic factor for the development of pneumonia, the leading cause of death in nursing homes [2]. The lower airways are protected against aspiration by the Laryngeal Adductor Reflex (LAR) [3]. This reflex consists of a rapid adduction of the vocal folds after application of a laryngeal stimulus [3]. An absent LAR provides an explanation for the development of aspiration pneumonia, a potentially fatal lung inflammation caused by intrusion of foreign particles [4]. The LAR latency could be used to define a threshold between physiological and pathological LAR phenotypes. Thus, a simple LAR screening procedure yielding a quantitative result is highly desirable.

1.1 LAR stimulation methods

A LAR triggering method with high repeatability is indispensable to assess LAR performance in a standardized setting. Conventional LAR trigger methods rely on tactile or electrical stimulation [5, 6]. Recently, the novel method *Microdroplet Impulse Testing of the Laryngeal Adductor Reflex* (MIT-LAR) has been developed for LAR triggering and latency investigation [7]. By shooting a fluid droplet onto the laryngeal mucosa, the LAR is provoked noninvasively [7].

1.2 Image processing applications in laryngoscopy

Image processing has previously been applied for segmentation and tracking of the glottis or the vocal folds [8]. Vibration parameters of the vocal folds have been obtained from endoscopic image sequences [9]. Vocal fold motion has been reconstructed using laser projection and a high-speed camera system [10]. However, to our knowledge, no image processing approach has been developed for the automatic quantification of LAR latencies based on high-speed frame sequences recorded during and after LAR stimulation by a water droplet.

2 Materials and methods

The performance of an image processing algorithm highly depends on the quality of the data provided. In this chapter, we elaborate on the acquisition process that was used to obtain laryngoscopic high-speed sequences. We outline the currently applied, manual LAR latency determination procedure and present a novel LAR latency determination algorithm.

2.1 Manual lar latency evaluation procedure

We based this work on sequences showing LAR onset after triggering the reflex with a water droplet. The sequences were recorded with a high-speed laryngoscopy system (HRes Endocam 5562, R. Wolf GmbH, Knittlingen, Germany) at a frame rate of 4 000 fps. After acquisition of a high-speed image sequence, the clinician has to determine the LAR latency manually by visual frame-by-frame inspection. Two key frame numbers have to be defined in a time-consuming procedure. Typical time-points of an exemplary sequence are depicted in Fig. 1. First, frame number n_{imp} corresponds to the point in time t_{imp} at which the

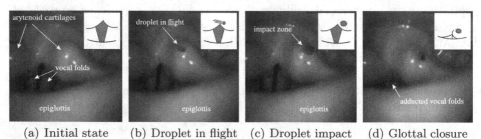

(a) Initial state   (b) Droplet in flight   (c) Droplet impact   (d) Glottal closure

Fig. 1. Laryngeal reaction to droplet impact.

stimulus is applied by water droplet impact. Second, frame number n_{on} corresponds to LAR onset time t_{on}. Thus, with a known laryngoscopic recording frame rate f_{rec} in frames per second, the LAR latency Δt_{LAR} in seconds can be calculated as follows

$$\Delta t_{LAR} = \frac{1}{f_{rec}} \left(n_{on} - n_{imp} \right) \tag{1}$$

To establish the described LAR assessment procedure as a commonly employed diagnostic method, the time spent to generate a valid LAR latency value from endoscopically gathered image data as well as the requirements concerning the examiner's qualification have to be reduced. We therefore aimed to develop an image processing algorithm for automatic LAR latency determination.

To evaluate the results obtained with our prototype algorithm, we asked two phoniatricians experienced in the evaluation of swallowing disorders and vocal fold movement to quantify LAR latencies by providing frame indices n_{imp} and n_{on} in a total of $n = 10$ laryngoscopic example sequences using a video playback tool capable of framewise visualization (Avidemux 2.7.0, www.avidemux.org). We assessed the inter-rater reliability for the latency-defining instants t_{imp} and t_{on} in each frame sequence.

2.2 Outline of lar latency determination workflow

Algorithmic LAR determination can be divided into two sub-problems: identifying frame number n_{imp} that marks the beginning of the reflex latency period in a given laryngoscopy sequence and determining frame number n_{on} that shows LAR onset. As both timestamps can be characterized by a change in the amount of motion in the high-speed sequence, we identified the optical flow to be a suitable tool for their automated identification. We selected the Horn-Schunck method implementation in MatLab R2016b (The MathWorks Inc., Natick, MA, USA) for optical flow calculation with iteration limit $max_{iter} = 10$, smoothness regularization term $\alpha = 1$ and minimum residual absolute velocity difference $\Delta v_{min} = 0$ as those settings produced satisfactory results for our purpose. The optical flow vector fields at the instant of droplet impact are presented in Fig. 2 for an exemplary set of sequences (vectors scaled by factor 800). The method yields a dense velocity vector field for each frame containing vectors $\mathbf{v}_i$ associated with

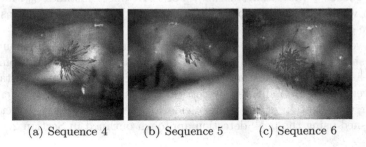

(a) Sequence 4   (b) Sequence 5   (c) Sequence 6

Fig. 2. Optical flow vector fields at droplet impact.

the frame pixels. In each frame, only regions that differ from the initial configuration of the larynx contain valuable motion information. Thus, we applied a difference image operation to each frame by pixel-wise subtraction of the mean intensity value based on the first five frames of each sequence. This was preceded by conversion of the originial sequence from RGB to grayscale colorspace and subsequent contrast adjustment and median filtering with a 3-by-3 neighborhood for noise reduction (total frame resolution 256×256 px). The absolute amount of motion $F(n)$ in a given frame n is given by the sum of vector norms

$$F(n) = \sum_i \|\mathbf{v_i}\| = \sum_i \left\| \left(v_{x,i}, v_{y,i} \right)^T \right\| \tag{2}$$

This sum will be susceptible to sensor noise added to the laryngoscopic image data by the acquisition system. Assuming the noise to be of Gaussian type, we defined flow entity Φ that we expected to be more robust to noise-induced optical flow as it is not affected by symmetric motion. For a given frame number n, $\Phi(n) \in \mathbb{R}_{\geq 0}$ is calculated by adding the absolute values of the signed component sums of flow vectors $\mathbf{v_i}$

$$\Phi(n) = \left\| \sum_i v_{x,i} \right\| + \left\| \sum_i v_{y,i} \right\| \tag{3}$$

To reduce remaining noise in $\Phi(n)$, we applied strong smoothing by means of an extremum-preserving Savitzky-Golay filter (polynomial order 1, frame length 23, applied twice). Finally, the double-filtered signal was examined by a peak detection procedure with a minimum peak prominence of 0.1. The first peak in each sequence satisfying this condition was retained as an indicator for droplet impact frame number n_{impact}. The given parameters were found to allow robust LAR stimulation instant detection based on available endoscopic image data.

3   Results

Inter-rater deviation for LAR stimulation instants t_{imp} was zero for all sequences except sequence 1 (deviation 0.25 ms). For LAR onset instants t_{on}, inter-rater deviation was found to be substantially higher at an average of 8.5 ms. Mean values are given in Tab. 1.

The evolution of Φ, normed via division by the respective maximum value Φ_{max}, is shown in Fig. 3 for all $n = 10$ sequences together with automatically detected and rater-given instants t_{imp} and rater-given LAR onset instants t_{on}. Rater-given values are indicated by vertical marks connected by gray crosslines for better visualization of inter-rater deviation. Automatic t_{imp} detection was accomplished using the peak detection approach outlined in Section 2.

Table 1. Mean LAR measurement results for $n = 10$ sample sequences.

Inter-expert t_{imp} deviation	Expert-algorithm t_{imp} deviation	Inter-expert t_{on} deviation	Expert-given LAR latency
0.02 ms	1.03 ms	8.5 ms	90.31 ms

4   Discussion

In this paper, we outline an algorithmic approach to support diagnosticians in calculating LAR latencies based on laryngoscopic high-speed sequences. Our results show a very good agreement between rater- and algorithm-given LAR stimulation time-points t_{imp} (mean deviation 1.03 ms). Automatic LAR onset instant determination has proven to be more challenging since the reflexive motion of the laryngeal structures can be described as a smooth and slowly accelerated process. This result is in line with the inter-rater agreement results for t_{imp} and t_{on}. In fact, mean inter-rater deviation for t_{imp} was only 0.02 ms with a maximum deviation of 0.25 ms, whereas inter-rater deviation for t_{on} was as high as 8.5 ms with a maximum deviation of 35.3 ms.

Overall, our algorithm shows a high performance in detecting t_{imp} and yields a distinct increase in Φ corresponding to LAR onset for 80 % of the sequences studied in this work. This is a remarkable result, taking into account the low quality of available image data and the optical aberrations induced by endoscopic image acquisition. Notably, initial vocal fold configuration, endoscopic angle of view and duration of the sequences used in this work varied strongly. We are confident that our algorithm could be a helpful and timesaving tool for

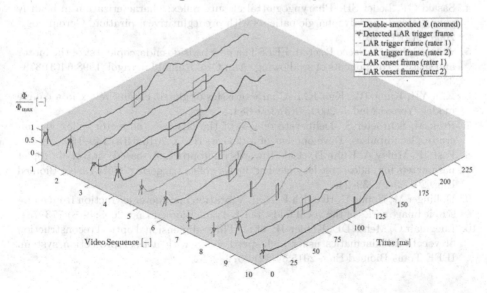

Fig. 3. Evolution of normed, double-smoothed Φ with detected and rater-given latency-defining instants.

clinical LAR latency assessment as it reliably identifies LAR trigger time-points in high-speed sequences. LAR onset is marked by a smooth increase in Φ calculated for all pixels of the endoscopic frame. Medical research focusing on LAR physiology could be supported by our algorithm that detects laryngeal motion very sensitively. Further studies should be based on a higher number of sample sequences as well as a larger expert base to increase statistical significance. Radial optical flow could be used in order to reduce errors introduced by endoscope translation. Finally, a machine learning approach could be used to segment laryngeal structures and thus, to achieve robustness against motion activity of non-LAR-related regions, e.g. of the epiglottis.

Acknowledgement. This work has been funded by the German Research Foundation (grants no. KA 2975/6-1 and PT 2/5-1). The authors would like to thank Mrs. Sarah Schroeter for the acquisition of the sequences that this work is based upon.

References

1. Eurostat. Causes of death statistics - people over 65; accessed: 25/10/2017. goo.gl/36wJqU.
2. Marik PE, Kaplan D. Aspiration pneumonia and dysphagia in the elderly. Chest. 2003;124(1):328–336.
3. Sinclair CF, Téllez MJ, Tapia OR, et al. Contralateral R1 and R2 components of the laryngeal adductor reflex in humans under general anesthesia. Laryngoscope. 2017;127(12):E443–E448.
4. Sasaki CT, Leder SB. Pharyngoglottal closure reflex: characterization in healthy young, elderly and dysphargic patients with predeglutitive aspiration. Gerontology. 2003;49(1):12–20.
5. Aviv JE, Kim T, Sacco R, et al. FEEST: a new bedside endoscopic test of the motor and sensory components of swallowing. Ann Otol Rhinol Laryngol. 1998;64(3):378–387.
6. Kim YH, Kang JW, Kim KM. Characteristics of glottic closure reflex in a canine model. Yonsei Med J. 2009;50(3):380–384.
7. Ptok M, Schroeter S. Deliberate release of the laryngeal adductor reflex via microdroplet impulses: Development of a device. HNO. 2016;64(3):149–155.
8. Fast JF, Muley A, Kühn D, et al. Towards microprocessor-based control of droplet parameters for endoscopic laryngeal adductor reflex triggering. Curr Direct Biomed Eng. 2017;3(2):239–243.
9. Dollinger M, Hoppe U, Hettlich F, et al. Vibration parameter extraction from endoscopic image series of the vocal folds. IEEE Trans Biomed Eng. 2008;49(8):773–781.
10. Luegmair G, Mehta DD, Kobler JB, et al. Three-dimensional optical reconstruction of vocal fold kinematics using high-speed video with a laser projection system. IEEE Trans Biomed Eng. 2015;34(12):2572–2582.

Fourier-based Reduction of Directed Streak Artifacts in Cone-Beam CT

Julia Gawellek[1], Bastian Bier[1], Garry Gold[2], Andreas Maier[1]

[1]Pattern Recognition Lab, Friedrich-Alexander-University Erlangen-Nuremberg
[2]Radiological Sciences Laboratory, Stanford University
julia.gawellek@fau.de

Abstract. Due to its adjustable scan trajectory, C-arm cone-beam CT has been used recently to acquire knee scans in an upright position. However, stabilization devices located outside the FOV introduce streak artifacts in the reconstructed images. This paper proposes a method to remove those streak artifacts. Using selective filtering of the Fourier transforms of the reconstructions, we propose a filter design that attenuates the frequencies that are responsible for the streak artifacts. The filter is constructed by taking both the frequency and the orientation of the introduced streaks into account. We compare our approach to a bandpass-filter. Our proposed method is able to reduce the streaks in the reconstruction remarkably while preserving edge information, whereas the bandpass-filter is not capable of preserving sharp edges in the filtered image. Moreover, our method yields an improved SSIM when comparing both filter techniques to simulated ground truth data.

1 Introduction

C-Arm Cone-Beam Computed Tomography (CBCT) is a versatile acquisition technique. There is a large scope of applications due to its flexible construction and big field of view (FOV) ranging from interventional to diagnostical applications. Nonetheless, several artifacts are present in CBCT scans such as scatter, beam hardening, truncation or ring artifacts.

To further improve the understanding of the knee function during loaded situations, CBCT scans under weight-bearing conditions are acquired [1]. Stabilization pipes for the patients are part of the acquisition set-up for those scans. However, since those pipes are located outside the FOV, vertical directed streak artifacts are present in the scans (Fig. 4(a)). In this case, only a fraction of the acquired projections contains information about this object, which is thus not sufficiently sampled and causing streak artifacts in the reconstructed images. Streak artifacts, which mostly appear from metal or sharp objects outside the FOV, are commonly reduced by metal artifact reduction algorithms [2] or view-alias alleviation techniques [3]. Spectral inpainting in the gradient domain was used to remove streaks in CT projections [4].

This paper proposes a technique to remove directed streaks artifacts by applying selective filtering in the frequency domain of the reconstructed images.

Compared to a standard bandpass-filter, our approach yields improved SSIM values compared to a simulated reconstruction.

2   Materials and methods

2.1   Fourier transform

For filtering in the frequency domain, the Fourier Transform of the respective image has to be computed. However, since an image $f(x, y)$ can be considered as a matrix containing discrete values, a 2D discrete Fourier Transform (DFT) is applied, where $F(u, v)$ is the frequency domain representation. Only the magnitude image $|F(u, v)|$ of the complex valued DFT result is relevant for our task, since each pixel represents a particular frequency contained in the spatial domain image. Consequently, if one wants to eliminate certain frequencies from an image, the corresponding pixels in the magnitude image $|F(u, v)|$ have to be attenuated before it is transformed back to spatial domain. In order to find the pixels responsible for the streaks artifacts in our CBCT knee scans, basic properties of the Fourier transformation have to be pointed out [5]. The magnitude image $|F(u, v)|$ is shifted so that its center is the origin of the frequency coordinate system. At this point, the horizontal component u and the vertical component v are zero. The value at this point $F(0, 0)$ represents the offset of the spatial image. As Fig. 1 illustrates, the further away a point is from the center in frequency domain, the higher the corresponding frequency. If the spatial image has vertically oriented streaks, its DFT is located near the horizontal axis u (right image in Fig. 1). Hence, points in the frequency domain image are perpendicular to edges in the spatial image.

2.2   Wedge-Filter

With these properties in mind, we design a custom tailored frequency selective filter, which aims at eliminating the streak artifacts in the CBCT reconstructions described before. A bandpass passes frequencies within a defined range and attenuates frequencies outside that range. For our application this represents a coarse solution. High frequencies should be attenuated, since they represent the streak artifacts. Moreover, low frequencies are rejected in order to sharpen the filtered image. In Fig. 2(b) the frequency domain representation of a bandpass-filter is depicted. We introduce a more thorough approach by defining a frequency selective filter referred to as wedge-filter, attenuating

Fig. 1. Visual comparison of DFTs from two periodic signals with different frequency and orientation.

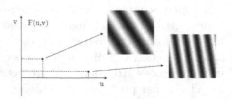

only a defined frequency range. A possible configuration of a wedge-filter is displayed in Fig. 2(a). A wedge-filter consists of two point symmetric wedges and attenuates only pixels in the magnitude image $|F(u, v)|$ that are located in the defined wedge. Each wedge-filter can be customized based on the respective CBCT data that features streak artifacts. If the spatial domain image features vertical streaks, the customized wedges are rotated such that they will attenuate frequency on and near the horizontal axis (Fig. 2(a)). Moreover, the frequency of the streak artifacts is also regarded by defining the radius of the wedge. The bigger the radius of the wedges, the higher frequencies are eliminated. The attenuation in each wedge is modeled with a Gaussian distribution, where the mean values are located along the frequencies causing the most common streaks. Hence, if the streaks' orientation is not constant but slightly varying, one can set a standard deviation value that defines how strong the attenuation is in the neighborhood of the mean value, so that also frequencies similar to the dominant ones are attenuated.

For each scan, we selected the filter parameters empirically. For a filter size of 512 x 512 pixels, the bandpass attenuates intensities in a circle with an inner radius of 2 and an outer radius of 250 pixels (Fig. 2 (b)). Consequently, high frequencies representing streaks are suppressed, whereas the offset of the spatial image is only slightly modified. The radius of the wedges is set accordingly. Due to vertical streaks in coronar and sagittal views, the wedges are located on the horizontal axis in the filter. For axial slices, the orientation of the wedges was rotated by an angle of $\pi/3$, since the streaks have the same angle in the reconstructions with respect to the vertical axis. The mean value of the Gaussian distribution in a wedge was set to 0.3 and the standard deviation to 50 pixels, in order not to fully suppress to targeted frequencies and to allow a certain variation of the streaks' direction.

2.3 Experiments

To test our proposed filter, we evaluated four subjects whose knees were scanned in an upright position under weight-bearing conditions. Additionally, a simu-

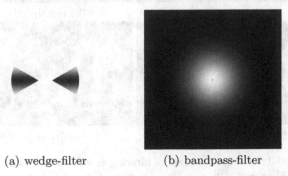

(a) wedge-filter   (b) bandpass-filter

Fig. 2. Comparison of a wedge- and a bandpass-filter.

lated dataset consisting of one ground truth acquisition and a simulated streak image generated by [4] was used for evaluation purposes.

3   Results

3.1   Qualitative results

First, we compare the filtering results of our proposed filter to the results of the bandpass-filter on a simulated data slice. The results are depicted in Fig. 3. One can see that the wedge-filtered image features less streaks than the corrupted image. The bandpass-filtered image also eliminates the streaks, but is not able of preserving sharp edges, since the bandpass-filter attenuates edges independent of their orientation.

In Fig. 4, filtering results of a wedge- and bandpass-filter for a axial and sagittal slice of a real data set are compared with respect to their difference images. For panels (b), (c), (g) and (h) customized wedge- and bandpass-filtered were applied to each respective original image. The difference image (d) between the original slice and the wedge-filtered image reveals that the streaks from the dominant direction were filtered, while high frequency information is preserved. The difference image (f) between the original axial slice and the bandpass approach indicates that the bandpass-filter is also capable of filtering streaks, but not of preserving edge information. Looking at the filtering results from the sagittal slice that mostly features vertical streaks, one can detect that the bandpass approach is not able to remove those streak, whereas our proposed wedge-filter approach can filter the streaks, as shown in the difference image (i).

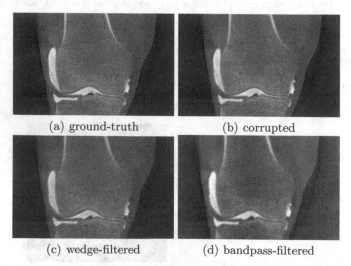

(a) ground-truth   (b) corrupted

(c) wedge-filtered   (d) bandpass-filtered

Fig. 3. Simulated data: Comparison of filtering results of a coronar slice when filtered with a wedge-filter and a bandpass. (a) shows the ground-truth streak-free coronar slice; (b) the streak-corrupted data; (c) the wedge-filtered; (d) the bandpass-filtered slice.

3.2   Quantitative results

For a quantitative analysis, a simulated ground truth and a corrupted image that contains simulated streaks were generated in order to compare the SSIM of the wedge-filter to the bandpass approach. For an axial, coronar and sagittal view the SSIM of the wedge-filter, bandpass and simulated streak data are depicted in

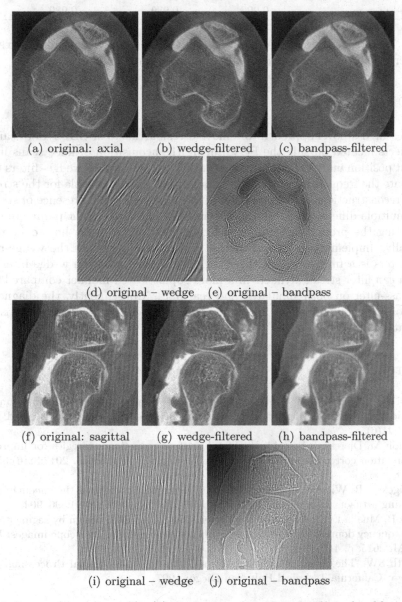

(a) original: axial   (b) wedge-filtered   (c) bandpass-filtered

(d) original – wedge   (e) original – bandpass

(f) original: sagittal   (g) wedge-filtered   (h) bandpass-filtered

(i) original – wedge   (j) original – bandpass

Fig. 4. Images (a) - (c) and (f) - (h) display the original, wedge-filtered and bandpass-filtered slice of a axial and sagittal view. Images (d), (e), (i) and (j) are difference images obtained by subtracting the filtered images from the original slice.

Table 1. SSIM of a simulated streak image, a bandpass- and wedge-filtered image against ground truth data.

Method	axial	coronar	sagittal
Simulated streaks [4]	0.898	0.889	0.894
Bandpass	0.967	0.877	0.901
Wedge-Filter	0.996	0.989	0.989

Tab. 1. The results reveal that the wedge-filter approach yields superior results for every view when compared to a bandpass-filter on simulated data.

4 Discussion

We presented a novel approach to remove streak artifacts in CBCT data caused by objects located outside the FOV during the acquisition of knee scans in an upright position under weight-bearing conditions. We applied wedge- filters that attenuate the frequencies in the FFT images that are responsible for the streaks in the reconstructions. One limitation of our approach is the presence of streaks with multiple different orientations. Moreover, finding the right parameters for generating the proper wedge-filter for each view and subject has to be done manually. Implementing a method that automatically defines the wedge-filter parameters is a future task in this field. We showed that the wedge-filter approach can filter streak artifacts in a more sophisticated manner compared to a bandpass-filter on both simulated and real data. Consequently, the diagnostic value of the acquired images increases, since further post-processing steps are facilitated.

References

1. Choi JH, Maier A, Keil A, et al. Fiducial marker-based correction for involuntary motion in weight-bearing c-arm ct scanning of knees. II. experiment. Med Phy. 2014;41(6).
2. Abdoli M, Dierckx RA, Zaidi H. Metal artifact reduction strategies for improved attenuation correction in hybrid PET/CT imaging. Med Phys. 2012;39(6):3343–3360.
3. Galigekere R, Wiesent K, Holdsworth D. Techniques to alleviate the effects of view aliasing artifacts in computed tomography. Med Phys. 1999;26(6):896–904.
4. Bier B, Mualla F, Steidl S, et al.; Springer. Band-Pass filter design by segmentation in frequency domain for detection of epithelial cells in endomicroscope images. Proc BVM. 2015; p. 413–418.
5. Smith SW. The Scientist and Engineer's Guide to Digital Signal Processing. San Diego: California Technical Pub. San Diego; 1997.

An Open Source Tool for Creating Model Files for Virtual Volume Rendering in PDF Documents

Julian Brandner[1], Axel Newe[1], Wolfgang Aichinger[2], Linda Becker[3]

[1]Chair of Medical Informatics, Friedrich-Alexander-Universität Erlangen-Nürnberg
[2]Method Park Engineering GmbH, Erlangen
[3]Chair of Health Psychology, Friedrich-Alexander-Universität Erlangen-Nürnberg
axel.newe@fau.de

Abstract. Volume rendering is an important technique for medical imaging where many modalities produce three-dimensional (3D) images. An appropriate three-dimensional rendering leads to a better perception of the image content. A major problem is exchangeability: Usually, only two-dimensional, static snapshots of a volume-rendered scene can be distributed electronically. The Portable Document Format (PDF) provides the possibility to embed 3D objects. With suitable reading software, these objects can be displayed interactively. This article presents an open-source implementation of a software tool that is based on the MeVisLab imaging framework and that can convert volume images into model files which can be embedded into PDF files to create a virtual volume rendering.

1 Introduction

Volume Rendering is a procedure to project three-dimensional (3D) volumetric image data onto a two-dimensional (2D) plane (e.g., a computer monitor). This is especially important in Medical Imaging where many modalities (e.g., X-Ray Computed Tomography or Magnetic Resonance) provide 3D images that need to be visualized in order to be accessible for their consumers.

This 3D visualization eases the user's perceptual processing and facilitates shape understanding [1]. It has many advantages over 2D such as better visualizing complex spatial structures, leading to a greater information density and, therefore, to less information loss than with 2D projections. Furthermore, the 3D structure generally better matches the user's mental representation of the visualized object and is generally closer to the object's real-world appearance [2].

The 3D visualization makes use of the user's cognitive perceptual abilities. During the perceptual processing of the real 3D world, it's image is projected onto a 2D retinal image. This 2D representation is, however, re-transformed into a 3D representation. The major cues for 3D depth perception of surfaces are either texture gradients, shading or gradients of binocular disparity [3].

Die Original-Version des Kapitels wurde korrigiert. Ein Erratum finden Sie unter
https://doi.org/10.1007/978-3-662-56537-7_97

The advantages of 3D versus 2D visualization can be further enhanced when additionally including the possibility to interactively manipulate or interact with the 3D object [4]. This is especially important for medical image perception, where e.g., the possibility to rotate a 3D object can bring a previously occluded structure to the foreground [5]. For laparoscopic surgeons it has been found that they prefer 3D versus 2D visualizations [6] and that they work more efficiently with 3D than with 2D applications [7]. A major problem of the Volume Rendering technique, however, is exchangeability. The rendering process requires a lot of computational resources and interaction with the rendered image usually requires specialized software. This impedes a simple distribution of truly interactive volume-rendered images. A usual workaround is to create 2D snapshots and to distribute these instead.

The well-known Portable Document Format (PDF) is the de-facto standard for the exchange of electronic documents. An extension to this format is the Portable Document Format-Healthcare (PDF/H) [8] which describes how to use the PDF as a trusted means to exchange, to preserve and to protect digital healthcare information.

A standard feature of PDF is the ability to embed 3D objects. The usefulness of this feature for publications and for the exchange of medical data has been proven [5]. This feature can also be used to mimic volume rendering in electronic documents [9]. The difference of this virtual volume rendering compared to real volume rendering is the fact that the volume is prerendered and limited to a fixed windowing, so that no actual rendering takes place. However, previously presented solutions [9] are rather cumbersome to implement and require programming skills which cannot be expected from scientists in the medical domain.

MeVisLab is a medical imaging platform and visual development environment, maintained by MeVis Medical Solutions AG and Fraunhofer MEVIS in Bremen, Germany. It is available for all major platforms and offers a variety of licensing options, including a license which is free for use in non-commercial organizations and research.

Every algorithm or library offered by MeVisLab is wrapped into a module. Modules can be connected and inserted into Networks using the graphical user interface (GUI), allowing the user to create complex procedures without programming experience. The actual functionality is provided by dynamically linked libraries (DLLs).

A community-created add-on to MeVisLab provides an application and several modules for the creation of PDFs with embedded 3D models [10]. Based on this PDF add-on, a module has been implemented that can be used to create model files in Universal 3D (U3D) format [10] which contain all the data needed to embed volume renderings into PDF documents. The solution is simple to use and requires no programming.

2   Material and methods

MeVisLab offers its own build system, which is based on QMake, to create the DLLs platform-independently. For this work, Microsoft Visual Studio 2013 was used in combination with MeVisLab 2.8.2. The module itself was developed using C++11, whereas the GUI could be described by the MeVis Definition Language (MDL).

The aim of this work led to the need of texture support for U3D files within the PDF add-on, which turned out to be a main goal of this project. One new module (U3DAddVolumeFromView) needed to be created within the scope of the MLU3D project [11] in order to provide the desired volume rendering functionality. Furthermore, modifications to an existing module (U3DSave) were necessary. In order to demonstrate the newly gained texture functionality, an additional module called U3DAddTextureFromFile was developed as well.

Since MLU3D is an open source project, aimed towards easy accessibility of its functionality, the code was annotated referencing the official U3D standard to allow for further developments. The newly created user interfaces were created with the medical use case in mind.

For validation of the U3D output, the Scientific3DFigurePDFApp of the PDF add-on [11] was used to embed the model data into a PDF file. This PDF was then visually inspected by means of the standard PDF renderer Adobe Reader (versions X and XI).

3   Results

The new module U3DAddVolumeFromView takes a 3D volume image as input and adds all necessary U3D elements for a virtual volume rendering (VVR) to an U3D file. It is available as part of the MLU3D project within the MeVisLab Community Modules on GitHub [12].

The functionality of the entire MLU3D project is built around an internal data structure representing the U3D file format. All previously available features write their data into this internal format first. As soon as the data has been modified to the satisfaction of the user, it can be written to the actual file using the U3DSave module. This module and the internal format are now extended to allow the embedding of textures in the files produced by MLU3D. A new data structure, containing the image data itself as well as required meta data, can now be stored in the internal format. Upon execution of U3DSave this data is read and used to write two data blocks per texture into the final file. The first data block declares the texture resource, the second one describes it. The texture itself is stored as a Portable Network Graphic (PNG) with four color channels and a bit depth of 32 bits.

The intermediate result module U3DAddTextureFromFile, additionally created, attaches an image from the local file system to an existing geometry. The respective U3D data structure has to be provided via the MeVisLab network GUI and needs to contain a mesh geometry, which can easily be created with the pre-existing U3D modules. After selecting the image which shall be used as texture, further adjustments can be made using a text field in the GUI of U3DAddVolumeFromFile. An idiom of the widely prevalent Extensible Markup Language (XML) is used to specify which meshes the texture shall be applied to. Optionally, texture coordinates can be assigned to the mesh in the same way. If no coordinates are provided, an example mapping is generated for testing purposes. The module itself converts the given data to the supported format and stores it with any additional data in the internal U3D representation to be used by U3DSave later. Since any changes made this way are persistent, it is possible to add an arbitrary amount of textures by repeating this process several times.

The sought volume rendering itself is completely texture based. The three-dimensional image data is cut into slices along one coordinate axis. For each slice a rectangular mesh is created and textured with the corresponding two-dimensional image. The Portable Network Graphics (PNG) format is used for those textures due to its lossless compression and its optional transparency channel. This leads to three different views of the same volume (one for each Cartesian axis). Using the JavaScript support of PDF, the most suitable view can be determined and enabled based on the viewing angle. This technique has been used conceptionally by a prior publication [9] and is well suited for usage in PDF due to its easy representation in U3D.

The main result module U3DAddVolumeFromView combines all newly created features. It uses the texturization support to implement the previously described volume rendering technique. The user has to provide a three-dimensional image in addition to an U3D structure. Via the module GUI a representing name has to be entered for the volume data. If multiple volumes are to be added to one file, the names have to be unique. As the module is executed, two-dimensional PNG files are constructed from the given three-dimensional image and stored in memory. For each of those a rectangular mesh is built and textured. This process is repeated three times (once for each axis) and the results are organized in U3D's own tree-like path system. Since the whole technique is based on already developed functionalities, no additional adaptation of U3DSave was required.

4   Discussion

The implemented solution extends the previously described PDF add-on for MeVisLab by the possibility to add textures to a U3D model and by the possibility to convert a volume image into a textured U3D model. This model can then be embedded into a PDF file in order to realize a virtual volume rendering in an electronic document. The solution requires no programming, the necessary network can be assembled in an easy and straightforward way. An example network is provided for reference (Fig. 1).

This solution requires MeVisLab which calls for a considerable effort regarding download an installation. On the other hand, MeVisLab is available for all major desktop operating-systems (MS Windows, Linux and MacOS) and allows

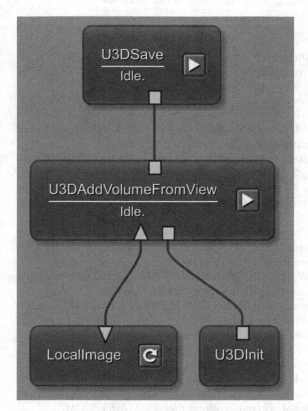

Fig. 1. Simple module network for adding a volume image to an U3D file.

integrating the creation of VVR PDFs into a comprehensive image processing network.

The resulting U3D (and thus the PDF) provides a pre-rendered virtual volume which is limited to a fixed windowing. It can be manipulated interactively by rotating, panning and zooming the volume. Windowing would be desirable, but the PDF specification does not allow to manipulate the image content itself.

For performance reasons it is recommended to limit the resolution to roughly one million voxels to maintain portability of the final result even on outdated or mobile hardware.

As a spillover result, texturization of traditional mesh geometries in U3D files is possible as well now with the MevisLab PDF add-on.

Acknowledgement. Linda Becker was supported by the Bavarian Equal Opportunities Sponsorship – Förderung von Frauen in Forschung und Lehre (FFL) – Promoting Equal Opportunities for Women in Research and Teaching.

References

1. St John M, Cowen M, Smallman HS, et al. The use of 2D and 3D displays for shape-understanding versus relative-position tasks. Hum Factors. 2001;43(1):79–98.
2. Teyseyre A, Campo M. An overview of 3D software visualization. IEEE Trans Vis Comput Graph. 2009;15(1):87–105.
3. Sakata H, Tsutsui K, Taira M. Toward an understanding of the neural processing for 3D shape perception. Neuropsychologia. 2005;43(2):151–61.
4. Bowman DA, Chen J, Wingrave CA, et al. New directions in 3D user interfaces. Int J Virtual Real. 2006;5(2):3–14.
5. Newe A, Becker L, Schenk A. Application and evaluation of interactive 3D PDF for presenting and sharing planning results for liver surgery in clinical routine. PLoS ONE. 2014;9(12):e115697.
6. Tanagho YS, Andriole GL, Paradis AG, et al. 2D versus 3D visualization: impact on laparoscopic proficiency using the fundamentals of laparoscopic surgery skill set. J Laparoendosc Adv Surg Tech. 2012;22(9):865–70.
7. Storz P, Buess GF, Kunert W, et al. 3D HD versus 2D HD: surgical task efficiency in standardised phantom tasks. Surg Endosc. 1984;26(1):1454–60.
8. American Society for Testing and Materials. Portable Document Format-Healthcare (PDF) A Best Practices Guide. [Online]. 2008 [Cited 2017 Oct 30]. . Available from: http://www.astm.org/cgi-bin/resolver.cgi?AIIMASTM.
9. Ruthensteiner B, Baeumler N, Barnes DG. Interactive 3D volume rendering in biomedical publications. Micron. 2010;41(7):886.
10. ECMA International. Standard ECMA-363, universal 3D file format, 4th edition (June 2007). [Online]. [Cited 2017 Oct 30].   Available from: https://www.ecma-international.org/publications/files/ECMA-ST/ECMA-363%204th%20Edition.pdf.
11. Newe A. Enriching scientific publications with interactive 3D PDF: an integrated toolbox for creating ready-to-publish figures. Peer J Comput Sci. 2016;2(3):e64.
12. The meVisLab community. meVisLab community modules. [Online]. [Cited 2017 Oct 30]. Available from: https://github.com/MeVisLab/communitymodules.

Comparison of Divergence-Free Filters for Cardiac 4D PC-MRI Data

Mickaël Francisco Sereno[1], Benjamin Köhler[2], Bernhard Preim[2]

[1]Paris-Sud University
[2]Dept. of Simulation and Graphics, Magdeburg University
serenomickael@gmail.com

Abstract. 4D PC-MRI enables the measurement of time-resolved blood flow directions within a 3D volume. These data facilitate a comprehensive qualitative and quantitative analysis.However, noise is introduced, e.g., due to inhomogeneous magnetic field gradients. Blood is commonly assumed as a non-Newtonian fluid, thus, incompressible, and divergence should be zero. Divergence-free filters enforce this model assumption and have been shown to improve data quality. In this paper, we compare binomial smoothing and three of these techniques: The finite difference method (FDM), divergence-free radial basis functions (DFRBF) and divergence-free wavelets (DFW). The results show that average and maximum velocities tend to decrease, while average line lengths tend to increase slightly. We recommend FDM or DFW divergence-free filtering as an optional pre-processing step in 4D PC-MRI processing pipelines, as they have feasible computation times of few seconds.

1 Introduction

4D phase-contrast magnetic resonance imaging (4D PC-MRI) [1] allows to acquire blood flow information as a 3D+time velocity vector field. Unfortunately, the data are prone to noise for various reasons. Proper pre-processing is essential to improve both subsequent qualitative and quantitative data analysis. Yet, simple image smoothing methods do not provide a sufficient correction. Therefore, customized methods were developed for each type of noise. For instance, the expected maximum velocity is a pre-scan parameter that has to be estimated based on experience and literature. If chosen too low, image values may flip and blood seemingly runs in the opposite direction (called phase wrap). If chosen too high, the measured vectors' accuracy and angular resolution suffers. Another cause for noise are inhomogeneous magnetic field gradients.

Blood is typically modeled as non-Newtonian, incompressible, laminar fluid. Divergence should be zero and a fluid element's density constant over time. However, noise in the data causes that the obtained divergence is non-zero. A specialized group of filters was established for 4D PC-MRI named divergence-free filters [2]. As the name suggests, they try to enforce this model assumption, which results in a smoother, theoretically more correct flow field.

139

In this work, we assess the results of three selected methods while using simple binomial smoothing as reference. The finite difference method (FDM) [3] reduces noise by projecting the data to a divergence-free vector field. The projection is reduced to a 7-point stencil Laplacian problem (two points on x, y and z plus the center) and is solved with a fast Poisson solver using fast Fourier transformations. Divergence-free radial basis functions (DFRBF) [4] employs a combination of normalized convolution and divergence-free radial basis functions in an iterative least-squares algorithm [5]. Divergence-free wavelets (DFW) [6] propose a soft divergence-free enforcement since it might be non-zero at the vessel boundaries due to partial volume effects.

Our comparison of 15 diverse datasets is based on both quantitative and qualitative criteria. We evaluate resulting pathlines according to different criteria, such as their length. Moreover, we assess measures, e.g., average velocities, for measuring planes in the vessels' cross-sections and perform side-by-side comparisons of the vector fields. Our results suggest that divergence-free filters perform better than binomial smoothing and might be a useful addition in a corresponding 4D PC-MRI pre-processing pipeline.

2   Methods

2.1   Data acquisition and pre-processing

Our 15 datasets were obtained with a 3 T Magnetom Verio MR at the Heart Center in Leipzig, a hospital specialized in diagnosis and treatment of heart diseases. The data comprise both healthy volunteers as well as patients with different cardiovascular diseases, such as aneurysms and aortic valve defects. The image sizes and scales are about $140 \times 190 \times 15\text{--}70$ ($1.8 \times 1.8 \times 1.8\text{--}3.5\,\text{mm}$) with 15–20 temporal positions (40–60 ms). The expected maximum velocity was chosen between 1.5–3.0 m/s, depending on the patient-specific situation, and phase unwrapping was performed [7]. A vessel surface is extracted from a binary segmentation via marching cubes and then smoothed. Centerlines were extracted [8] with the Vascular Modeling ToolKit (VMTK). Blood flow-representing pathlines are integrated using Runge-Kutta-4. Köhler et al. [2] provide a comprehensive overview about the general 4D PC-MRI data processing pipeline.

2.2   Implementation and parameters

All methods were implemented in C++. The three divergence-free filters are based on MATLAB code provided by Ong et al. [6]. OpenMP was used to parallelize the computation of individual time steps (each algorithm considers one temporal position at a time). Optimization was set to -O3.

For binomial smoothing (Binom) we used an isotropic kernel size of 3. Analogous to the divergence-free filters, each temporal position is processed separately. The finite difference method (FDM) requires no further settings. SureShrink [9] was used as threshold for Divergence-free Wavelets (DFW) with $spin = 2$, both as suggested by the authors [6]. For divergence-free radial basis functions (DFRBF) we used an isotropic convolution kernel of size 3. This rather small size limits the smoothing effect that comes with RBF. In our examples, convergence was observed experimentally at about 20 iterations, which we use as default.

2.3   Comparison

We calculate all of the criteria below for each dataset in every configuration (original, different filterings) and then calculate ratios where the original is the reference. The ratios indicate whether the corresponding criterion decreases (values < 100 %) or increases (values > 100 %) after filtering. The ratios' distribution (one ratio per dataset per filtering) will be presented as box plots. The criteria were inspired by divergence-free papers [3, 4, 6].

Our first employed measure is the average divergence within the vessel segmentation. For this, we manually chose the time step that represents peak systole (when the blood is pumped).

Four equidistant measuring planes were placed, starting inside the ascending and ending in the descending aorta, where higher and lower velocities are expected, respectively. Besides a qualitative comparison of the in-plane vector fields, we evaluated the average and maximum velocity vector magnitudes. To increase robustness, we use the 95 % quantile as maximum.

We integrate one pathline for each voxel of the vessel segmentation in 3 temporal positions: peak systole and its predecessor and successor. For these pathlines, we calculate their absolute length as accumulation of Euclidean distances between subsequent line segments. The temporal components are ignored. Also, we calculate their relative length by projecting all pathline points onto the vessel's centerline and then determining the centerline's arc length between the two projected points closest to the beginning and end of the centerline. This measure resembles the distance of end points while taking into account the curved vessel as domain. If there is a significant deviation of absolute and relative line length, this is an implicit indicator for increased curvature, e.g., due to vortex flow. The last measure reuses the measuring planes. It describes how many pathlines connect the first and the last plane. An increase of this measure indicates that less lines prematurely abort because they run out of the segmentation due to noisy flow directions.

3   Results and discussion

This section starts with a performance assessment of the employed divergence-free methods. We proceed by comparing results of 15 datasets according to the previously described criteria. Fig. 1 illustrates the ratios how each criterion increases or decreases relative to the unfiltered dataset.

The tests were performed on an Intel i5-6400 quad core with 3.4 GHz. Generally, computational effort depends on the image size. DFRBF additionally depends on the number of iterations. DFW computation time increases with higher spin values. On average, FDM was performed in 1–3 s, DFW in 15–45 s, and DFRBF in 5–15 min. We consider up to 1 min as feasible for integration in a processing pipeline of a corresponding evaluation tool. Thus, DFRBF is not appropriate in this respect.

Fig. 2 shows an exemplary comparison of resulting divergence fields. Binomial smoothing consistently lowers the divergence as velocities and their derivatives become smaller. To our surprise, FDM increases the divergence by median +16.3 % (Fig. 1(c)). DFW and DFRBF both have decreased the divergence for every dataset by median −11.3 % and −28.1 %, respectively. The comparably strong decrease of DFRBF might be due to the general smoothing that comes with using RBF. For DFM and DFW the decrease is not as strong as we expected. The high remaining divergence values at the segmentation boundaries are a known problem in the corresponding papers [4].

The results from Figs. 1(a)–(b) indicate that both the mean and maximum velocities are decreasing for all methods, though, not as strongly as with simple binomial smoothing. There are mostly minor changes up to 10 %. This seems plausible since a certain degree of smoothing comes with application of the filters. The smoothness of DFRBF is comparable to binomial filtering, FDM has the least degree of smoothing and DFW is in between. Fig. 3 shows an exemplary measuring plane. Velocity changes can be crucial, since velocities directly influence quantitative measures, such as net flow volumes, that assess the flow passing a measuring plane.

FDM significantly increases both the pathlines' absolute and relative length up to +36.4 % and +34.7 % maximum and +15.1 % and +10.1 %, respectively (Figs. 1(d)–(e)). DFW produces approximately the same absolute and relative line lengths as the unfiltered datasets (median −1.9 % and −0.4 %), so does DFRBF (median −1.1 % and +2.7 %). For the latter two approaches, visual

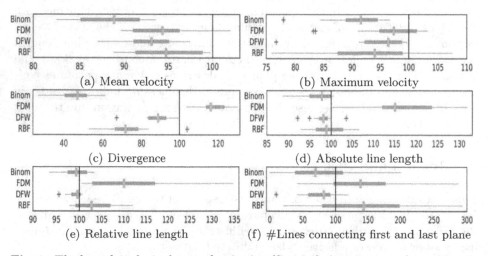

(a) Mean velocity

(b) Maximum velocity

(c) Divergence

(d) Absolute line length

(e) Relative line length

(f) #Lines connecting first and last plane

Fig. 1. The box plots depict how each criterion (Sec. 2.3) changes w.r.t. the unfiltered original. Black vertical lines mark the reference at 100 %. Orange lines are median values. Blue boxes are interquartile ranges. Red crosses are outliers.

Fig. 2. Divergence field of a healthy volunteers aorta during systole in sagittal orientation. Binomial smoothing (b) decreases, FDM (c) slightly increases, DFW (d) slightly decreases, and DFRBF (e) strongly decreases the divergence field. The divergences at the vessel boundaries remains comparably high (c-e), which is a known behavior in the corresponding papers.

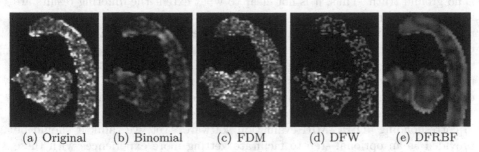

   (a) Original   (b) Binomial   (c) FDM   (d) DFW   (e) DFRBF

pathline changes are not noticeable. For FDM we could observe situations where laminar pathlines, starting in the ascending aorta, followed the vessel course longer than before, i.e., they reached farther into the descending aorta, which is physiologically expected. This is underlined by the number of lines connecting the first and last measuring plane (Fig. 1(f)). Here, FDM achieves a median improvement of +38.5 %. Interestingly, DFRBF even reaches +43.4 % improvement although the line lengths were not significantly increased. This could be explained by a straightening of the pathlines. DFW had a decline of −18.1 %. For all three line-related criteria, DFW is closest to the binomial smoothing result.

4 Conclusion and future work

In this work we have evaluated three state-of-the-art divergence-free filters (FDM, DFW, DFRBF) for their influence on the resulting flow field and pathlines. Velocity values decreased up to 10 % with all methods, which we consider as a reasonable margin. The pathline quality improved in many cases, which was observable via increasing line lengths and more lines being able to follow the vessel course correctly. Divergence did not decrease as strongly as we expected

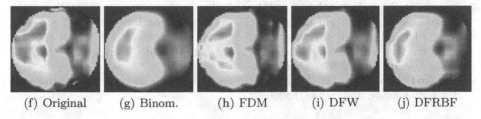

   (f) Original   (g) Binom.   (h) FDM   (i) DFW   (j) DFRBF

Fig. 3. Velocities (rainbow color scale) of a measuring plane inside the ascending aorta of a patient during systole. The general velocity distribution is preserved in all approaches, however, the degree of smoothing strongly varies. The DFRBF result is the smoothest, which is confirmed by the highest decline of average velocities.

and even increased using FDM. However, standard binomial smoothing, which was used as a reference, produced worse results, e.g., by strongly altering vortex flow patterns. This underlines the value of divergence-free filters.

A drawback of our comparison and 4D PC-MRI data in general is that there is no ground truth. Thus, it is not clear to what extent the differing results are improvements or not. A future work could be to employ 2D PC-MRI, which measures only one slice over time within the vessel, but with a higher spatio-temporal resolution. One could argue that this should produce more accurate results than the same measuring plane in 4D PC-MRI. Hence, if quantification results, e.g., for net flow volumes, come closer to the 2D PC-MRI reference after divergence-free filtering, this should indicate a definite improvement.

We cannot recommend divergence-free filtering as a mandatory pre-processing in corresponding 4D PC-MRI evaluation software. Yet, we think it should be provided as an optional step to facilitate getting more experiences with these techniques. With respect to the computation times, FDM (≤ 3 s) and DFW (≤ 45 s) are feasible, whereas DFRBF (≥ 5 min) is not.

Acknowledgement. This work was funded by the German Research Foundation (PR 660/18-1).

References

1. Dyverfeldt P, Bissell M, Barker AJ, et al. 4D flow cardiovascular magnetic resonance consensus statement. J Cardiovasc Magn Reson. 2015;17(1):1–19.
2. Köhler B, Born S, Van Pelt RFP, et al. A survey of cardiac 4D PC-MRI data processing. Comput Graph Forum. 2017;36(6):5–35.
3. Song SM, Napel S, Glover GH, et al. Noise reduction in three-dimensional phase-contrast MR velocity measurements. J Magn Reson Imaging. 1993;3(4):587–96.
4. Busch J, Giese D, Wissmann L, et al. Reconstruction of divergence-free velocity fields from cine 3D phase-contrast flow measurements. J Magn Reson Imaging. 2013;69(1):200–10.
5. Paige CC, Saunders MA. LSQR: An algorithm for sparse linear equations and sparse least squares. ACM Trans Math Softw. 1982;8(1):43–71.
6. Ong F, Uecker M, Tariq U, et al. Robust 4D flow denoising using divergence-free wavelet transform. J Magn Reson Imaging. 2015;73(2):828–42.
7. Loecher M, Schrauben E, Johnson KM, et al. Phase unwrapping in 4D MR flow with a 4D single-step Laplacian algorithm. J Magn Reson Imaging. 2015;43(4):833–42.
8. Antiga L, Iordache EB, Remuzzi A. Computational geometry for patient-specific reconstruction and meshing of blood vessels from MR and CT angiography. IEEE Trans Med Imaging. 2003;22(5):674–84.
9. Donoho DL, Johnstone IM. Adapting to unknown smoothness via wavelet shrinkage. J Am Stat Assoc. 1995;90(432):1200–24.

Employing Spatial Indexing for Flexibility and Scalability in Brain Biopsy Planning

Lukas Pezenka[1], Stefan Wolfsberger[2], Katja Bühler[1]

[1]VRVis Center for Virtual Reality and Visualization, 1220 Vienna, Austria
[2]Medical University of Vienna, 1090 Vienna, Austria
pezenka@vrvis.at

Abstract. Planning of deep brain tumor biopsy is a time intensive task and the result highly dependent on tumor position and patient individual anatomy. The decision on the best needle trajectory is generally based on expert knowledge on optimal entry points and angles as well as trajectory length and rigid rules in respect to avoidance of and safety margins to risk structures. The increasing availability of more detailed data on brain anatomy further increases the complexity of the planning task. However, current computer supported planning systems generally work with fixed rules and a limited set of structures at risk. We propose BrainXPlore, a visual analytics based planning tool allowing neurosurgeon to interactively explore and refine the space of possible trajectories in the context of different quality measures and to define custom rules. To ensure interactivity and performance even for a high number of anatomical structures, we employ a spatial index allowing to access distance information for trajectories in real time. We evaluated BrainXPlore on real brain biopsy planning tasks and conclude that our system can decrease the time needed for biopsy planning and aid novice users in their decision-making process.

1 Introduction

A brain tumor biopsy is a neurosurgical intervention extracting a sample of tumor tissue using a navigation systems and a tracked biopsy needle. In general, a needle trajectory is defined by an entry point in the skull and a target point/region on or inside the tumor.To prevent severe damage to the patient, vital tissues must be avoided by the trajectory and hence, protected from damage caused by the needle. Several systems have been proposed to plan and visualize needle trajectories [1, 2, 3, 4, 5]. While some aspects of the planning process are partially solved by previously proposed systems, other issues, namely scalability and flexibility, remain unaddressed. Recent advances in high resolution brain imaging will create more and more detailed brain atlases [6]. Orringer et al. [7] point out that advances in MRI imaging have enabled the possibility of incorporating functional data (fMRI) into the neuro-navigational datasets. Thus, the number of structures and functional areas that can be considered for optimal needle trajectories is constantly increasing. To the best of our knowledge, existing systems with acceptable performance are technically restricted to a limited number of structures [1, 2, 5] and do not provide the possibility of flexible definition of rules for trajectory filtering.

In this paper we propose BRAINXPLORE, an interactive planning system to support neurosurgeons in decision finding for optimal needle trajectories. BRAINXPLORE allows a flexible definition of custom rules to optimally support the planning process. An initial set of automatically computed candidate trajectories can be incrementally and interactively refined until an optimum has been found. We solve the issue of scalability by using an out-of-core spatial index as intermediate data structure for fast distance computation of spatial objects [8]. This component allows us, in contrast to existing solutions, to access distance information on a very high number of structures at risk (SAR) and to apply changing custom distance rules to a large number of structures and trajectories in reasonable time.

2   Concept and implementation

Major steps for planning a brain biopsy can be summarized as follows: 1) Data pre-processing and segmentation, 2) target point definition, 3) entry point or region definition, 4) trajectory generation, 5) trajectory inspection and filtering, 6) trajectory refinement, and 7) final decision. Steps 5 and 6 can be repeated iteratively, until a suitable candidate trajectory has been found. BrainXplore supports all steps despite the data pre-processing and segmentation step. In our study, segmentation of cortical and subcortical regions was performed using FreeSurfer [9]. The tumor was manually segmented, blood vessels were semi-automatically segmented with MeVisLab, using the built-in vesselness module. While most existing brain biopsy and DBS planning systems [1, 2, 4] use surface meshes for trajectory planning presenting an additional pre-processing step and a potential loss of precision, BRAINXPLORE works directly on original binary segmentation masks. We have implemented our system using MeVisLab. Custom functionality was implemented in Python, the interactive Visual Analytics views were implemented using Matplotlib.

A single needle trajectory is defined by an entry point and the target point in a user defined target region. The minimal distance of a trajectory to the SAR included into the planning process defines a trajectory's risk signature (RS). Potential entry points are generated by creating a set of sampling points on the skull surface. To prevent trajectories that would pass through the eyes, ears or mouth to be created, the number of crossed bone layers is counted, similar to the approach presented by Beyer et al. [10]. Trajectories that do not cross exactly one layer are discarded. For all remaining trajectories defined by entry-target point couples, RS are computed using a spatial indexing scheme [8] providing fast access to point-object distances/intersection. When building the spatial index, all distances above a feasible threshold are discarded. In this way, only the structures in close proximity to a queried trajectory are considered and a higher number of structures has only limited impact on computation times. The index is out-of-core, i.e. not limited by available CPU or GPU RAM and can in principle store spatial information for an unlimited number of SAR at arbitrary resolution.

Rules work similar as presented by Essert et al. [2]. Trajectories resulting from the above described sampling process are filtered with respect to a set of hard rules, defining mandatory quality criteria for candidate trajectories, like a safety distance to vessels. Trajectories that do not satisfy these hard rules are discarded. Hard rules can be defined in the user interface by setting slider controls to the desired values. The quality Q of acceptable trajectories is an aggregated cost function and calculated as described in Eq. 1. Soft rules $R_{r_1 \ldots r_n}, r_i \in [0,1]$ describe either the spatial relationship between the trajectory and a structure at risk (e.g., the minimal distances to the vascular and ventricular system, overlap with the tumor) or a geometric property of the trajectory (trajectory length and insertion angle at the skull). In order to use them in a unified quality measure, values are normalized by considering the respective data range. A value of 1 is considered optimal quality, e.g., the shortest path or largest safety margin above a pre-defined threshold. On the contrary, 0 is considered the worst quality with respect to the given rule. Each rule r_i has an associated weight $w_i^{>0}$ chosen by the expert. Candidate trajectory bundles related to a single entry point but different target points are further filtered. Only the best trajectory from each bundle is kept. This reduction of a bundle to a singular best reference path is similar to the work presented by Mastmeyer et al. [11].

$$Q = \sum_{i=1}^{n} r_i * w_i, \quad w_i \in \mathbb{R}_{>0} \tag{1}$$

BrainXplore's interactive user interface consists of four parts, as illustrated in Fig. 1. The Main View (Fig. 1(a)) presents potential trajectories in their spatial anatomical context and risk structures, color coded with respect to their quality. The Main View allows the user to interactively explore the scene and to pick specific trajectories for further investigation. Green markers denote the best entry points, red show the worst entry points and shades of yellow and orange represent entry points of medium quality. Existing trajectories can be interactively refined by either moving the entry point, target point, or both. The spatial index is queried and provides distance information on the altered trajectory in real time. A Supporting 3D View (Fig. 1(b)) offers further contextual information, i.e., the trajectories proximity to vessels or other SAR. The Augmented Slice View shows slices through the volume perpendicular to the needle trajectory and highlights SAR. Finally, the Visual Analytics View (Fig. 1(c)) presents quantitative and qualitative information of the risk structure of either a single trajectory or all available trajectories. In this view, the neurosurgeon can interactively explore and filter the current set of trajectories. Parallel coordinates (PC) show quantitative trajectory attributes (Fig. 1). Brushing in this view filters selected trajectories and allows the neurosurgeon to find the best trajectory in an iterative manner. A histogram view illustrates the distribution of trajectory attributes and conveys a heuristic how subsequent filtering operations will impact the search space. Trajectories are binned with regards to the distance to SAR. Bins of trajectories can be either included for further consideration or filtered. A scatterplot view allows the neurosurgeon to select trajectories in a coordinate system defined by two user-defined attributes (e.g., trajectory length vs minimal distance to nearest vessel). Finally, a RS view visualizes the trajectory quality and serves the purpose of comparing individual trajectories.

Both hard and soft rules can be refined and re-evaluated expanded at runtime. A small number of rules (e.g., only minimal distances to vessels and ventricles) can be used as a starting point and iteratively increases (by e.g., distances to sulci, maximum path length). In the case of hard rules, the introduction of new rules will filter the candidate trajectories and yield increasingly better results. Refining soft rules will not filter the result, but result in a different color coding. In our case study, four soft rules were defined for trajectory quality evaluation: 1) maximization of distances to vessels, 2) maximization of distances to cortical sulci, 3) maximization of distances to the left lateral ventricle, and 4) minimization of trajectory length.

3   Results

We evaluated the usefulness of our application based on a real dataset from a past biopsy. In cooperation with our domain expert, we used BRAINXPLORE to produce a biopsy trajectory for the dataset and evaluated the quality of the result. 178 SAR were segmented, 15 target points were defined on the tumor. Initial sampling and trajectory generation took approximately 6 minutes and yielded 89376 potential entry points. 17 hard rules regarding minimal distances to SAR and maximal path length constraints were defined. Hard rule application took approximately 0.6 seconds and reduced the number of trajectories by 93% to

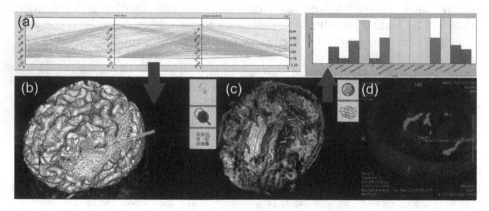

Fig. 1. Components of the user interface. (a) The Visual Analytics view offers color coded parallel coordinates for trajectory filtering and represents single trajectories in different formats such as bar charts indicating their RS. (b) Main View. (c) Supporting 3D View. (d) Augmented Slice View.

6080. Soft rule evaluation for those trajectories took approximately 0.7 seconds and identified the best candidate.

Fig. 2(a) presents the RS of the generated trajectory. Red bars indicate low distances, i.e., high risk. Green bars indicate high distance, i.e., a safe trajectory. We have reconstructed the reference trajectory from the post-operation MRI and evaluated it using our system. The corresponding RS is presented in Fig. 2(b). As can be seen, the reference trajectory exhibits a higher distance to the cortical sulci and the pyramid tract than the solution computed by our system. On the other side, distances towards the vessels and the left lateral ventricle are higher in our solution.

4   Discussion

BRAINXPLORE presents a brain biopsy planning framework that allows interactive exploration and adaptation of possible needle trajectories as well as customized rule definition and fast re-evaluation of trajectories due to an optimized access to spatial distance information for registered SAR.

A unique feature of BRAINXPLORE is the possibility to include an very high number of structures at arbitrary resolution. Out-of-core spatial indexing allows our system to run on consumer-grade hardware and even laptops with no GPU support and limited memory while maintaining reasonable performance and interactivity. We have built our test case on 178 different SAR. To the best of our knowledge, no other system has been shown to be able to consider such a high number. Another distinguishing feature of BRAINXPLORE is the possibility to define custom rules for the evaluation of trajectory qualities. Zombori et al. [1] employ a risk metric that calculates a trajectory's total risk as a function of the insertion angle, angle and the distance towards the nearest structure. All structures are considered to be of equal importance. In contrast, BRAINXPLORE allows the neurosurgeon to assign different safety margins and weights to different structures. We have implemented interaction techniques based on established Visual Analytics techniques. All potential trajectories are presented to the neurosurgeon in an intuitive manner that supports interaction techniques such as picking and brushing. This allows the neurosurgeon to select suitable trajectory candidates in a very efficient manner and at each point, gives an estimate of how subsequent filtering operations will impact the search space.

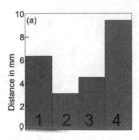 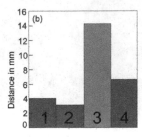

Fig. 2. (a) Risk Signature for resulting trajectory. (b) Risk Signature for reference trajectory. All specified quality criteria have been met. Shown from left to right are the distances to: 1) Vascular system, 2) cortical sulci 3) pyramid tract, and 4) the left lateral ventricle.

Acknowledgement. This work was enabled by the Competence Centre VRVis. VRVis is funded by BMVIT, BMWFW, Styria, SFG and Vienna Business Agency in the scope of COMET - Competence Centers for Excellent Technologies (854174) which is managed by FFG. We thank MeVisLab for providing an extended evaluation license for the implementation of our project.

References

1. Zombori G, Rodionov R, Nowell M, et al. A computer assisted planning system for the placement of sEEG electrodes in the treatment of epilepsy. Proc IPCAI. 2014; p. 118–127.
2. Essert C, Haegelen C, Jannin P. Automatic computation of electrodes trajectory for deep brain stimulation. Proc MIAR. 2010; p. 149–158.
3. Zelmann R, Bériault S, Mok K, et al. Automatic optimization of depth electrode trajectory planning. In: Workshop on Clinical Image-Based Procedures. Springer; 2013. p. 99–107.
4. Gao C, Chen L, Hou B, et al. Precise and semi-automatic puncture trajectory planning in craniofacial surgery: A prototype study. Proc BMEI. 2014; p. 617–622.
5. Herghelegiu P, Manta V, Perin R, et al. Biopsy planner: visual analysis for needle pathway planning in deep seated brain tumor biopsy. Comput Graph Forum. 2012;31(3):1085–1094. Presented at EuroVis 2012.
6. Amunts K. Human Brain Project: Aufbau eines multimodalen Gehirnatlas. Dtsch Arztebl Int. 2017;114(37):[26].
7. Orringer DA, Golby A, Jolesz F. Neuronavigation in the surgical management of brain tumors: current and future trends. Exp Rev Med Dev. 2012;9(5):491–500.
8. Bruckner S, Šoltészová V, Gröller E, et al. BrainGazer: visual queries for neurobiology research. IEEE Trans Vis Comput Graph. 2009 Nov;15(6):1497–1504.
9. Reuter M, Schmansky NJ, Rosas HD, et al. Within-Subject template estimation for unbiased longitudinal image analysis. NeuroImage. 2012;61(4):1402–1418.
10. Beyer J, Hadwiger M, Wolfsberger S, et al. High-Quality multimodal volume rendering for preoperative planning of neurosurgical interventions. Trans Vis Comput Graph. 2007;13(6):1696–1703.
11. Mastmeyer A, Fortmeier D, Handels H. Evaluation of direct haptic 4D volume rendering of partially segmented data for liver puncture simulation. Sci Report. 2017;7(1):671.

Measuring Finger Lengths from 2D Palm Scans

Alexander Twrdik[1], Ulf-Dietrich Braumann[2,3], Franziska Abicht[1],
Wieland Kiess[1,4], Toralf Kirsten[1]

[1]LIFE Research Center for Civilization Diseases, University of Leipzig
[2]Faculty of Electrical Engineering and Information Technology, HTWK Leipzig
[3]Fraunhofer Institute for Cell Therapy and Immunology, Leipzig
[4]Hospital for Children and Adolescence, University of Leipzig
atwrdik@life.uni-leipzig.de

Abstract. A goal of Life Child is to study the development of children
and adolescents. The growth of fingers and other palm compartments
in this age group has been received little attraction so far. Usually,
finger lengths are measured manually even when 2D palm images have
been produced. This is often cumbersome for very large studies. In this
paper, we introduce an approach to automatically segment palm and
finger compartments of scanned 2D palm scans. The scans were taken by
a single document scanner with the goal to measure finger lengths. Our
algorithms are rotation invariant, automatically recognize hand objects
in images using a skin color model, determine the finger segments for
that the length from the fingertip to the crease is derived. We outline
steps of the image processing pipeline and show first evaluation results.

1 Introduction

The goal of epidemiological studies and medical surveys is to review the current
state and to recognize trends of diseases but also to discover new aspects in the
human development, both using a population of interest, e.g., the population of
a city or country. LIFE Child [1] is an epidemiological study in the described
context. The goal of LIFE Child is to determine the development of children
and adolescents from the beginning (prenatal phase in pregnancy) to the age of
18. Each study participant is determined by multiple examinations including
interviews, questionnaires, physical examinations and samplings (e.g., blood,
urine, etc.). In one examination, the hands of the participants are scanned in
order to survey the geometry of hand compartments such as fingers and the
palm of the hand. The goal is twofold. On the one hand, we aim to relate such
measures to diseases and other participant phenotypes (properties) in a way to
use finger lengths as a predictor candidate; see for example [2, 3]. On the other
hand, we tend to derive normative data about the development of fingers (e.g.,
finger lengths) during childhood and adolescent years.

From image processing perspective, hand measuring is often used in security
related applications, e.g., [4, 5], taking geometrical and biometrical properties
into account. In medical studies, hand measuring often requires image processing

151

when hand compartments including fingers need to be automatically determined. Available segementation approaches rely on geometrical properties of hand objects [6, 7] whereas others additionally leverage the object's color information, e.g., [8, 9], making the process more accurate. We reused and adpated some of these approaches to automatically segment hand compartments and to determine finger lengths of children and adolescents in LIFE Child.

2   Materials and methods

All data capturing processes according to scanning hands take place in the LIFE Child ambulance. The process is standardized and described by a standard operating procedure. The scan device is an office combi print and scan system TA DCC 2725. Both hands of a study participant are scanned at once; hands are completely scanned in a way that the crease between arm and hand is always in the scanned image. Both hands lie flat on the scanner glass, are ensured to be clearly separated from each other and the scanner top cover is closed during the scan process. The scanner generates a PDF file including the image (20cm x 20cm, 300 DPI resolution). The scan image is extracted from the PDF file and stored into a JPEG file without adding additional loss using the publicly available poppler utilities (pdfimages, version 0.41).

The process of measuring finger lengths consists of 5 steps. Figure 1 shows a high-level overview of the process together with exemplified input and output. The goal of the first step is to segment the image and to detect hand objects. We assume that two hands are scanned of every study participant. Hence, the algorithm tries to detect the two largest objects. The assumption for detecting hand objects is that the skin color of the palmar hand side is similar for most humans, even for humans of different ethnicities. We adopted the approach for detecting skin color as described by [10] using a color model in the YC_bC_r color space. In this way, we firstly randomly selected a sample set of 20 images. Subsequently, several sample areas showing human skin were manually extracted from these images and collected in a single image file. Finally, after converting the file from RGB to the YC_bC_r color space the histogram analysis focusing on C_b and C_r channels showing that human skin color of the palmar hand side can be described within the bounds: $97 \leq C_b \leq 123$ and $135 \leq C_r \leq 170$.

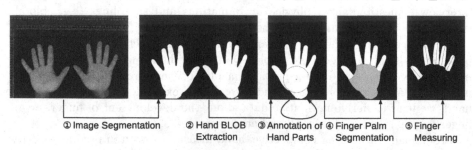

① Image Segmentation   ② Hand BLOB Extraction   ③ Annotation of Hand Parts   ④ Finger Palm Segmentation   ⑤ Finger Measuring

Fig. 1. Overview of the Finger Segmentation and Measurement Process.

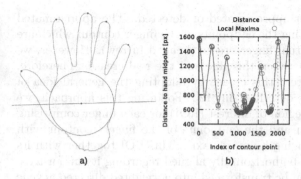

Distance ———
Local Maxima ○

Fig. 2. Fingertip detection.

a) b)

By applying a pixel-based segmentation using these bounds as thresholds skin colored objects within the scan image can be detected resulting in a binary mask. The two largest contiguous parts that could be detected are assumed to be the left and right hand of the study participant. We also experienced artifacts within the binary mask (i.e. gaps), in particular, when the palm or fingers are stained (e.g., from using a pen) or when the skin contains a liver spot. To compensate for these artifacts the gaps in the mask can be removed using the outer object contour as a closed polygon chain and marking every point inside the polygon as skin color.

In the second step, we extract the recognized hand objects from the image and manage them in separate binary images. The goal of step three is to annotate the result images of the previous step with information required by subsequent steps. Firstly, we calculate the location of each finger valley as described by [11]. We adjusted this approach by adding an angle constraint in a way that the angle between the two vectors formed by a possible valley location and its two surrounding neighbouring convex hull points has to be less than 100°. This describes the limits a human is easily able to achieve regarding the spreading of his fingers while simultaneoulsy suppressing erroneous detection of finger valleys in the region around the wrist. This is followed by the detection of fingertip locations using an adjusted version of the approach described by [9] allowing us to use it on hand shaped objects including the forearm as a visible part. In this case, all possible fingertip locations have to be filtered in a way that only those locations are kept laying on the same side of the hand as the fingers. The idea is to use a 2D-hyperplane separating the hand object into two sides; one side comprises all fingers whereas the other side contains none. The hyperplane is a straight perpendicular to a longitudinal axis of the hand with the hand's midpoint on the hyperplane (Fig. 2a). The vector of such a longitundinal axis is pointing from the hand's midpoint to the centroid of all four finger valley locations that have previously been calculated. Since this reference location is known to be on the same side as fingers, the side of the hand comprising the fingers can be detected.

The goal of step four is to segment a hand object to extract individual fingers as separate objects. A finger object itself can be described by its boundary (i.e. its contour and the crease visibly separating it from the palm). The contour can easily be calculated leveraging the information calculated in step three.

The finger crease can be either approximated or detected. The approximated crease is a straight line connecting the endpoints of the finger contour which are roughly located next to the actual finger crease (bended furrow). However, we experienced large differences between this line and the real crease. Therefore, we developed a method to detect this crease by adopting the general idea of the seam carving algorithm as described in [12]. Following this approach, we firstly calculate a rectangular region of interest (ROI) for each finger comprising its finger crease near the palm and the endpoints of the fingers contour with the approximated crease line being its major axis. This ROI together with its content is then transformed to be horizontally aligned regarding its major axis. This aligned sub-image can then be transformed into a weighted directed acyclic graph in which each pixel is a node. Edges (p_1, p_2) connect pixel p_1 at position (x, y) with pixels p_2 at positions $\{(x + 1, y + 1), (x + 1, y), (x + 1, y - 1)\}$. Each edge is associated with a weight taking the RGB-vectors of both corresponding pixels into account. Let $RGB(p_{x,y})$ be the RGB-vector associated with the pixel p at position (x, y) within the horizontally aligned sub-image. Then the weight W of an edge pointing from node $p_{a,b}$ to node $p_{c,d}$ is calculated as $W = \|RGB(p_{c,d})\| - \|RGB(p_{a,b})\|$. Using this graph, we search for the shortest path connecting endpoints of the left finger contour with those of the right contour. The created graph implies that the shortest path is along the darkest pixels within the ROI representing the finger crease which is always darker than its surroundings (this holds true if the fingers are spread). After decoding the nodes that are part of the path their associated pixel positions can be transformed back into the coordinate system of the original image.

Finally, in step five, we measure the length of each finger segment. In this way, we identify the centre of the finger crease (approximated or detected) which is connected to the fingertip of a particular finger using a straight line. The length of this line is a good measure for the finger length being measured in number of pixels.

3   Results

We got a data set for developing and testing the detection and measuring algorithms by the data usage proposal PV0292 of the LIFE Research Center for Civilization Diseases. The data set includes both, 5,177 images and finger lengths of the index and ring fingers of the left and right hand. These measurements correspond to the set of images, i.e., for each image a measurement is available, vice versa. Prior to the development of our solution the finger lengths were measured in a manual process using the software AutoMetric (version 2.2). This manual process was run by a single person of the LIFE Child staff.

We developed the algorithms using a sample of 50 images. We then applied the image processing pipeline to all received images and derived the finger lenghts of all fingers of the left and right hand according to each image. Next, we comparatively evaluate the automatically derived measurements of index and ring fingers according to manually measured finger lengths taking the full set of images into account. This way, we use the manually measured finger lengths as gold standard for evaluating our image processing pipeline. Figure 3 a)-d) show Bland-Altman plots for each finger (index, ring) on both hands comparing manually and automatically derived finger lengths. These plots show that measured finger lengths are very close for most individuals. Hence, taking the image processing pipeline we can reproduce the manually measured finger lengths in most cases. There are few outliers where the image processing pipeline generates a much larger (lower) value than manually measured. Most outliers are generated when the algorithm detects the finger crease on the wrong position. In these cases, the contour is very fringed influencing selecting start and end points of the shortest path search in the graph. This affects the centroid detection of the finger crease and, finally, measuring the finger length.

4   Discussion

We designed and implemented an image processing pipeline that automatically derives finger lengths from 2D palm images. The images were produced in the LIFE Child study running in Leipzig. The evaluation shows that for most individuals the manually measured finger lengths can be reproduced by the image

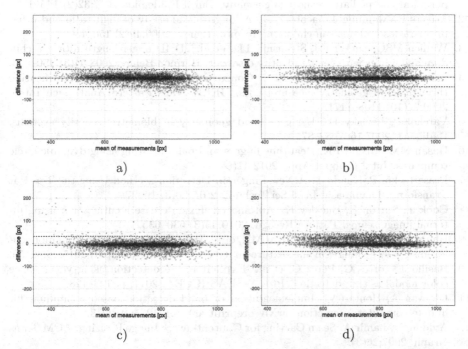

a)   b)

c)   d)

Fig. 3. Evaluation Results (Bland-Altman plots) for index fingers of the left a) and right hand c) and for the ring fingers of the left b) and right hand d). The upper and lower dashed line represent the boundary of the confidence interval with a confidence level of 95%.

processing pipeline. However, our evaluation assumes that all manually measured values are always correct and, thus, can be used as gold standard, i.e., the image processing results are only as good as the manually measured finger lengths. This is true for many individuals but we experienced images with curved fingers. We will improve our algorithms to recognize finger lengths of such "outliers" in future. Moreover, we will work on deriving the length of thumbs to capture lengths of all fingers. An important feature of our segmentation algorithms is that they are rotation invariant. Thus we can avoid to place hands of study participants in an aligned position resulting in a more complicated and error-prone scan process.

Acknowledgement. This publication is supported by LIFE - Leipzig Research Center for Civilization Diseases, University of Leipzig. LIFE is funded by means of the European Union, by the European Regional Development Fund (ERFD) and by the Free State of Saxony within the framework of the excellence initiative.

References

1. Poulain T, Baber R, Vogel M, et al. The life child study: a population-based perinatal and pediatric cohort in germany. Eur J Epidemiol. 2017;32(2):145–158.
2. Trivers R, Manning J, Jacobson A. A longitudinal study of digit ratio and other finger ratios in Jamaican children. Hormon Behav. 2006;49(2):150–156.
3. Wallien MSC, Zucker KJ, Steensma TD, et al. 2D:4D finger-length ratios in children and adults with gender identity disorder. Hormon Behav. 2008;54(3):450–454.
4. Sanchez-Reillo R, Sanchez-Avila C, Gonzalez-Marcos A. Biometric identification through hand geometry measurements. IEEE Trans Pattern Anal Mach Intell. 2000;22(10):1168–1171.
5. Varchol P, Levicky D. Using of hand geometry in biometric security systems. Radioeng. 2007;16(4):82–87.
6. Hasan MM, Mishra PK. Real time fingers and palm locating using dynamic circle templates. Int J Comput Appl. 2012;41(6).
7. Prasertsakul P, Kondo T. A New Fingertip Detection Method Using the Top-Hat Transform. Thammasat Int J Sci Technol. 2015;20(3):19–27.
8. Cook T, Sutton R, Buckley K. Automated flexion crease identification using internal image seams. Pattern Recogn. 2010;43(3):630–635.
9. Bhuyan MK, MacDorman KF, Kar MK, et al. Hand pose recognition from monocular images by geometrical and texture analysis. J Vis Lang Comput. 2015;28:39–55.
10. Basilio J, Torres G, Pérez G, et al. Explicit image detection using ycbcr space color model as skin detection. Proc WSEAS ICCEA. 2011; p. 123–128.
11. Dhawan A, Honrao V. Implementation of hand detection based techniques for human computer interaction. arXiv preprint arXiv:13127560. 2013.
12. Avidan S, Shamir A. Seam Carving for Content-aware Image Resizing. ACM Trans Graph. 2007;26(3).

Towards Analysis of Mental Stress Using Thermal Infrared Tomography

Marcin Kopaczka, Thomas Jantos, Dorit Merhof

Institute of Imaging and Computer Vision, RWTH Aachen University, Germany
marcin.kopaczka@lfb.rwth-aachen.de

Abstract. A number of publications has focused on detecting and measuring mental stress using infrared tomography as it is a noninvasive and convenient monitoring method. Several potential facial regions of interest such as forehead, nose and the upper lip in which stress may potentially be detectable have been identified in previous contributions. However, these publications are not comparable since they all rely on different approaches regarding both experiment design (stressor, ground truth/reference measurements) as well as evaluation methodology such as either average temperature monitoring or advanced image processing methods. We therefore focus on two aspects: Designing an experiment that allows a reliable induction of mental stress and measuring temperature changes in all aforementioned regions as well as on introducing and evaluating a GLCM-based method for quantitative analysis of the recorded image data. We show that signals extracted from the upper lip region correspond well with high stress levels, while no correspondence can be shown for the other regions. The suggested GLCM-based method is shown to be more specific towards stress response than established measurements based on average region temperature.

1 Introduction

Answering sociological or socio-medical questions regarding stress in humans requires reliable measuring methods for assessing mental or social stress. Workpace stress and scientific analysis of stressful social situations are examples of scientific research fields where stress measurements are desirable. Established methods use contact-based measurements such as electrocardiography (ECG) [1], electroencephalography (EEG) [2] or skin resistance measurements (galvanic skin response, GSR) [3] to assess stress levels live. When live measurement is not required or available and the amount of stress a person has experienced during the last 30 minutes provides sufficient information, then measuring salivary cortisol levels is considered as most reliable stress indicator [4]. Even with these methods available, human stress researchers are constantly searching for a noninvasive and contactless stress measurement method. Thermal infrared imaging has been identified as a potential novel approach due to the supposed correlation between parameters such as skin temperature or transpiration and stress.

In our work, we first provide a review of several previous attempts of thermal infrared stress monitoring together with the respective methodology used. We then describe the design of our own stress invoking procedure and perform data analysis on different ROIs using both established and novel methods.

2   Previous work

In addition to the traditional methods described above, thermal reaction as immediate stress response has been investigated by several authors utilizing different methods used to invoke stress as well different evaluation methodology:

- Puri et al. [5] used the Stroop Color Word Conflict[1] method to inflict stress on 12 subjects. The thermal response was recorded and a region of interest on the forehead was analyzed to gain stress information. The reference values for the experiment were gained by measuring oxygen uptake, assuming that oxygen uptake is correlated with stress. A correlation between forehead temperature and oxygen uptake was reported.
- Or and Duffy [6] combine a driving simulator with arithmetic problem solving to invoke stress. 30 subjects were tested and a correlation of self-reported stress and nasal temperature was analyzed. Temperature changes of the nose were found to correlate with stress.
- Merla and Romani [7] used a modified Stroop test as stressor and recorded several ROIs such as forehead and upper lip. Reference measurements were acquired by measuring GSR and heart rate. The authors found a correlation between reference measurements and increased transpiration in the upper lip region.
- Pavlidis et al. [8] analyze the impact of a challenging manual task. Expert and novice surgeons were instructed to perform simulated laparoscopic surgery and the transpiration in the upper lip region was evaluated using wavelet analysis. The study revealed that transpiration in this region was much stronger in the novice group than in the expert group, indicating a correlation between stress and thermal response.

3   Materials and methods

In this section, we motivate our experiment design and give detailed information on the image processing methods applied to the data. All recordings were performed using an Infratec HD820 camera with a spatial resolution of 1024 x 768 pixels and a thermal resolution of 0.03K.

3.1   Experiment design

The goal of our experiment was to invoke stress reliably. Additionally, the stress perceived by the participants should be as high as possible. Preliminary ex-

---

[1] In this method, a word describing a color is shown in a different color, for example the word 'red' is shown in green. The participant is asked to name the actual color (green) instead of reading the word. This conflict is assumed to induce mental stress.

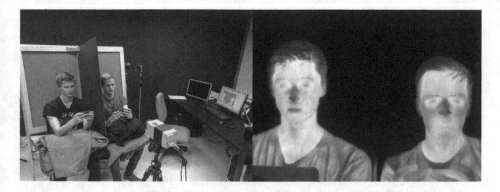

Fig. 1. Experimental setup. Left: Photograph of the setting with both participants recorded by the thermal camera against a neutral background. Right: actual infrared frame from the recording.

periments performed at our lab using the Stroop color word test and different mathematical challenges had shown that none of the methods was stressing the subjects in a sufficient manner. Therefore, combinations of several tests have been evaluated. We picked the test routine that allowed best stress induction according to self-reports. This is the final routine:

1. There were two new participants in each run. Both participants had to sit down in front of our thermal camera at a distance of about 1m. They were put against a thermally neutral backdrop, separated by a barrier and given cell phones running a software for the Stroop color word conflict that had been designed for this study. Both participants were wearing headphones and were allowed to listen to comforting music of their own choice. This allowed the study coordinator to communicate with one of the participants without disturbing the other. Both participants were asked to minimize their head movement if possible in order to allow for better image analysis. Fig. 1 shows the actual setup.
2. The experiment was described in detail to the participants, giving them the chance to ask questions. This time frame of about 10 minutes was also used to allow the subjects to adjust to the room's temperature.
3. (0:00 - 2:00) The participants were asked to put on their headphones and recording was started. No stressor was put on the participants for the first two minutes, this part of the recording was the baseline.
4. (2:00 - 3:30) After two minutes, both participants were given a signal to start the Stroop test. Stress response was recorded.
5. (3:30 - 4:00) After three and a half minutes, one randomly picked participant received a signal from the study coordinator to remove their headphones. The coordinator explained to the person that he/she will be asked to perform an additional task: On top of continuing with the Stroop test, the person was asked to perform basic arithmetic operations by adding or subtracting two two-digit numbers. None of the participants had been informed about

this part of the experiment beforehand. The second participant remained fully unaware of this additional task, continuing the Stroop test.

6. (4:00 - 6:00) Four minutes after the recording had been started the additional stress test was started for the selected participant. The study coordinator asked the person arithmetical questions, giving five seconds to respond. Wrong answers resulted in the same question being asked a second time, if a question was not answered within five seconds then the participant was told to answer faster and given a new question. Both strategies aimed at increasing the participant's stress.

7. (6:00 - 10:00) After six minutes, the stress test period for both participants ended. Both were asked to put down the phones and to remain still for four additional minutes, allowing to record relaxation effects.

Recording two subjects simultaneously made it possible to use the person that had to perform only one task as reference and comparing them to the person that was given the additional task. This was necessary as no ground truth measurement using one of the established methods had been performed. Additionally, recording both participants under identical conditions allowed to minimize recording-related bias.

3.2   Image processing methods

Even with the participants being asked to minimize head movement, minimal movement still needed to be corrected first. To this end, a tracker based on thermal active appearance models [9] was used. Subsequently, all ROIs that had been used in at least one of the previous publications were analyzed: Forehead, nose tip and upper lip region. The ROIs were defined using landmarks detected by the tracker. ROI analysis itself was performed using two methods: First, we computed each ROI's average temperature as this was the most commonly used analysis method used in literature. Additionally, we computed the gray-level-co-occurence-matrix (GLCM) for each ROI and derived the values for contrast, correlation and energy as defined in standard literature and also used in [10] for emotion detectionin thermal infrared images.

4   Experiments and results

The experiment described above was performed ten times with twenty different participants over the course of several days. AAM tracking, ROI extraction and analysis were performed as described. In the analysis, we compare the temperature curves of the double-stressed participants with their corresponding reference counterparts.

Analysis was performed by computing average ROI temperature and comparing both groups qualitatively. Analysis revealed no qualitative differences between the temperature values for both groups for the forehead and nose tip region. A small difference in the temperature curves can be seen in the upper lip region, where the peaks show higher variance for the simultaneous Stroop part and especially the double-stressed time frame. The curves for the upper lip region analysis are shown in Fig. 2.

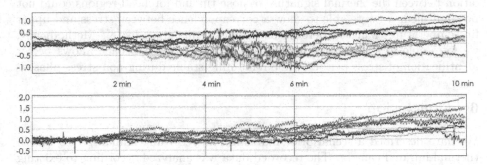

Fig. 2. Average temperature change in °C in the upper lip region of stressed (top) and non-stressed participants (bottom) over time. Same colors belong to corresponding pairs.

Similarly, GLCM analysis of the nose tip and forehead regions returned no visible differences between both groups. However, the analysis of the upper lip region using the contrast measure showed a strong difference between both groups exclusively during the double-stressed period. While only minimal contrast changes were visible in the other time ranges, a strong contrast increase can be seen in most of the recordings. Also, the recordings show a highly similar relaxation behavior with the contrast gradually returning to normal levels over less than 30 seconds (Fig. 3).

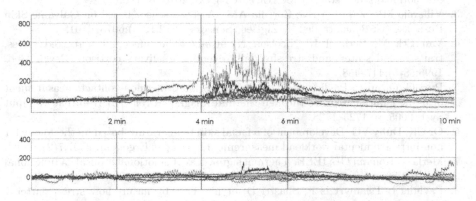

Fig. 3. GLCM contrast curve of the upper lip region of stressed (top) and non-stressed participants (bottom). Same colors belong to corresponding subject pairs.

5   Discussion

Our experiments show a partial confirmation of existing literature. While correlation between the thermal signature of nose tip and forehead regions could not be confirmed, we were able to show a correspondence between stress and upper lip temperature changes, thereby confirming results given by [8]. Methodically, we were able to show that our proposed GLCM-based approach allows better identification of stress periods while remaining stable during non-stress phases.

6   Conclusion

We have described a scenario for inducing and recording human stress with a thermal infrared camera. The recorded data was analyzed according to existing literature and using a GLCM-based method. Results show that the upper lip region shows temperature patterns that are temporarily linked to invoked stress. The changes can be visualized using established average temperature monitoring and show even higher distinctness when using the new GLCM approach.

References

1. Karthikeyan P, Murugappan M, Yaacob S. ECG signal denoising using wavelet thresholding techniques in human stress assessment. Int J Electric Eng Inform. 2012;4(2):306.
2. Hosseini SA, Khalilzadeh MA; IEEE. Emotional stress recognition system using EEG and psychophysiological signals: Using new labelling process of EEG signals in emotional stress state. Proc IEEE ICBECS. 2010; p. 1–6.
3. Villarejo MV, Zapirain BG, Zorrilla AM. A stress sensor based on Galvanic Skin Response (GSR) controlled by ZigBee. Sensors. 2012;12(5):6075–6101.
4. Van Eck M, Berkhof H, Nicolson N, et al. The effects of perceived stress, traits, mood states, and stressful daily events on salivary cortisol. Psych Med. 1996;58(5):447–458.
5. Puri C, Olson L, Pavlidis I, et al.; ACM. StressCam: non-contact measurement of users' emotional states through thermal imaging. Proc CHI Hum Fac Comput Syst. 2005; p. 1725–1728.
6. Or CK, Duffy VG. Development of a facial skin temperature-based methodology for non-intrusive mental workload measurement. Occupat Ergonom. 2007;7(2):83–94.
7. Merla A, Romani GL; IEEE. Thermal signatures of emotional arousal: a functional infrared imaging study. Proc IEEE EMBS. 2007; p. 247–249.
8. Pavlidis I, Tsiamyrtzis P, Shastri D, et al. Fast by nature-how stress patterns define human experience and performance in dexterous tasks. Sci Report. 2012;2.
9. Kopaczka M, Acar K, Merhof D. Robust Facial Landmark Detection and Face Tracking in Thermal Infrared Images using Active Appearance Models. Proc VISIGRAPP. 2016; p. 150–158.
10. Latif M, Sidek SN, Rusli N, et al. Emotion detection from thermal facial imprint based on GLCM features. ARPN J Eng Appl Sci. 2016;11(1):345–350.

Preliminary Study Investigating Brain Shift Compensation using 3D CBCT Cerebral Vascular Images

Siming Bayer[1], Roman Schaffert[1], Nishant Ravikumar[1], Andreas Maier[1], Xiaodong Tong[2], Hu Wang[2], Martin Ostermeier[3], Rebecca Fahrig[3]

[1]Pattern Recognition Lab, FAU Erlangen-Nuremberg, Germany
[2]Tianjin Huanhu Hospital, Tianjin, China
[3]Siemens Healthcare GmbH, Forchheim, Germany
siming.bayer@fau.de

Abstract. During a neurosurgical procedure, the exposed brain undergoes an elastic deformation caused by numerous factors. This deformation, also known as brain shift, greatly affects the accuracy of neuronavigation systems. Non-rigid registration methods based on point matching algorithms are frequently used to compensate for intraoperative brain shift, especially when anatomical structures such as cerebral vascular tree are available. In this work, we introduce a pipeline to compensate for the volumetric brain deformation with Cone Beam CT (CBCT) image data. Point matching algorithms are combined with Spline-based transforms for this purpose. The initial result of different combination is evaluated with synthetical image data.

1 Introduction

Image guided navigation systems (IGNS) have become an essential part of neurosurgical procedures due to their ability to maximize the extent of tumor resection and minimize surgical trauma. However, the accuracy of image guided neurosurgery is greatly affected by the so-called brain shift phenomenon. This time dependent elastic deformation of brain tissue during surgery is not recovered by conventional navigation systems, as they typically assume rigid behavior of the head and its contents [1]. Without any intraoperative image update procedure, the anatomical information captured by preoperative MRI is no longer useful for surgical guidance as it does not account for the induced soft tissue deformation. Hence, updating the preoperative image data based on intraoperative images is a major challenge in image guided neurosurgery. Different intraoperative modalities such as MR, Ultrasound, Laser Range Image and Stereo Vision are used to update the preoprative image [2]. In this work, we introduce a new pipeline to compensate intraoperative brain shift by using 3D vascular tree captured with cone beam CT (CBCT). Generally, we use the bifurcations on the vascular tree geometries as anatomical landmarks to calculate a sparse displacement field, which is transformed to a dense displacement field reflecting the

163

deformation between preoperative brain image and its intraoperative state. We implemented state-of-the-art point matching algorithms [3, 4] and spline-based transformations [5, 6] in the context of brain shift compensation.

2   Materials and methods

The overall brain shift compensation pipeline presented in this study includes the following steps: extraction of anatomical landmarks from the 3D vascular image, use point set registration to identify homologous points, and finally, interpolate the sparse displacement field on to a dense grid and updating the undeformed (preoperative) image using the estimated deformation field. The proposed method is evaluated using synthetic CBCT data. An elastic deformation is introduced to the prefrontal part of our digital phantom in the way described in [7]. Since the clinical data is not free of noise, the landmarks selected as described in section 2.1 contains outliers. Thus, we added 20% random outliers to the selected landmarks to evaluate the robustness of the methods.

2.1   Feature extraction

The bifurcation points on the vessel tree were segmented automatically with vesselness filter [8] and Otsu's method [9]. The centerline is extracted by using an octree data structure which examines the neighborhood of a pixel [10]. We use a 3x3x3 window centered at each voxel lying on the centerline to detect the bifurcation points. A bifurcation point is defined as the voxel which has more than two neighboring voxels on the centerline.

2.2   Point matching and spline based transformation

After the segmentation and feature extraction, the resulting two 3D point sets act as sparse anatomical landmarks on undeformed (pre-) and deformed (intraoperative) images. In order to find one-to-one correspondence between the two point sets and reduce the impact of noise and outliers, we investigated the Robust Point Matching (RPM) [3] and Coherent Point Drift (CPD) [4] for non-rigid registration. Robust Point Matching was formulated as a joint estimation of pose and correspondence using the softassign and deterministic annealing algorithm. The core idea is to optimize a fuzzy assignment least squares energy function which includes a smoothness term, an entropy term which controls the fuzziness and a regularization term that controls the proportion of points considered as outliers. In contrast to Iterative Closest Point (ICP) where the correspondence of two points is binary, softassign allows the correspondence of two points to be anywhere from zero to one. This enables fuzzy, partial matches between the source and target point sets. Coherent Point Drift was introduced as a probabilistic approach for both rigid and nonrigid point set registration. The authors consider the alignment of two point sets as a probability density estimation problem where

Table 1. Relative overlap rate of the complete brain tissue and region of interest (ROI) after using different point matching and interpolation techniques.

Scenario		Before	CPD-B	CPD-TPS	RPM-B	RPM-TPS
(1)	Full Brain	0.9178	0.9371	0.9376	*0.9532*	0.9272
(2)	ROI	0.8864	0.9316	0.9229	*0.9374*	0.9028
(3)	Full Brain (with outlier)	0.9178	0.8531	0.6622	0.8523	0.6494
(4)	ROI (with outlier)	0.8864	0.8793	0.8171	*0.9230*	0.8248

the source point set represents the GMM centroids and the target point set represents the data points [4]. Two point sets are registered by estimating a set of transformation and model parameters that maximize the posterior probability of target point set. In order to preserve the topology of the shape being registered, the GMM centroids are forced to move coherently. For the nonrigid point matching, a displacement regularization term based on the motion coherent theory [11] is incorporated into the cost function that is optimized (Matlab implementation available at https://sites.google.com/site/myronenko/research/cpd). Thin Plate Spline transformation [5] belongs to the family of Radial Basis Function and interpolates n-dimensional scattered data to continuous space. The concept of Thin Plate Splines is based on the theory of deformation of thin elastic plates, where the bending forces are orthogonal to the surface. For each control point (source point), the distance to all points on the homologous point set (target point set) is calculated. The weighted sum of the distances is used to formulate the TPS at each point, which implies a control point, which is far away from a certain point, still has influence on the position of this point. Another popular choice to interpolate the deformation between control points is to use B-spline. In context of medical image registration, this approach was first proposed in [6]. In order to estimate an accurate and smooth dense displacement field based on the control points, we used the multi-resolution approach provided in [6]. B-splines are locally controlled, which means the position of a certain control point only affects the transformation of the points in its neighborhood.

3   Results

Four approaches to brain shift compensation were investigated in this study: CPD with Bspline transformation (CPD-B), CPD with TPS transformation (CPD-TPS), RPM with Bspline transformation (RPM-B) and RPM with TPS transformation (RPM-TPS). The point set registration results for CPD and RPM are visualized by the plots shown in Fig. 1. For the quantitative evaluation, the brain tissue on the source, target and result images were segmented manually with 3D Slicer. The Relative Overlap Metric described in [12] was used as evaluation metric. We calculated it both for the complete brain tissue and the region where we introduced elastic deformation (ROI) to compare the global and local impact of TPS and Bspline tranformations.

Fig. 1. Scatter plot of the point matching result for both data sets : (a) with 20% random outliers and (b) bifurcation points estimates as described in section 2.1. The hyperparameters for CPD was set as follows: $\beta = 0.2$, $\lambda = 10$, outlier weight $= 0.2$ in (a), $\beta = 0.2$, $\lambda = 10$, outlier weight $= 0$ in (b). For RPM, we used the default parameter setting suggested in the original paper.

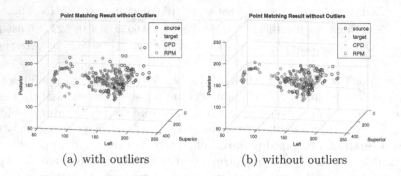

(a) with outliers   (b) without outliers

The relative overlapping rates are shown in Tab. 1. In the fourth scenario, only RPM-B is able to cover the deformation in ROI. However, for the data set containing outliers, there was no improvement in the overlap metric for the entire brain region (relative to the baseline). With the exception of the third scenario, where the combination of CPD and B-spline transformation achieved a slightly better result than the combination of RPM and B-spline transformation, RPM-B always outperforms the other three methods. Although the highest overlapping rate is calculated in the first scenario, the most improvement can be observed in the second scenario.

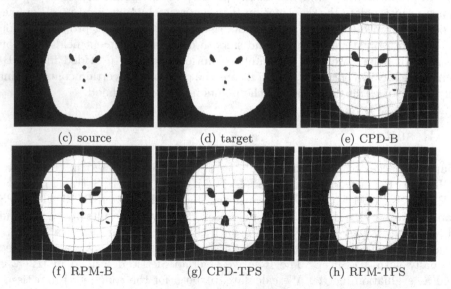

(c) source   (d) target   (e) CPD-B

(f) RPM-B   (g) CPD-TPS   (h) RPM-TPS

Fig. 2. An example axial slice with displacement field overlay. (a) and (b) are the source and target images. (c) - (f) are registration result of different methods.

4   Discussion

In this work, we introduced a new pipeline for brain shift compensation with intraoperative image data from CBCT. State-of-the-art point matching methods and spline based transformation techniques are employed for this purpose. Initial result on synthetic image data shows RPM combined with B-spline transformation is basically a good choice. It is the most robust combination against outliers and keeps the deformation localized. Table 1 shows, outliers affect the accuracy of the methods greatly, especially for TPS based methods in our experiments. A common practice to improve the performance of TPS transformation is to insert extra landmarks manually where no deformation is expected to occur. Overall, the TPS based methods are less accurate than their B-spline counterparts. Compared with baseline, both CPD-TPS and RPM-TPS achieved better results in the two cases where outliers are absent. With the introduction of outliers, the results are reversed. This behavior is consistent with the theory of TPS: it is a globally controlled transformation and sensitive to the choice of control points. This characteristic can be also observed in Fig. 3. B-spline transformation affects changes only in the neighborhood while TPS introduces deformation to the entire image volume. The result in Fig. 1 shows, RPM behave more robust against outliers but CPD is able to find the right correspondence for the points where RPM could not find correspondence. This is based on the different outlier handling strategies: RPM is rejecting outliers per se with a regularization to avoid too much rejections. CPD includes a hyperparameter which controls the relative importance of outliers compared to the Gaussian components in the mixture model. Another qualitative finding obtained from Fig. 3 is, that in comparison with RPM based methods, CPD tend to introduce more undesirable deformation to the subsurface structure (e.g. ventricle). This observation will be further investigated and quantified in furture work. Since there is, rarely if ever a Gold Standard to evaluate image registration results, no metric alone is sufficient to evaluate the performance of a nonrigid registration method [12]. Hence, other evaluation metrics such as target registration error should also be considered in the further experiments. A possible approach is to calculate the ground truth deformation of the volumetric meshes by comparing the deformed and non-deformed meshes at first, then interpolate this vector field into the image volume. Based on this ground truth deformation field, the exact difference between the displacement calculated with our proposed pipeline and actual displacement at each voxel can be obtained. Another important aspect of intraoperative brain shift compensation is the computational expense and numerical stability of the algorithm. B-splines are locally controlled, which makes them computationally efficient even for a large number of control points. In contrast, TPS transformation is computational expensive for large number of control points, since it considers every control point for each voxel. Our experience also shows the calculation of the inverse of L Matrix (see original paper [5]) is very crucial for the accuracy and numerical stability of TPS transformation. Since the L Matrix is often not invertable, numerical tricks such as pseudo inverse or Tikonov regularization are used to solve this problem. This is at the expense of the accuracy of the calculation result. In context of TPS transformation, a minimal error of each value in the inverse L Matrix leads to a summation of the error which produces implausible deformations. Due to these reasons, we propose to use B-spline transformation instead of TPS in subsequent studies.

Disclaimer. The concepts and information presented in this paper are based on research and are not commercially available.

References

1. Hill DLG, Maurer CR, Maciunas RJ, et al. Measurement of intraoperative brain surface deformation under a craniotomy. Neurosurgery. 1998;43(3):514–526.
2. Bayer S, Maier A, Ostermeier M, et al. Intraoperative imaging modalities and compensation for brain shift in tumor Resection Surgery. Int J Biomed Imaging. 2017;2017:18.
3. Chui H, Rangarajan A. A new point matching algorithm for non-rigid registration. Comput Vis Image Underst. 2003;89(2):114 – 141.
4. Myronenko A, Song X. Point set registration: coherent point drift. IEEE Trans Pattern Anal Mach Intell. 2010;32(12):2262–2275.
5. Bookstein FL. Principal warps: thin-plate splines and the decomposition of deformations. IEEE Trans Pattern Anal Mach Intell. 1989;11(6):567–585.
6. Rueckert D, Sonoda LI, Hayes C, et al. Nonrigid registration using free-form deformations: application to breast MR images. IEEE Trans Med Imaging. 1999 Aug;18(8):712–721.
7. Bayer S, Maier A, Ostermeier M, et al. Generation of synthetic Image Data for the Evaluation of Brain Shift Compensation Methods. Proc IGIC. 2017.
8. Frangi AF, Niessen WJ, Vincken KL, et al. Multiscale vessel enhancement filtering. Proc MICCAI. 1998; p. 130–137.
9. Otsu N. A threshold selection method from gray-level histograms. IEEE Trans Syst Man Cybern. 1979;9(1):62–66.
10. Lee TC, Kashyap RL, Chu CN. Building skeleton models via 3-D medial surface axis thinning algorithms. Comput Vis Graph Image Process. 1994;56(6):462 – 478.
11. Yuille AL, Grzywacz NM. A mathematical analysis of the motion coherence theory. Int J Comput Vis. 1989 Jun;3(2):155–175.
12. Christensen G, Geng X, G Kuhl J, et al.. Introduction to the non-rigid image registration evaluation project (NIREP); 2006.

Abstract: Patches in Magnetic Particle Imaging

Mandy Ahlborg[1], Christian Kaethner[1], Patryk Szwargulski[2,3],
Tobias Knopp[2,3], Thorsten M. Buzug[1]

[1]Institute of Medical Engineering, Universität zu Lübeck
[2]Section for Biomedical Imaging, University Medical Center Hamburg-Eppendorf
[3]Institute for Biomedical Imaging, Hamburg University of Technology
ahlborg@imt.uni-luebeck.de

Magnetic Particle Imaging (MPI) is a tracer-based imaging technology [1] with which superparamagnetic nanoparticles can be detected and located using specific magnetic fields. The selection field, a gradient field in form of a field free point (FFP), restricts the area in which particles can be remagnetized. The drive field, a homogeneous and time-varying magnetic field, remagnetizes the particles and moves the FFP. As a result a time dependent signal can be measured and then reconstructed to the actual spatial distribution of the tracer.

The movement of the FFP is specified by the frequency and the amplitude of the drive field and is referred to as trajectory. The ratio of amplitude and gradient particularly defines the size of the field of view (FOV) of a trajectory. In theory, the trajectory size can be chosen arbitrarily to meet the requirements of the (medical) imaging application. However, technical as well as physiological aspects limit the actual amplitude of the drive field and thus the FOV size. A possible solution to this constraint are imaging patches. Patches are multiple FOVs at different positions that need to be combined to obtain one large image.

In [2], the influence of overlaps between patches and different reconstruction techniques were investigated. The main focus was the reduction of truncation artifacts that occur on the edges of individual patches. It was shown that it is necessary to choose the MPI system matrix larger than the applied trajectory resulting in an inherent system matrix overlap. Further, a small trajectory overlap between patches significantly reduces artifacts. The data redundancy resulting from the overlapping areas has to be considered in the image reconstruction step. The two superior methods identified in [2] are (i) reconstruction of the individual patches and consecutive combination of the images by cutting off the patch edges and (ii) combination of the patch data in one system of equations and joint reconstruction.

In this contribution, we will validate the results of [2] with different experimental settings to demonstrate the robustness of the proposed methods.

References

1. Gleich B, Weizenecker J. Tomographic imaging using the nonlinear response of magnetic particles. Nature. 2005;435(7046):1214–1217.
2. Ahlborg M, Kaethner C, Knopp T, et al. Using data redundancy gained by patch overlaps to reduce truncation artifacts in magnetic particle imaging. Phys Med Biol. 2016;61(12):4583.

Phasenkontrast Röntgen mit 2 Phasengittern und medizinisch relevanten Detektoren

Johannes Bopp[1], Michael Gallersdörfer[2], Veronika Ludwig[2], Maria Seifert[2], Andres Maier[1], Gisela Anton[2], Christian Riess[1]

[1]Lehrstuhl für Mustererkennung, Friedrich-Alexander-Universität Erlangen-Nürnberg, Martensstr. 3, 91058 Erlangen
[2]Erlangen Centre for Astroparticle Physics (ECAP), Erwin-Rommel-Straße 1, 91058 Erlangen
Johannes.Bopp@fau.de

Kurzfassung. In den letzten Jahren hat die Forschung zu gitterbasierter Phasenkontrast-Bildgebung mittels Röntgenstrahlen große Fortschritte gemacht. Neueste Ergebnisse zeigen, dass das Absorptionsgitter G_2, durch ein zweites phasenschiebendes Gitter ersetzt werden kann und somit die Absorption hinter dem Patienten vermieden wird. Durch die Überlagerung des Selbstabbildes des ersten Phasengitters mit dem zweiten Phasengitter wird eine Schwebung erzeugt, deren Periode ausreichend groß ist, um mit dem Detektor direkt aufgelöst zu werden. In diesem Beitrag wollen wir diesen sogenannten zwei Phasengitteraufbau analysieren. Insbesondere untersuchen wir die Möglichkeiten, solche Aufbauten mit medizinisch relevanten Detektoren zu realisieren. Einen großen Einfluss auf die Ergebnisse hat hierbei die Impulsantwort des Detektors. Mit diesem Wissen wurde die Schwebungsfrequenz bestimmt, die eine möglichst hohe Visibilität liefert. Um die simulierten Ergebnisse zu validieren, wurden Messungen analog zu den Simulationen durchgeführt. Die Ergebnisse der Simulation und der Messungen stimmen sehr gut überein.

1 Einleitung

Phasenkontrast-Röntgenbildgebung ist eine vielversprechende Technik für Anwendungen in der Medizin und in der zerstörungsfreien Materialprüfung. Es gibt unterschiedliche Möglichkeiten um die Phaseninformation der Röntgenwelle auszulesen. Eine breitere Übersicht über die vielfältigen Methoden gibt zum Beispiel Endrizzi [1]. In dieser Arbeit beschränken wir uns auf Phasenkontrast-Röntgen mit Gittern. Die erfolgversprechendste Variante ist hier das sogenannte Talbot-Lau-Interferometer (TLI) (Abb. 1a). Es besteht aus drei Gittern und kann mit einer herkömmlichen medizinischen Röntgenröhre betrieben werden [2]. Es können die drei Bildinformationen Absorptionsbild, differentielles Phasenbild, sowie das Dunkelfeldbild rekonstruiert werden. Ein Nachteil des TLI ist das Absorptionsgitter G_2 direkt vor dem Detektor. Es absorbiert etwa 50% der Strahlung hinter dem Patienten. Dies hat zur Folge, dass ungenutzte Dosis im Patienten deponiert wird, welche nicht für die Bildgebung verwendet werden kann. Es wäre daher wünschenswert, keine Strahlung nach dem Patienten zu verlieren. Miao *et al.* haben gezeigt, dass es grundsätzlich möglich ist, das absorbierende G_2 durch ein zweites Phasengitter G_1' mit einem längeren Propagationsabstand zu ersetzen (Abb. 1 b) [3]. Da Phasengitter transparent für Röntgenstrahlen sind, kommt es zu keiner Absorption hinter dem Patienten. Kagias *et al.* zeigten, dass zwei Phasengitter eingesetzt werden können, um die Sensitivität des Dunkelfeldsignales zu variieren [4]. Allerdings haben beide Gruppen Detektoren verwendet, die nicht für eine Anwendung im klinischen Alltag geeignet sind. In dieser Arbeit wollen wir die Möglichkeiten von gitterbasierter Phasenkontrast-Bildgebung mit zwei Phasengittern für die Anwendung mit klinischen Detektoren analysieren. Dafür haben wir für die Abmessungen vorhandener Gitter einen geeigneten Aufbau in der numerischen Wellenfeldsimulation CXI [5] gesucht und diesen anschließend mit Messungen validiert.

2 Material und Methoden

Der Effekt der beiden phasenschiebenden Gitter auf die Welle Φ kann approximiert werden als

$$\Phi\left[\cos\left(2\pi\frac{x}{p_1^{\text{proj}}}\right) + \cos\left(2\pi\frac{x}{p_1'}\right)\right]$$

$$= 2\Phi\cos\left[\pi x\left(\frac{1}{p_1^{\text{proj}}} - \frac{1}{p_1'}\right)\right]\cos\left[\pi x\left(\frac{1}{p_1^{\text{proj}}} + \frac{1}{p_1'}\right)\right] \quad (1)$$

Hierbei ist p_1^{proj} die durch den Kegelstrahl leicht vergrößerte Periode des G_1 Gitters in der G_1' Ebene und p_1' ist die Periode des G_1' Gitters. Da beide Cosinus Funktionen leicht unterschiedliche Frequenzen haben entsteht eine Schwebung. Diese Schwebung kann durch die Positionierung der beiden Gitter zueinander variiert werden. Ein Gütemaß eines phasen-sensitiven Aufbaus ist die sogenannte Visibilität. Bei klassischen TLI Aufbauten wird die periodische Struktur, die

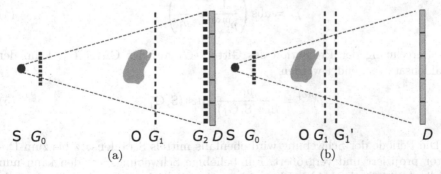

S G_0 O G_1 G_2 D S G_0 O G_1 G_1' D
(a)   (b)

Abb. 1. Vergleich eines herkömmlichen TLI mit einem zwei Phasengitteraufbau, bei dem das Absorptionsgitter G_2 durch ein zweites Phasengitter G_1' und eine längere Propagationsdistanz ersetzt wurde.

durch das G_1 erzeugt wird, mittels des G_2 Gitters abgetastet. Als Ergebnis erhält man eine sogenannte Phasestepping-Kurve, die einer Sinusschwingung entspricht. Aus einem Sinus-Fit $\mathbf{r}$ an die Phasestepping-Kurve kann die Visibilität aus dem Verhältnis der Amplitude zum Mittelwert des Sinus berechnet werden

$$v = \frac{\max(\mathbf{r}) - \min(\mathbf{r})}{\max(\mathbf{r}) + \min(\mathbf{r})} \qquad (2)$$

Alternativ kann die Visibilität mittels der harmonischen Schwingungen der Fourier-Transformierten des Fits errechnet werden

$$v = 2\frac{\hat{\mathbf{r}}[1]}{\hat{\mathbf{r}}[0]} \qquad (3)$$

Für Aufbauten mit zwei Phasengittern kann man entweder ebenfalls Phasestepping mit einem der Gitter durchführen oder auf Kosten von Ortsauflösung direkt die periodische Schwebung auswerten. Daraus können analog zum Standard TLI die drei Bildmodalitäten Absorption, differentielle Phase und Dunkelfeld berechnet werden.

Für traditionelle TLI mit einem Absorptionsgitter G_2 existieren bereits Formeln, um gute Parametrierungen zu bestimmen [6, 7]. Wir stellen im Folgenden eine Erweiterung dieser Formeln auf zwei Phasengitter vor. Der Parametersuchraum wurde für die Optimierung der Parameter dahingehend eingeschränkt, dass wir uns auf vorhandene Komponenten beschränken. Das sind zum einen eine Mikrofokus-Röntgenröhre mit einem Fokus von $9.5\,\mu m$ bei einem Spektrum von $40\,kVp$, und ein medizinischer Detektor mit $50\,\mu m$ Pixelgröße und einer Gadolinium-Oxysulfid Konverterschicht (Gd_2O_2S). Bei den Gittern handelt es sich um Nickel Gitter, die jeweils eine Höhe von $8.7\,\mu m$, und Perioden p von 4.12 und $4.37\,\mu m$ haben. Auf Grund des geringen Flusses der Röhre wurde der gesamte Aufbau (Fokus-Detektor Abstand) auf eine Länge von $1.5\,m$ beschränkt.

Die Schwebungsperiode ist eine Funktion der beiden Gitterperioden p_1' und p_1 projiziert auf das zweite Phasengitter G_1'

$$p_s = \text{abs}\left(\frac{1}{p_1^{\text{proj}}} - \frac{1}{p_1'}\right) \qquad (4)$$

Zur Berechnung der Projektion des Gitters G_1 auf das Gitter G_1', kann der Strahlensatz verwendet werden

$$p_1^{\text{proj}} = \frac{p_1}{\text{dist}(S, G_1)} \cdot \text{dist}(S, G_1') \qquad (5)$$

Die Periode der Schwebung wird ebenfalls mittels Strahlensatz bis zum Detektor projiziert und vergrößert. Für beliebige Schwebungsperioden kann nun auf die Abstände der beiden Phasengitter innerhalb des Strahlengangs, für jede beliebige Position, zurück gerechnet werden. Hierbei gibt es durch die Mehrdeutigkeit der Betragsfunktion in Gleichung 4 zwei mögliche Gitterabstände, welche die gleiche Schwebung erzeugen. Diese zwei möglichen Gitterabstände ergeben sich aus dem Abstand zum Detektor und der vorgegebenen Schwebungsperiode. Innerhalb der Simulation wurde die Position des G_1' Gitters variiert, die zu erzeugende Schwebungsperiode, sowie die beiden dafür möglichen Positionen des G_1. Aufgrund der geringen Periode der Schwebung im Verhältnis zur Pixelgröße, hat die Impulsantwort des Detektors einen großen Einfluss auf das Ergebnis. Durch die Konverterschicht werden eingehende Photonen auch auf benachbarten Pixeln detektiert. Dadurch kommt es zu einem Verwaschen der hohen Frequenzen. In der Simulation kann die gemessene PSF h mit der Detektorantwort F gefaltet werden um die tatsächliche Detektorantwort

$$I = F \star h + n \qquad (6)$$

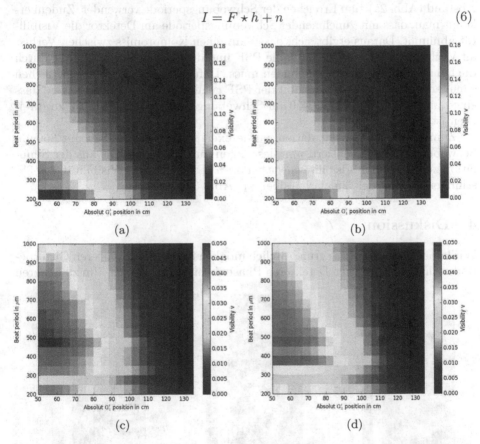

(a) (b)

(c) (d)

Abb. 2. Ergebnisse der Simulation. Bei allen Abbildungen ist auf der X-Achse die absolute Position des G_1' Gitters von der Quelle gemessen variiert. Auf der Y-Achse wird die erzeugte Schwebungsperiode in μm angegeben und die Farbskala kodiert die Visibilität. Die obere Reihe zeigt die Ergebnisse ohne und die untere Reihe die Ergebnisse mit Faltung mit der detektorspezifischen PSF. In der linken Spalte ((a) und (c)) ist der kleinere mögliche Gitterabstand zu erkennen, in der rechten Spalte ((b) und (d)) der größere. Für jeden simulierten Aufbau sind diese Abstände unterschiedlich. Es ist zu sehen, dass mit dem kleineren Gitterabstand höhere Visibilitäten erzeugt werden.

zu errechnen. Hierbei bezeichnet $\star$ den Faltungsoperator und n das Rauschen, welches hier nicht simuliert wurde.

3 Ergebnisse

Die Messung der PSF ergab, dass sie hinreichend genau mit einem Gaußfilter mit einer Standardabweichung σ von 1.48 Pixeln approximiert werden kann. Die Ergebnisse der Simulation ohne die PSF zeigen, dass ein größerer Propagationsabstand zwischen G_1' und dem Detektor zu besseren Visibilitäten führt, unabhängig davon, ob man den größeren (Abb. 2b) oder den kleineren möglichen Abstand (Abb. 2a) zum Erreichen der Schwebungsperiode verwendet. Zudem erkennt man, dass mit zunehmender Schwebungsperiode am Detektor die Visibilität abnimmt. Daraus ergibt sich, dass man einen Kompromiss zwischen Verlust an Visibilität am Detektor durch die PSF und den Verlust der Visibilität durch die höhere Schwebungsperiode finden muss. Dafür wurden die unterschiedlichen simulierten Detektorantworten mit der PSF gefaltet. Die Ergebnisse zeigen, dass eine optimale Visibilität bei 450 μm Schwebungsperiode mit etwa 5% zu erreichen ist.

Zum Validieren der Simulation wurde exemplarisch ein Aufbau mit 350 μm Schwebungsperiode realisiert, um Messungen durchzuführen. Die aus der Simulation zu erwartende Visibilität liegt bei 3.8%. Die gemessene Visibilität von 3% stimmen gut mit der Simulation überein (Abb. 3).

4 Diskussion

Wir haben gezeigt, dass es grundsätzlich möglich ist, auch mit größeren Gitterperioden und medizinischen Detektoren Phasenkontrast zu messen. Um zu höheren

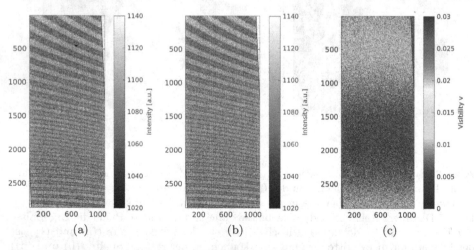

(a)   (b)   (c)

Abb. 3. Ergebnisse der Messung. (a) und (b) zeigen zwei einzelne Phasenschritte. (c) zeigt die rekonstruierte Visibilitätskarte. In den Randbereichen oben rechts und unten links endet der Gitterbereich.

Visibilitäten zu kommen ist es notwendig entweder die Gesamtlänge des Aufbaus zu vergrößern oder die Gitterperiode zu verkleinern. Der limitierende Faktor für die Gitterperioden bei herkömmlichen TLI ist das Aspektverhältnis des G_2 Gitters. Dies wird in den zwei Phasengitteraufbauten nicht verwendet, weswegen deutlich kleinere Perioden hergestellt werden können. Noch mehr als bei herkömmlicher Röntgenbildgebung ist hier die Impulsantwort (PSF) des Detektors von Bedeutung. Mit dem jetzt validierten Simulationstool können weitere Optimierungen für zwei Phasengitteraufbauten durchgeführt werden und zukünftige Aufbauten vorab analysiert bzw. optimiert werden.

Danksagung. Wir danken Siemens Healthineers für die finanzielle Unterstützung dieser Arbeit.

Literaturverzeichnis

1. Endrizzi M. X-ray phase-contrast imaging. Nuclear Instruments and Methods in Physics Research Section A: Accelerators, Spectrometers, Detectors and Associated Equipment. 2017.
2. Pfeiffer F, Weitkamp T, Bunk O, et al. Phase retrieval and differential phase-contrast imaging with low-brilliance X-ray sources. Nature Phys. 2006;2(4):258–261.
3. Miao H, Panna A, Gomella AA, et al. A universal moiré effect and application in X-ray phase-contrast imaging. Nature Phys. 2016;12:830–834.
4. Kagias M, Wang Z, Jefimovs K, et al. Dual phase grating interferometer for tunable dark-field sensitivity. Appl Phys Lett. 2017;110(1):014105.
5. Ritter A, Bartl P, Bayer F, et al. Simulation framework for coherent and incoherent X-ray imaging and its application in Talbot-Lau dark-field imaging. Optics Expr. 2014;22(19):23276–23289.
6. Thuering T, Stampanoni M. Performance and optimization of X-ray grating interferometry. Philosoph Trans Royal Soc London A: Math Phys Eng Sci. 2014;372(2010):20130027.
7. Weitkamp T, David C, Kottler C, et al. Tomography with grating interferometers at low-brilliance sources. Proc SPIE. 2006;6318:63180S.

CT-basiertes virtuelles Fräsen am Felsenbein

Bild- und haptischen Wiederholfrequenzen bei unterschiedlichen Rendering Methoden

Daniela Franz[1], Maria Dreher[1,2], Martin Prinzen[1], Matthias Teßmann[2],
Christoph Palm[3], Uwe Katzky[4], Jerome Perret[5], Mathias Hofer[6],
Thomas Wittenberg[1,7]

[1]Fraunhofer Institut für Integrierte Schaltungen IIS, Erlangen
[2]Hochschule Nürnberg Georg Simon Ohm
[3]Regensburg Medical Image Computing (REMIC), Ostbayerische Technische
Hochschule Regensburg
[4]szenaris GmbH, Bremen [5]Haption GmbH, Aachen
[6]Klinik und Poliklinik für Hals-, Nasen-, Ohrenheilkunde, Universität Leipzig
[7]Lehrstuhl für Graphische Datenverarbeitung LGDV, Universität Erlangen-Nürnberg
daniela.franz@iis.fraunhofer.de

Kurzfassung. Im Rahmen der Entwicklung eines haptisch-visuellen Trainingssystems für das Fräsen am Felsenbein werden ein Haptikarm und ein autostereoskopischer 3D-Monitor genutzt, um Chirurgen die virtuelle Manipulation von knöchernen Strukturen im Kontext eines sog. Serious Game zu ermöglichen. Unter anderem sollen Assistenzärzte im Rahmen ihrer Ausbildung das Fräsen am Felsenbein für das chirurgische Einsetzen eines Cochlea-Implantats üben können. Die Visualisierung des virtuellen Fräsens muss dafür in Echtzeit und möglichst realistisch modelliert, implementiert und evaluiert werden. Wir verwenden verschiedene Raycasting Methoden mit linearer und Nearest Neighbor Interpolation und vergleichen die visuelle Qualität und die Bildwiederholfrequenzen der Methoden. Alle verglichenen Verfahren sind sind echtzeitfähig, unterscheiden sich aber in ihrer visuellen Qualität.

1 Einleitung

Das chirurgische Einsetzen eines Cochlea-Implantats (CI) erfordert das Üben der notwendigen Operationsschritte, sowie intensives Studium der umgebenden Anatomie. Der operative Zugang zur Cochlea (Hörschnecke im Innenohr) für eine CI verläuft durch das Felsenbein und wird mit einer Fräse eröffnet. Das Felsenbein ist der Teil des Schädels, der das Innenohr umfasst. Die Schwierigkeit des Eingriffs liegt dabei in der komplexen, dreidimensionalen Anordnung der angrenzenden Risikostrukturen, bspw. Gesichtsnerv, Chorda Tympani, Dura. Während des Fräsvorgangs gilt es, deren Verletzung unbedingt zu vermeiden. Dafür muss der Chirurg die komplexe Anatomie des Felsenbeins genau kennen und zu jedem Zeitpunkt des Fräsvorgangs wissen, welche Struktur sich hinter den Knochen befindet [1].

Konventionell lernen HNO-Chirurgen eine CI Implantation durch das Beobachten erfahrener Chirurgen im Operationssaal, durch das Üben an 3D-Drucken [2] oder Leichenpräparaten [3] und später durch begleitetes Operieren am Patienten. Die Verfügbarkeit tierischer und menschlicher Präparaten ist jedoch beschränkt, die Nutzung von 3D-Drucken des Felsenbein immer noch kostspielig. Eine mögliche Ergänzung der chirurgischen Ausbildung ist daher die virtuelle Simulation. Auf der Basis von patientenspezifischen CT-Datensätzen des Kopfes wird ein dreidimensionales Modell des Felsenbeins und der darin eingebetteten Ziel- und Risikostrukturen generiert. Mit Hilfe eines Haptikarms können angehende Ärzte und Chirurgen das Fräsen in virtuelle Knochen üben und dabei auch rückwirkende Kräfte erfahren [4, 5]. Die Güte und Glaubwürdigkeit einer virtuellen Simulation liegt dabei u.a. auch in der realitätsgetreuen Darstellung, Haptik und Aufbereitung des simulierten Eingriffs.

2 Material und Methoden

Im Rahmen des bestehenden Systems laufen das haptisches und graphisches Rendering in jeweils einem eigenen Thread als Endlosschleife. Das haptische Rendering wird dabei mit der Chai3d-Bibliothek realisiert. Der Haptik-Thread prüft anhand der Position des Haptikarms kontinuierlich, ob eine Kollision der Fräse mit dem virtuellen Felsenbein (oder Risikostrukturen) vorliegt. Liegt eine Kollision vor, wird das Modell des Felsenbeins durch Eliminierung der Betroffenen Voxel aktualisiert und dass modifizierte Modell an die Grafikkarte übergeben. Wir berechnen die Interaktionskräfte zwischen Fräse und Knochen mit dem Finger Proxy Algorithmus aus Chai3D [6].

Um eine Kollision zu erkennen prüfen wir zunächst eine Kollision mit der Bounding Box des Modells und, wenn diese vorliegt, berechnen wir den genauen Kollisionspunkt. Abb. 2 (rechts) zeigt ein gefrästes Loch.

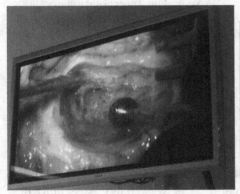 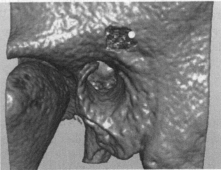

Abb. 1. Mikroskop-Ansicht des ausgefrästen Felsenbein während einer Cochlea Implantation in der HNO-Klinik Leipzig (links) und Visualisierung des Fräsens am Felsenbein mit Direct Volume Rendering (rechts).

Das graphische Rendering wird mit OpenGL realisiert. Hat eine Kollision der Fräse mit dem Knochen stattgefunden, wird die Opazität der Voxel im Kollisionsbereich (Bounding Box um den Kollisionspunk) transparent gesetzt. Eine Bounding Box um den betroffenen Voxel markiert den Kollisionsbereich. Nachdem die 3D-Textur auf der CPU aktualisiert wurde, wird der Kollisionsbereich mit Hilfe des glTexSubImage3D Befehls an die GPU übergeben und damit nur ein kleiner Teil des Bildes neu berechnet.

Volumendaten können einerseits mit Surface Rendering einer Isofläche, andererseits mit Direct Volume Rendering visualisiert werden. Folgende Rendering Methoden werden verwendet und im Folgenden vorgestellt: Direct Volume Rendering, Voxel Colormap, Isosurface Colormap, Isosurface Colors, Isosurface Material. Bei Direct Volume Rendering werden die Voxel direkt in die Bildebene projiziert. Implementiert wird Direct Volume Rendering oft mit Volume Raycasting, bei dem pro Pixel der Bildfläche ein Sichtstrahl durch das Volumen geschickt wird. Der Farbwert des Pixel ergibt sich durch aufsummieren der Farb- und Opazitätswerte aus einer Lookup Tabelle an Abtastpunkten entlang des Sichtstrahls. Erreicht die Summe die maximale Opazität bevor der Sichtstrahl das Volumen verlässt, kann die Berechnung des Pixelwertes vorzeitig abgebrochen werden (Early Ray Termination). Der Farbwert wird nun noch mit einem Beleuchtungsterm multipliziert und der Pixel dargestellt. Voxel Colormap summiert hingegen nur die Farbwerte aus der Lookup Tabelle auf, die Opazitätswerte sind fest vorgegeben, der Beleuchtungsterm wird nicht berücksichtigt. Beim Surface Rendering wird entlang eines Isoflächenwertes ein Polygongitter erzeugt und als Oberfläche dargestellt. Isosurface Colormap betrachtet die Farbwerte entlang des Sichtstrahls. Bei ersten Wert größer dem Isoflächenwert, wird anhand einer Lookup Tabelle der Farbwert des aktuellen Pixels bestimmt. Isosurface Colors hingegen verwendet direkt die Grauwerte des Volumendatensatzes und keine Lookup Tabelle, Isosurface Material zusätzlich noch Materialeigenschaften.

Bei allen Verfahren treffen die Abtastpunkte nicht zwingend einen der diskreten Voxel, sondern liegen zwischen den Voxeln. Die Interpolationsmethode bestimmt, wie der Zwischenwert bestimmt wird. Bei der Nearest Neighbor Interpolation wird dem Abtastpunkt der Wert des nähsten Voxels zugewiesen. Bei der linearen Interpolation wird der Wert anhand der linear gewichteten Werte aller Nachbarvoxel berechnet.

3 Ergebnisse

Nachfolgend evaluieren die Autoren die visuelle Qualität und Wiederholfrequenzen des Grafik- und Haptik-Thread. Die Evaluation wurde mit einem Desktoprechner mit i7-3770 Prozessor (CPU 3.40GHz, 8GB RAM) und deiner Nvidia GeForce GTX 750Ti Grafikkarte durchgeführt. Der verwendete Ausschnitt des genutzten CT-Datensatzes umfasst ein Volumen von $60 \times 30 \times 40$mm mit einer Voxelgröße von $0.2604^2 \times 0.3$mm^3 und insgesamt 280000 Voxeln.

Die Rendering Methoden werden einerseits anhand ihrer Wiederholfrequenz, andererseits anhand der visuellen Qualität ihrer Darstellung bewertet. Sie soll die Darstellung im OP nachbilden (Abb.2, links). Sowohl die haptische als auch die graphische Wiederholfrequenz wird mit linearer und Nearest Neighbor Interpolation für die fünf evaluierten Rendering Methoden und unter drei Randbedingungen (im Stillstand, bei Bewegen der virtuellen Kamera und beim Fräsen) 30 mal, 30 Sekunden lang gemessen und gemittelt.

Die gemessenen mittleren Wiederholfrequenzen und Standardabweichungen des Grafik-Thread sind in Abb. 2 und des Haptik-Thread in Abb. 3 dargestellt.

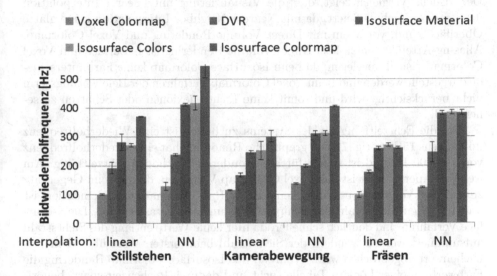

Abb. 2. Mittlere Wiederholfrequenz des graphischen Rendering unter den verschiedenen Randbedingungen (NN=Nearest Neighbor).

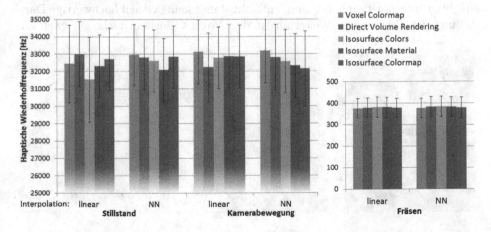

Abb. 3. Mittlere Wiederholfrequenz des haptischen Rendering unter den verschiedenen Randbedingungen (NN=Nearest Neighbor).

Der visuelle Vergleich der Rendering Methoden beinhaltet Direct Volume Rendering, Voxel ColorMap und Isosurface Colormap, der abgesehen von der Farbe die gleiche Darstellung hervorbringt wie auch Isosurface Colors und Isosurface Material (Abb. 4).

4 Diskussion

Der visuelle Vergleich zeigt, dass die Visualisierung mit linearer Interpolation das bessere Ergebnis liefert, da mit Nearest Neighbor Interpolation keine glatte Oberfläche und, vor allem mit Direct Volume Rendering und Voxel Colormap, Aliasing-Artefakte entstehen. Direct Volume Rendering ist Isosurface und Voxel Colormap visuell überlegen, da beim Isosurface Colormap keine Farbunterschiede dargestellt werden und beim Voxel Colormap Verfahren der Beleuchtungsterm nicht berücksichtigt wird und somit keine Lichtreflexionen oder Schatten zu sehen sind.

Um die Echtzeitfähigkeit des Systems zu halten ist eine Wiederholfrequenz mindestens 15Hz nötig [7]. Das graphische Rendering hat eine Wiederholfrequenz von 100-500 Hz und ist damit für alle Rendering Methoden echtzeitfähig. Am wenigsten performant ist das Voxel Colormap Verfahren, da hier - im Gegensatz zum Direct Volume Rendering - keine Early Ray Termination implementiert ist und für jeden Sichtstrahl das komplette Volumen abgetastet wird. Die Isosurface Verfahren sind deutlich schneller, da hier keine Werte entlang des Sichtstrahl aufsummiert werden, sondern der Sichtstrahl beim ersten Wert über dem Isoflächenwert abgebrochen wird. Während das Isosurface Colormap Rendering die Farbwerte in einer Lookup Tabelle sucht und dadurch Rechenzeit spart, benötigen Isosurface Colors und -Material einen zusätzlichen Zugriff auf die Grauwerte des CT-Volumen und verlangsamt damit diese Verfahren.

Obwohl die Bildwiederholfrequenz aller Rendering Methoden mit Nearest Neighbor Interpolation höher sind, entsteht damit keine visuell hochwertige Darstellung des Felsenbeins. Weiterhin ist das Voxel Colormap nicht geeignet für

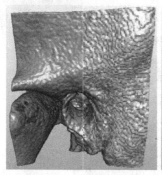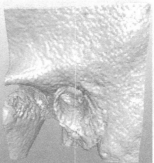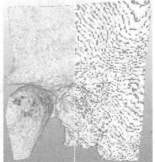

Abb. 4. Visueller Vergleich von linearer (jeweils links) und Nearest Neighbor Interpolation (jeweils rechts) und der Rendering Methoden Direct Volume Rendering (links), Isosurface Colormap (mitte) und Voxel Colormap (rechts).

die Visualisierung in diesem Kontext: es liefert sowohl das visuell schlechteste Ergebnis, als auch die geringste Bildwiederholfrequenz. Das visuelle Ergebnis von Direct Volume Rendering ist dem von Isosurface Colormap/-Material leicht überlegen, die Bildwiederholfrequenzen aber dafür leicht unterlegen.

Das haptische Rendering ist unabhängig von der Rendering- und Interpolationsmethode. Im Stillstand und bei Kamerabewegung wird eine Wiederholfrequenz von 31000-33000 Hz erreicht, beim Fräsen 370-390 Hz. Die enorme Reduktion der Wiederholfrequenz entsteht durch die aufwändigen Kräfteberechnungen im Haptik-Thread im Falle einer Kollision.

Graphisches und haptisches Rendering sind also ausreichend performant, die visuelle Qualität bei Surface Rendering und mit Direct Volume Rendering ausreichend. Um die Simulation aber noch realitätsnäher zu gestalten, muss im Folgenden weitere Materialien simuliert werden. Beim Fräsen bildet sich Knochenstaub, der simuliert werden muss. Da am Kochen nass gefräst wird, muss das Wasser simuliert und visualisiert werden. Im Operationsgebiet austretendes Blut muss simuliert und die Veränderung der Farbe simuliert werden: Blut wird dunkeler, wenn es gerinnt. Des Weiteren müssen verschiedene Oberflächeneigenschaften simuliert werden. Das Berühren des Knochens mit der Fräse sollte sich anders anfühlen als das Berühren von Weichgewebe [8].

Literaturverzeichnis

1. Boenninghaus H, Lenarz T. Hals-Nasen-Ohren-Heilkunde. Springer-Verlag; 2006.
2. Strauß G, Bahrami N, Pößneck A, et al. Evaluation eines Trainingssystems für die Felsenbeinchirurgie mit optoelektrischer Detektion. Hno. 2009;57(10):999–1009.
3. Mason T, Applebaum E, Rasmussen M, et al. Virtual temporal bone: creation and application of a new computer-based teaching tool. Otolaryngology–Head and Neck Surgery. 2000;122(2):168–173.
4. Franz D, Katzky U, Neuman S, et al. Haptisches Lernen für Cochlea Implantationen Konzept–HaptiVisT Projekt. Proc CURAC. 2016; p. 21.
5. Maier J, Haug S, Huber M, et al. Development of a haptic and visual assisted training simulation concept for complex bone drilling in minimally invasive hand surgery. Proc CARS. 2017.
6. Ruspini DC, Kolarov K, Khatib O. The haptic display of complex graphical environments. In: Proc. Comput graph interact tech; 1997. p. 345–352.
7. Akenine-Möller T, Haines E, Hoffman N. Real-time rendering. CRC Press; 2008.
8. Fortmeier D, Mastmeyer A, Handels H. An image-based multiproxy palpation algorithm for patient-specific VR-simulation. In: Proc MMVR; 2014. p. 107–113.

Segmentierung von Brustvolumina in Magnetresonanztomographiedaten unter der Verwendung von Deep Learning

Thomas G. Jentschke[1], Katrin Hegenscheid[2,3], Henry Völzke[3],
Florentin Wörgötter[1], Tatyana Ivanovska[1]

[1]Institut für Biophysik, Georg-August Universität Göttingen
[2]Sana Klinikum Lichtenberg Berlin
[3]Universitätsmedizin Greifswald
tiva@phys.uni-goettingen.de

Kurzfassung. Die Segmentierung von Hintergrund und Brustgewebe
ist ein wichtiger Teil der Auswertung von Magnetresonanztomographie-
Daten der Brust. Normalerweise wird diese von Ärzten manuell durchgeführt. In dieser Arbeit wurde die Segmentierung hingegen mit einer
U-net Architektur realisiert. Dabei wurden zwei Netzwerke trainiert und
anschließend auf ein unbekanntes Testset, bestehend aus 8 Probandinnen,
angewendet. Die so berechneten Segmentierungen wurden dann mit von
Ärzten manuell vorgenommenen verglichen. Das erste U-net nutzt keine
weitere Vorverarbeitungsmethode und erreicht einen DSC von 0.91 ± 0.09
(Mittelwert $\pm$ Standardabweichung). Beim zweiten Netzwerk wurde der
N4ITK Bias Correction Algorithmus als Vorverarbeitungsmethode verwendet. Die Masken für N4ITK können sehr grob sein und daher in
einer späteren Anwendung von einem Arzt schnell erstellt werden. In
dieser Konstellation wurde bei der Segmentierung des Testsets ein DSC
von 0.98 ± 0.05 erreicht. Die Segmentierungen benötigen darüber hinaus
nach Anfertigung der Masken für den Vorverarbeitungsalgorithmus 14s.
Die Methode hat somit das Potential, Anwendung in der medizinischen
Diagnostik zu finden.

1 Einleitung

Die Bedeutung der bildgebenden Diagnostik im Bereich der Medizin nimmt immer weiter zu. Eines der wichtigsten Verfahren ist dabei neben der Computerto-
mographie (CT) die Magnetresonanztomographie (MRT). Diese ist sowohl zeit-
als auch kostenintensiv, da die erzeugten Bilder heutzutage noch überwiegend
manuell von Spezialisten ausgewertet werden müssen. Seit geraumer Zeit wird
daher versucht dies mittels spezieller Algorithmen durchzuführen.

Bei der Auswertung von MRT-Bildern der Brust ist einer der wichtigsten
Schritte die Segmentierung von Brustgewebe. Die so erhaltenen Daten können
dann von anderen Algorithmen weiter ausgewertet werden. Darüber hinaus lässt
sich direkt aus den Segmentierungen von Brustvolumina und Parenchym die

Die Original-Version des Kapitels wurde korrigiert. Ein Erratum finden Sie unter
https://doi.org/10.1007/978-3-662-56537-7_97

Brustdichte bestimmen. Diese ist ein wichtiger Indikator zur Einschätzung des Risikos einer Brustkrebserkrankung.

Es gibt viele vergleichbare Arbeiten zu diesem Thema, in denen jeweils unterschiedliche Algorithmen verwendet wurden. Die von Ivanovska et al. [1] verwendete Level-Set-Methode mit simultaner Bias-Korrektur erreichte einen durchschnittlichen Dice Koeffizient von 0.960 ± 0.017 von 37 MRT-Scans. Ein anderes Beispiel ist die Methode von Gubern-Mérida et al. [2], bei der ein DSC von 0.94 erreicht wurde.

Alle diese Algorithmen sind mehr oder weniger stark abhängig von den verschiedenen Charakteristika der verwendeten MRT-Bilder.

In dieser Arbeit sollen Deep Learning Methoden zur Segmentierung der Brust verwendet werden. Diese sind in der Lage, die entsprechenden Charakteristika der jeweiligen MRT-Bilder zu lernen, und somit unabhängiger von den erhobenen Daten. Wie in der Arbeit von Dalmış et al. [3] soll hierfür eine sogenannte U-net Architektur [4] verwendet werden. Diese wurde schon in anderen Arbeiten sehr erfolgreich zur Lösung von biomedizinischen Segmentierungsproblemen verwendet. Wie in der medizinischen Diagnostik notwendig, ist das fertig trainierte U-net darüber hinaus in der Lage, die MRT-Bilder sehr schnell zu verarbeiten.

2 Material und Methoden

2.1 Eigenschaften der Daten

Das Datenset umfasst Brust-MRT Untersuchungen von 40 weiblichen Probanden aus der Study of Health in Pomerania [5] mit jeweils 128 Bildschichten, die im Abstand von 1.5 mm aufgenommen wurden. Je 10 Probanden gehören den 4 verschiedenen ACR Klassifikationen ACR0 - ACR3 an. Diese Klassifikation gibt an, wie groß der Anteil des Drüsengewebes jeweils ist, und wurde von einem Arzt vorgenommen. Die Bilder sind in axialer Richtung aufgenommen worden und verfügen über eine Auflösung von 512×512 Pixeln. Die Aufnahmen wurden mittels eines 1.5 Tesla MRT-Geräts erstellt. Zu jedem Bild existiert außerdem eine von Ärzten mit mehr als 8-jähriger Berufserfahrung erstellte Maske mit korrekten Segmentierung von Brust und Hintergrund. Ein solches MRT-Bild mit der Maske ist beispielhaft in Abb. 1(a) dargestellt.

Wie man sehen kann, weisen die Daten einen starken Helligkeitsgradienten in y-Richtung, sowie Helligkeitsinhomogenitäten an den Brusträndern auf. Dies ist problematisch, da der Algorithmus schneller lernt, die hellen Bereiche richtig zu segmentieren und die dunklen unter Umständen gar nicht. Auch der Kontrast zwischen Drüsen- und Fettgewebe ist in den dunklen Bereichen deutlich verringert. Ein Ziel der Datenvorbereitung wird es daher sein, diese Helligkeitsdifferenzen auszugleichen und den Kontrast zwischen den zu segmentierenden Klassen zu vergrößern.

2.2 Datenvorbereitung und Netzwerkarchitektur

Ein wichtiger Faktor für die Qualität des trainierten Netzwerkes ist die Menge der Daten. Um diese zu erhöhen, ist es sinnvoll beide Bildhälften einzeln für das Training zu verwenden und so die Anzahl der Bilder zu verdoppeln. Hierfür können die MRT-Bilder in der Mitte zerschnitten und die eine Hälfte, in diesem Fall die Rechte, gespiegelt werden. Da die MRT-Bilder bereits symmetrisch sind, ist dafür keine weitere Vorbereitung notwendig.

Darüber hinaus wurde für die Vorverarbeitung der Daten der sogenannte N4ITK Bias Correction Algorithmus [6] verwendet, um die im vorherigen Abschnitt beschriebenen Helligkeitsinhomogenitäten auszugleichen. Hierbei wurde der Algorithmus nur auf eine Maske angewendet, die durch Vergrößern und Verzerren der manuell erzeugten Segmentierungsmasken erzeugt wurde. Der Umriss der Brust ist dabei sehr grob und könnte leicht und unter geringem Zeitaufwand von einem Arzt erstellt werden.

Wie in Abb. 2 zu sehen ist, konnte auf diese Weise die Helligkeit im Vergleich zum Original im gesamten Bereich der Brust deutlich erhöht werden und damit auch der Kontrast zwischen Brust und Hintergrund. Auch die Helligkeitsdifferenz zwischen den Maxima und Minima und damit der Kontrast zwischen Drüsen- und Fettgewebe konnte durch die Verwendung der Maskierung erhöht werden. Die Helligkeitsinhomogenitäten an den Brusträndern konnten ebenfalls behoben werden. Betrachtet man die in Abb. 2 dargestellten Helligkeitsverläufe, so ist zu erkennen, dass der Helligkeitsgradient in y-Richtung nach wie vor vorhanden jedoch gegenüber dem Original verringert ist. Der Algorithmus funktioniert am besten in den mittleren Schichten, bei denen die Brust wie in Abb. 2 sehr großflächig ist. In den äußeren Schichten wird die Brust jedoch schmaler. Wie in Abb. 1(b) zu sehen, gelingt es dem Algorithmus in diesem Bereich nicht mehr, den Gradienten in y-Richtung zu korrigieren.

Wir haben die 2 Klassen-Netzwerkarchitektur vom Dalmis et al. [3] übernommen und für unsere Daten adaptiert. Als Lossfunktion E wird der Inverse Dice Koeffizient verwendet: $E = 1 - DSC$. Der Dice Koeffizient ist wie folgt definiert: $DSC = 2|S_1 \cup S_2|/(|S_1| + |S_2|)$, wobei S_1 und S_2 die manuelle Segmetierung und das vom Netzwerk gelernte Ergebnis sind. Aus jeder ACR-Gruppe mit jeweils 10 Datensätzen wurden randomisiert 2 Probandinnen für das Testing ausgewählt. Die restlichen 32 Datensätze wurden als Trainingsset genommen. Das Validierungsset besteht aus ca. 20% der verbliebenen Daten, die vor jedem Trainings-

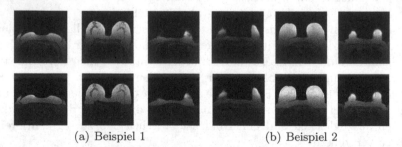

(a) Beispiel 1   (b) Beispiel 2

Abb. 1. Obere Reihe: Exemplarische Darstellung der Daten aus verschiedenen Bereichen der Brust. Untere Reihe: Links: die manuell erstellten Masken wurden in grüner Farbe über das Bild gelegt. Rechts: Ergebnisse von mit N4ITK Bias Correction Algorithmus.

durchlauf zufällig ausgewählt werden. Dabei werden die Daten der Probandinnen so gruppiert, dass sie jeweils vollständig in einem der Sets lagen.

3 Ergebnisse

In einem ersten Versuch wurde ein U-net ohne Vorverarbeitung der Daten mit dem N4ITK Bias Correction Algorithmus trainiert. Dieses erreichte jedoch nur einen DSC von 0.91 ± 0.09. Im zweiten Versuch wurden die Daten mit dem N4ITK Bias Correction Algorithmus vorverarbeitet und bei der Segmentierung der Daten aus dem Testset ein DSC von 0.98 ± 0.06 erreicht. In Abb. 3 sind exemplarisch 4 vorverarbeitete MRT-Bilder aus dem Testset und darunter die jeweils berechneten Segmentierungen dargestellt. Auf der linken Seite ist ein Bild aus einer der mittleren Schichten eines MRT-Scans dargestellt. Die berechnete Segmentierung stimmt bis auf einige Pixel am Rand genau mit der vom Arzt erstellten Maskierung überein. Die „Zebrastreifen", wie sie im dritten Bild von links zu sehen sind, werden ebenso korrekt als Hintergrund klassifiziert. Problematisch sind nach wie vor MRT-Scans von Probandinnen mit viel Drüsengewebe und geringer Abgrenzung zwischen diesem und dem Hintergrund, wie beispielhaft auf dem zweiten Bild von links zu sehen ist. In diesem Fall wird nahezu das komplette Drüsengewebe dem Hintergrund zugeordnet. Der DSC der Segmentierungen der MRT-Bilder dieser Probandin liegt nur bei 0.93 und ist damit der niedrigste im gesamten Testset. In den äußeren Schichten werden anders als im ersten Netzwerk nicht mehr zu viel Pixel der Brust zugeordnet sondern zu wenige. Dabei haben die Segmentierungen oft unrealistische Formen und es lassen sich keine Bildfehler erkennen, die dieses Verhalten erklären könnten.

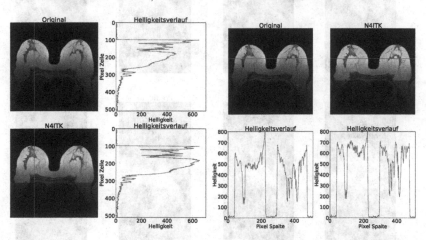

Abb. 2. Vergleich eines mit dem N4ITK Bias Correction Algorithmus mit Maskierung vorverarbeiten MRT-Bildes mit dessen Original. Auf der linken Seite sind dabei die Helligkeitsverläufe in y-Richtung abgebildet, auf der rechten die Helligkeitsverläufe in x-Richtung.

Der Zeitaufwand pro Proband, also in diesem Fall 128 MRT-Bilder, bei der Segmentierung mit dem betrachteten U-net beträgt auf einer Graphikkarte mit 12 GB durchschnittlich ca. 13.6 s.

4 Diskussion

Dalmış et al. [3] zeigten, dass die U-Nets die klassischen Ansätze übertrafen, und beobachteten, dass die U-Net-basierten Methoden minimal von Intensitätsinhomogenitäten betroffen wurden. Wir haben eine ähnliche Netzwerkarchitektur auf Daten mit sehr starker Inhomogenität angewendet und gezeigt, dass das Netzwerk in unserem Fall Probleme hatte, die starken Inhomogenitäten zu lernen. Wir haben auch gezeigt, dass die Intensitätsinhomogenitätskorrektur mit N4ITK [6] die Leistung des Netzwerks deutlich verbessert hat. Bei der Segmentierung wurde bei dem ohne weitere Vorverarbeitungsmethoden trainierten U-net ein DSC von 0.91 ± 0.09 erreicht. Dieses Ergebnis bleibt etwas zurück hinter dem von Dalmış et al. [3] erreichten DSC von 0.944 beim 2C-U-net zur selben Problemstellung, allerding mit einem anderen Datensatz. In der vorliegenden Arbeit war dabei, der einschränkendste Faktor der starke Helligkeitsgradient in y-Richtung, der zu deutlich schlechteren Segmentierungen in den dunkleren Bereichen der Brust

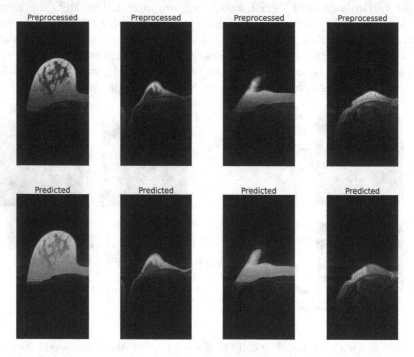

Abb. 3. Exemplarische Darstellung einiger Segmentierungen die mit dem U-net erstellt wurden. Dabei sind TP grün, FP rot und FN orange eingefärbt. Über den Segmentierungen ist jeweils zum Vergleich das vorverarbeitete Bild dargestellt.

führte. Unter Verwendung der mit dem N4ITK Bias Correction Algorithmus vorverarbeiten Daten wurde ein U-net trainiert, das einen DSC von 0.98 ± 0.05 bei der Segmentierung des Testsets erreichte.

Problematisch ist die Segmentierung von MRT-Scans mit sehr viel Drüsengewebe und geringer Abgrenzung zwischen diesem und dem Hintergrund, wie es in Abb. 3 zu sehen ist. Möglicherweise ließe sich dies durch Hinzufügen von Informationen der benachbarten Schichten verbessern, da diese zum Teil besser segmentiert werden konnten als im genannten Beispiel. In jedem Fall sinnvoll wäre das Hinzufügen der 3D-Informationen in den äußeren Schichten. In diesem Bereich ist es auch für Ärzte aufgrund eines einzelnen MRT-Bildes kaum möglich, dieses richtig zu segmentieren. Die manuelle Segmentierung erfolgt daher unter starker Berücksichtigung der umliegenden Schichten.

Sinnvoll wäre eine Verifizierung der Ergebnisse durch weitere Datensets. Ein Nachteil ist, dass die notwendigen groben Masken für N4ITK erstellt werden müssen. Zur Erstellung der Masken könnte beispielsweise ein Schwellenwert-Verfahren verwendet werden.

Abschließend lässt sich festhalten, dass die in dieser Arbeit erreichte Genauigkeit viel versprechend ist für einen Einsatz in der medizinischen Diagnostik. Darüber hinaus benötigt der Algorithmus im Durchschnitt lediglich eine Rechenzeit von 13.6 s pro Proband auf einer Graphikkarte mit 12 GB und ist somit für eine Anwendung in der Praxis geeignet.

Literaturverzeichnis

1. Ivanovska T, Laqua R, Wang L, et al. A level set based framework for quantitative evaluation of breast tissue density from MRI data. PLOS One. 2014 11;9(11):1–19.
2. Gubern-Merida A, Kallenberg M, Mann RM, et al. Breast segmentation and density estimation in breast MRI: a fully automatic framework. IEEE J Biomed Health Inform. 2015;19(1):349–357.
3. Dalmis MU, Litjens G, Holland K, et al. Using deep learning to segment breast and fibroglandular tissue in MRI volumes. Medical Physics. 2017;44(2):533–546.
4. Ronneberger O, Fischer P, Brox T. U-Net: Convolutional networks for biomedical image Segmentation. Proc MICCAI. 2015;9351:234–241.
5. John U, Hensel E, Lüdemann J, et al. Study of health in pomerania (SHIP): a health examination survey in an east german region: objectives and design. Sozial- und Präventivmedizin. 2001;46(3):186–194.
6. Tustison NJ, Avants BB, Cook PA, et al. N4ITK: Improved N3 bias correction. IEEE Trans Med Imaging. 2010;29(6):1310–1320.

Einfluss nicht-rigider Bildregistrierung auf 4D-Dosissimulation bei extrakranieller SBRT

Nik Mogadas, Thilo Sothmann, René Werner

Department of Computational Neuroscience, University Medical Center
Hamburg-Eppendorf, Hamburg, Germany
nik.mogadas@stud.uke.uni-hamburg.de

Kurzfassung. Das Ziel dieser Studie ist der Vergleich nicht-rigider Open Source-Registrierungsalgorithmen (DIR) in Bezug auf ihre Genauigkeit sowie ihren Einfluss auf korrespondenzmodellbasierte 4D-Dosissimulation bei extrakranieller Strahlentherapie (SBRT). Es wurden drei verbreitete DIR-Algorithmen ausgewählt und mittels der DIRLAB-4D-CT-Datensätze zunächst ihre Registrierungsgenauigkeit evaluiert sowie Korrespondenzmodelle (regressionsbasierte Korrelation von externen Atemsignalmessungen und internen Bewegungsfeldern) generiert und die Modellpräzision analysiert. Unter Verwendung von zehn Strahlentherapie-Planungs-4D-CT-Datensätzen von fünf Leber- und fünf Lungen-Tumorpatienten wurden dann Korrespondenzmodelle gebildet und im Rahmen einer modellbasierten 4D-Dosissimulation zur Abschätzung der Auswirkungen der patientenindividuellen Bewegungen während der Bestrahlung auf die applizierte Dosis eingesetzt. Berechnete Abweichungen zwischen geplanter und 4D-simulierter Dosisverteilung wurden verglichen und mit der Registrierungsgenauigkeit sowie bekannten klinischen Endpunkten (Lokalrezidiv ja/nein) in Beziehung gesetzt.

1 Einleitung

Die stereotaktische Strahlentherapie (SBRT) ist eine effektive Therapieform zur Behandlung von Lungen- und Lebertumoren. Als eine der größten Herausforderungen verbleibt jedoch die Berücksichtigung der atembedingten Tumor- und Risikoorganbewegungen und -verformungen während der Bestrahlungsplanung. In aktuellen klinischen Arbeitsabläufen der 4D-Strahlentherapie wird ein zeitaufgelöstes CT (4D-CT) aufgenommen, um den für die Bestrahlungsplanung relevanten Tumorbewegungsraum (sog. Internal Target Volume, ITV) zu definieren. Eine Integration der 4D-CT- oder weiterer Informationen zu Tumor- und Risikoorganbewegungen in die Dosisberechnung und -optimierung erfolgt mittels sogenannter 4D-Dosisakkumulation bzw. -simulation. Zur Extraktion von Tumor- und Risikoorganbewegungen bzw. -deformationen aus dem 4D-CT-Datensatz werden nicht-rigide Bildregistrierungsalgorithmen (deformable image registration, DIR) eingesetzt. Resultierende Bewegungsfelder zwischen einer vorher definierten Referenzphase und den anderen 4D-CT-Phasen können dann entweder direkt oder unter Verwendung von Bewegungsmodellen [1] zur Deformation der geplanten Dosisverteilungen bzw. -segmenten verwendet werden, um die zu erwartende Dosisverteilung unter Einbeziehung der patientenindividuellen Bewegung abzuschätzen. Die Genauigkeit der 4D-Dosissimulation ist somit von der Genauigkeit der DIR-basierten Bewegungsschätzung abhängig. Dies motiviert wiederum die Untersuchung von DIR-Genauigkeit und DIR-Einfluss auf 4D-Dosissimulationen sowie deren Zusammenspiel. In der vorliegenden Studie wurden drei Open Source- und in der initialen EMPIRE10 Studie [2] gut platzierte DIR-Algorithmen ausgewählt und im Kontext der 4D-Dosissimulation angewandt. Allgemeine DIR-Genauigkeit sowie DIR-basierte Korrespondenzmodell-Genauigkeit wurde mittels der DIRLAB-4D-CT-Daten analysiert [3]. Weiterhin wurde unter Verwendung von realen Patientendatensätzen der Einfluss der DIR-Algorithmen auf die korrespondenzmodellbasierte 4D-Dosissimulation untersucht und DIR-spezifische Resultate mit klinischen Endpunkten (Lokalrezidiv ja/nein) in Beziehung gesetzt. Sowohl die detaillierte Analyse der Auswirkung von DIR-Algorithmen auf 4D-Dosissimulationen als auch der Korrelation der Resultate mit klinischen Endpunkte sind unseres Wissens nach bislang nicht in der Literatur beschrieben worden.

2 Material und Methoden

2.1 DIR-Algorithmen

Für diese Studie wurden drei verbreitete, methodisch jedoch unterschiedliche Open Source-DIR-Algorithmen ausgewählt. Es wurden ein klassischer (Elastix [4]) und ein diffeomorpher B-Spline-basierter Algorithmus (ANTS [5]) sowie ein nicht-parametrisches Verfahren (VarReg [6]) ausgewählt. Zu minimierende Ähnlichkeitsmaße waren normalisierte Kreuzkorrelation (ANTS, Elastix) sowie eine normalisierte Version der Summe der quadrierten Differenzen (VarReg). Die Verfahren zeichneten sich durch gutes Abschneiden in der EMPIRE10-Studie [2] aus; ausgewählte Algorithmenparameter entsprechen den EMPIRE10-Angaben.

2.2 Datenkollektiv

Für die Beschreibung der DIRLAB-4D-CT-Daten sei auf diesbezügliche Publikationen [3] verwiesen. Das hierüber hinaus betrachtete Patientenkollektiv bestand aus zehn mittels volumenmodulierter Bogenbestrahlung (volumetric modulated arc therapy, VMAT) behandelten Lungen- und Lebertumorpatienten mit insgesamt 15 Metastasen (6 Lunge, 9 Leber). Neben einem 10-Phasen-Planungs-4D-CT mit einer Auflösung von $0.98 \times 0.98 \times 2\,mm$ beinhalteten die Datensätze den zugehörigen, nach ITV-Konzept geplanten VMAT-Bestrahlungsplan sowie während der Bestrahlung aufgezeichnete Atemkurven (anterior-posterior (AP)-Komponente des Varian RPM-Systems). Für jede Metastase war bekannt, ob zum Zeitpunkt der Studie bereits ein Lokalrezidiv aufgetreten war.

2.3   Korrespondenzmodellbasierte 4D-Dosissimulation

Ein Korrespondenzmodell repräsentiert einen patientenspezifischen funktionalen Zusammenhang zwischen externen Atemsignalmessungen und Atembewegungen von internen Strukturen (Zielvolumen, Risikoorgane) [1]. In dieser Studie wird ein multivariates lineares Korrespondenzmodell genutzt:

- *Input* 4D-CT-Datensatz, d.h. eine Serie von 3D-CT-Bilddaten $(I_i)_{i \in \{1,...,n_{\mathrm{ph}}\}}$, $I_i : \Omega \subset \mathbb{R}^3 \to \mathbb{R}$ mit $i \in \{1,\dots,n_{\mathrm{ph}}\}$ als Atemphase eines 3D-CT-Datensatzes und n_{ph} als Gesamtanzahl an Atemphasen (hier: $n_{\mathrm{ph}} = 10$). Die Messungen des während des 4D-CT aufgenommenen und zu den Bilddaten zugeordneten Atemsignals sind als $(\zeta_i)_{i \in \{1,...,n_{\mathrm{ph}}\}}$, $\zeta_i = (z_i, \partial_t z_i)^T \in \mathbb{R}^2$ bezeichnet. Hierbei sind z_i und ∂z_i AP-Komponente des Varian RPM-Systems und die zugehörige zeitliche Ableitung.
- *Bewegungsfeldschätzung* Annahme einer Referenzphase (hier: $i_0 = 3$, mittlere Expirationsphase) und zugehöriges 3D-CT-Bild I_{i_0} als DIR-Referenzbild. Der Registrierungsprozess resultiert dann in einer Serie von Transformationen $(\varphi_i)_{i \in \{1,...,n_{\mathrm{ph}}\}}$, $\varphi_i : \Omega \to \Omega$ mit $\varphi_{i_0} = $ id und zugehörigen Bewegungsfeldern $(u_i)_{i \in \{1,...,n_{\mathrm{ph}}\}}$, $u_i : \Omega \to \mathbb{R}^3$ mit $u_i = \varphi_i - id$ (d. h. $u_{i_0} = 0$).
- *Modellbildung mittels multivariater Regression* Die Atemsignalmessungen $(\zeta_i)_{i \in \{1,...,n_{\mathrm{ph}}\}}$ und Bewegungsfelder $(u_i)_{i \in \{1,...,n_{\mathrm{ph}}\}}$ sind die Basis für das Korrespondenzmodelltraining und werden hier als zufällige Variablen $\mathbf{Z}_i$ ($\equiv \zeta_i$) und $\mathbf{U}_i \in \mathbb{R}^{3m}$ mit m als die Voxelanzahl von I_{i_0} interpretiert. Das Korrespondenzmodell ist dann definiert über $\hat{\mathbf{U}} = \overline{\mathbf{U}} + \mathbf{B}\left(\hat{\mathbf{Z}} - \overline{\mathbf{Z}}\right)$. Dabei repräsentiert $\hat{\mathbf{Z}} \in \mathbb{R}^2$ eine Atemsignalbeobachtung und $\hat{\mathbf{U}} \in \mathbb{R}^{3m}$ das korrespondierende und gesuchte interne Bewegungsfeld. Die Koeffizientenmatrix $\mathbf{B} \in \mathbb{R}^{3m \times 2}$ basiert auf den oben genannten Tupeln $(\mathbf{U}_i, \mathbf{Z}_i)$ und wird mittels gewöhnlicher Kleinste-Fehlerquadrate-Regression berechnet.

Die korrespondenzmodellbasierte 4D-Dosissimulation kann unter Verwendung des funktionalen Zusammenhangs zwischen externer und interner Bewegungsdaten folgendermaßen beschrieben werden:

- *4D-Dosissimulation* Mittels der zeitabhängigen Dosisrate $\dot{D} : \Omega \times \mathcal{T} \subset \mathbb{R} \to \mathbb{R}_+$ während der Behandlung kann der dynamische Dosisapplikationsprozess und sein Zusammenspiel mit der Patientenbewegung sowie die resultierende Dosisverteilung $D_{4\mathrm{D}} : \Omega \to \mathbb{R}_+$ als $D_{4\mathrm{D}}(x) = \sum_{t \in \tilde{\mathcal{T}}} D_t(\varphi(x,t))$ beschrieben werden. Hierbei ist $\varphi : \Omega \times \mathcal{T} \to \mathbb{R}^3$ die Position $\varphi(x,t)$ des Voxels $x \in \Omega$ in der CT-Referenzphase I_{i_0} zum Zeitpunkt $t \in \mathcal{T} = [0; T) \subset \mathbb{R}$. Mit $\hat{\varphi} = id + \hat{u}$ und $\hat{\zeta} : \mathcal{T} \to \mathbb{R}^2$ als $\hat{\zeta}$ als im vorliegenden Fall während der Dosisapplikation aufgenommenes Atemsignal ergibt sich die korrespondenzmodellbasierte 4D-Dosissimulation als $D_{4\mathrm{D}}(x) = \sum_{t \in \tilde{\mathcal{T}}} D_t\left(x + \hat{u}\left(x, \hat{\zeta}_t\right)\right)$ mit $\hat{\zeta}_t = \hat{\zeta}(t)$.

2.4   Simulationen und Evaluationsstrategie

Die Registrierungsgenauigkeit der DIR-Algorithmen wurde mittels DIRLAB-4D-CT-Daten landmarkenbasiert evaluiert [3]. Neben der direkten Bestimmung von

Tabelle 1. DIR-basierte Registrierungs- (obere Hälfte) und Korrespondenzmodell-Genauigkeit (untere Hälfte), evaluiert anhand von 10 DIRLAB-4D-CT-Datensätzen.

Algorithmus	TRE, Registrierung (mm)					
	$00 \leftrightarrow 50$	$20 \mapsto 00$	$20 \mapsto 10$	$20 \mapsto 30$	$20 \mapsto 40$	$20 \mapsto 50$
ANTS	2.4 ± 1.3	1.5 ± 0.4	1.6 ± 0.3	1.6 ± 0.4	1.7 ± 0.5	1.9 ± 0.6
VarReg	2.5 ± 1.3	1.3 ± 0.3	1.5 ± 0.3	1.5 ± 0.4	1.7 ± 0.4	1.9 ± 0.4
Elastix	2.6 ± 1.2	1.7 ± 0.7	1.7 ± 0.5	1.6 ± 0.5	1.9 ± 0.7	2.2 ± 1.0
Ohne Reg.	8.5 ± 3.3	4.4 ± 1.4	3.2 ± 1.1	2.5 ± 1.1	3.9 ± 1.8	4.9 ± 2.4
	TRE, LOO Ansatz $20 \mapsto n$ (mm)					
	$\varnothing_n$	$n = 00$	$n = 10$	$n = 30$	$n = 40$	$n = 50$
ANTS	3.0 ± 0.8	2.9 ± 1.5	2.1 ± 0.7	2.7 ± 1.4	3.4 ± 2.1	3.9 ± 2.6
VarReg	2.0 ± 0.3	2.0 ± 0.9	2.0 ± 0.5	1.9 ± 0.6	2.1 ± 0.8	2.2 ± 0.7
Elastix	2.2 ± 0.4	2.2 ± 1.1	2.2 ± 0.6	1.9 ± 0.7	2.2 ± 1.0	2.4 ± 1.0

landmarkenbasierten Registrierungsfehlern (target registration errors, TRE) für die Registrierung von maximaler Inspirations- (Phase 00) zur maximalen Expirationsphase (Phase 50) wurde die DIR-Genauigkeit zwischen korrespondenzmodellbasierter Referenzphase und verbleibenden Phasen überprüft. Die Genauigkeit der DIR-spezifisch generierten Korrespondenzmodelle wurde mittels LOO (leave one phase out)-Ansatz analysiert. Basierend auf den 10 Patientendatensätzen wurden dann korrespondenzmodellbasierte 4D-Dosissimulationen für jeden ausgewählten DIR-Algorithmus durchgeführt. Der Vergleich zwischen geplanter und simulierter Dosisverteilung fand anhand von $\Delta D_{95} = D_{95,\text{Sim}} - D_{95,\text{Plan}}$ statt, mit D_{95} als der Dosis die 95% des Zielvolumens erhält.

3 Ergebnisse

3.1 DIRLAB-basierte Analyse der DIR-Genauigkeit

Die Registrierung der Extremphasen $00 \leftrightarrow 50$ sowie der Registrierung von Referenzphase 20 (= mittlere Expiration) auf verbleibende Phasen ergibt ähnliche TRE-Werte für die drei DIR-Algorithmen, siehe obere Hälfte von Tabelle 1. Der Vergleich zu Landmarkendistanzen vor Registrierung (Tab. 1, ohne Reg.) zeigt eine deutliche Verbesserung im Vergleich zum Ausgangszustand.

Für die LOO-Analyse nach Korrespondenzmodellbildung ergeben sich für VarReg und Elastix ähnlich niedrige TRE-Werte. Für ANTS werden die Fehler des Korrespondenzmodells vor allem bei weiter von der Referenzphase entfernten Phasen im Vergleich zur ursprünglichen Registrierung jedoch deutlich größer (vgl. untere Hälfte von Tab. 1).

3.2 Korrespondenzmodellbasierte 4D-Dosissimulation

Der Vergleich der für jeden Patientendatensatz und DIR-Algorithmus durchgeführten korrespondenzmodellbasierten 4D-Dosissimulation illustriert den Einfluss der Registrierungsansätze auf resultierende Dosisverteilungen. Berechnete

Tabelle 2. Vergleich von geplanter und simulierter 4D-Dosisverteilung über den Parameter ΔD_{95} für alle Metastasen/DIR-Algorithmen. * = Metastase mit Lokalrezidiv.

| Met. | $\Delta D_{95} = D_{95,4D\text{-sim}} - D_{95,Plan}$ (Gy) | | |
	ANTS	VarReg	Elastix
Lunge			
1	+0.47	+0.45	+0.44
2.1/2.2*	−0.13/−0.28	−0.12/−0.30	+0.02/−0.02
3	+0.35	+0.39	+0.26
4*	−0.51	−0.52	−0.56
5	−0.09	−0.06	−0.09
Leber			
6*	−2.73	−2.65	−8.40
7.1/7.2/7.3	−0.49/+0.17/+0.26	−0.47/+0.17/+0.32	−1.57/−3.40/+0.24
8.1/8.2/8.3*	+0.14/+0.17/−12.21	+0.12/+0.11/−13.17	+0.13/+0.20/−26.49
9	−0.43	−0.30	−1.48
10	−0.69	−0.85	−0.96

ΔD_{95}-Werte für die Lungenmetastasen (vgl. obere Hälfte von Tab. 2) weisen kaum Unterschiede zwischen den Algorithmen auf. Negative ΔD_{95}-Werte für Metastase 4 deuten auf eine mögliche Unterdosierungen während der Bestrahlung hin, die zum Teil das aufgetretene Lokalrezidiv erklären könnte.

Bei den Ergebnissen für die Lebermetastasen werden jedoch DIR-spezifische Unterschiede deutlich. Während ANTS und VarReg wieder ähnliche Resultate zeigen, unterscheiden sich für die Metastasen 6, 7.1/7.2, 8.3 und 9 die ΔD_{95}-Werte von etwa 1 Gy bis zu 13 Gy zwischen ANTS/VarReg und Elastix (vgl. untere Hälfte von Tab. 2). Zur Visualisierung dieser Differenzen sind in Abbildung 1, beispielhaft für Metastase 6, Bewegungsfelder und simulierte Dosisverteilungen dargestellt. Elastix zeigt, relativ zu ANTS/VarReg, starke Bewegungen in der superior-inferior-Achse. Folglich wird mittels Elastix ein wesentlicher stärkerer Bewegungseinfluss auf die applizierte Dosis berechnet. Da für Metastasen 6 und 8.3 jedoch sämtliche Verfahren in negativen ΔD_{95}-Werten resultieren, bleibt unklar, welches Verfahren die Realität am Besten repräsentiert. Anders als ANTS und VarReg führt Elastix jedoch auch für Metastasen 7.1 und 7.2 zu deutlichen negativen ΔD_{95}-Werten; ein Lokalrezidiv wurde jedoch bislang nicht beobachtet.

4   Diskussion

Die vorgestellte Studie untersucht den Einfluss von nicht-rigiden Bildregistrierungen auf die 4D-Dosissimulation für Lungen- und Lebermetastasen. Ergebnisse der DIRLAB-basierten DIR-Genauigkeitsanalyse lassen die Aussage zu, dass eine hohe DIR-Genauigkeit nicht zwangsläufig mit niedrigen TRE-Werten der DIR-basierten Korrespondenzmodelle einhergeht (vgl. Resultate für ANTS). Unterschiede in der Genauigkeit der Korrespondenzmodelle führen jedoch wiederum nicht zwangsläufig zu relevanten Unterschieden der abgeschätzten bewegungsbe-

Abb. 1. Visualisierung der geschätzten Bewegungsfelder zwischen Phasen 50 und 20 sowie simulierter bewegungsbeeinflusster Dosisverteilungen für Metastase 6.

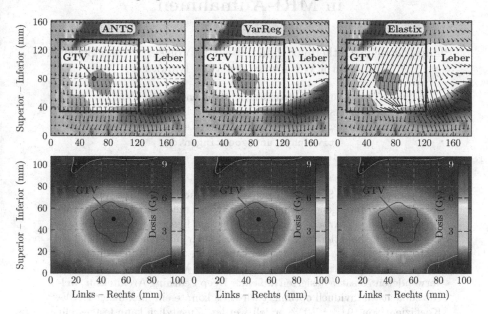

einflussten Dosisverteilungen. Dies wird insbesondere für die betrachteten Lungenmetastasen deutlich. Unterschiede der berechneten Bewegungsfelder sowie der ΔD_{95}-Werte für Lebermetastasen (Abb. 1) illustrieren jedoch Unsicherheiten bei der Anwendung rein intensitätsbasierter DIR-Algorithmen in kontrastarmen Bildbereichen wie der Leber; als Folge verbleiben weiter zu untersuchende Unsicherheiten im Kontext DIR- und modellbasierter 4D-Dosissimulationen.

Literaturverzeichnis

1. McClelland JR, Hawkes DJ, Schaeffter T, et al. Respiratory motion models: a review. Med Image Anal. 2013;17:19–42.
2. Murphy K, van Ginneken B, Reinhardt JM, et al. Evaluation of registration methods on thoracic CT: the EMPIRE10 challenge. IEEE Trans Med Imaging. 2011;30:1901–1920.
3. Castillo R, Castillo E, Guerra R, et al. A framework for evaluation of deformable image registration spatial accuracy using large landmark point sets. Phys Med Biol. 2009;54:1849–1870.
4. Klein S, Staring M, Murphy K, et al. Elastix: a toolbox for intensity-based medical image registration. IEEE Trans Med Imaging. 2010;29:196–205.
5. Tustison NJ, Cook PA, Klein A, et al. Large-scale evaluation of ANTs and FreeSurfer cortical thickness measurements. Neuroimage. 2014;99:166–179.
6. Werner R, Schmidt-Richberg A, Handels H, et al. Estimation of lung motion fields in 4D CT data by variational non-linear intensity-based registration: A comparison and evaluation study. Phys Med Biol. 2014;59:4247–4260.

Effiziente Segmentierung trachealer Strukturen in MRI-Aufnahmen

Philip Dietrich[1], Catherine Schmidt[2], Henry Völzke[2], Achim Beule[2,3],
Florentin Wörgötter[1], Tatyana Ivanovska[1]

[1]Georg-August-Universität Göttingen, Deutschland
[2]Universitätsklinikum Greifswald, Deutschland
[3]Universitätsklinikum Münster, Deutschland
tiva@phys.uni-goettingen.de

Kurzfassung. Die Segmentierung verschiedener Strukturen im Körper
ist eine der grundlegenden Operationen in der medizinischen Bildverarbeitung. In dieser Arbeit werden auf Machine Learning basierende Methoden zur Segmentierung medizinischer Bilder untersucht. Das Ziel ist
es, in MRI-Scans die Trachea zu segmentieren. Jedoch soll in dieser Arbeit speziell die Effizienz der Algorithmen im Vordergrund stehen. Die
verwendeten Ansätze basierten auf einer Deep Learning Architektur, welche zunächst individuell optimiert wird. Es konnte ein maximaler DICE-
Koeffizient von $(94.4 \pm 2.1)\%$ erzielt werden. Zusätzlich kann festgestellt
werden, dass die Segmentierung sehr effizient geschieht. Die Segmentierung von einmen Datensatz aus 40 Schichten dauert dabei weniger als
eine Sekunde, wobei bei bisherigen Methoden es über eine Minute benötigte.

1 Einleitung

Die Segmentierung medizinischer Bilddaten ist ein zentrales Problem der medizinischen Bildanalyse. Sie ist für die computergestützte ärztliche Diagnostik
und Therapie von besonderer Bedeutung, da sie die Grundlage für eine weiter-
gehende Analyse, Vermessung und 3D-Visualisierung medizinischer Bildobjekte
bildet [1].

In diesem Bereich konnten zuletzt mit Hilfe des Maschinellen Lernens große
Fortschritte erzielt werden. In den letzten Jahren brachten Neuronale Netzwerke
deutliche Verbesserungen im Bereich der Bildverarbeitung [2]. Speziell die sogenannten Convolutional Neural Networks konnten klassische Methoden deutlich
überbieten (zum Beispiel [3]). Im Bereich der Segmentierung wurden auch signi-
fikante Verbesserungen erzielt, wie z. B., durch die Methode von Ronneberger et
al. [4].

Die Untersuchung der Trachea in MRI-Aufnahmen spielt speziell bei Patien-
ten mit einem inspiratorischen Stridor eine große Rolle. Hierzu ist es nötig die
Trachea in den entschprechenden Aufnahmen zu segmentieren. Es gibt einige
Verfahren für automatische und semi-automatische Segmentierung der oberen
Atemwege. Ivanovska et al. entwickelte hierfür einen Algorithmus, welcher auf

Die Original-Version des Kapitels wurde korrigiert. Ein Erratum finden Sie unter
https://doi.org/10.1007/978-3-662-56537-7_97

Clustering-Methoden und Graph-Cuts basierte [5]. Shahid et al. [6] präsentierte einen Ansatz für Segmentierung von Pharynx und Fat Pads. Seifert et al. [7] schlug eine kombinierte Methode vor, um die Trachea und Wirbelsäule zu extrahieren. Das Problem von allen klassischen Ansätze ist allerdings in der fehlenden Effizienz. Die Segmentierung von einem MRI Datensatz benötigte damit über eine Minute und die Genauigket lag ung. bei $90-91\%$. Zu unserem Wissen wurde noch keine Deep Learning Methode bei der Trachea Segmentierung angewendet.

Das Ziel dieser Arbeit ist einen effizienten Deep Learning Algorithmus zur Segmentierung der Trachea in MRI-Aufnahmen zu finden.

2 Material und Methoden

2.1 Der Datensatz

Der Datensatz ist als Teil der Study of Health in Pomerania (SHIP) [8] aufgenommen worden. Sie wurde im Raum Vorpommern durchgeführt und dient der allgemeinen Untersuchung von Gesundheitsfaktoren und Risiken. Bei den verwendeten Daten handelt es sich um Aufnahmen aus MRT-Scans mit einem 1.5 Tesla MRT-Gerät (Magnetom Avanto, Siemens Medical Solutions, Erlangen, Deutschland). Ein einzelner Scan besteht aus 40 Bildern, welche jeweils mit 256×256 Pixeln aufgelöst sind. Speziell im unteren Bereich der Scans sind aufgrund der Atemluft der Patienten starke Artefakte zu erkennen, welche die Segmentierung deutlich erschweren.

Insgesamt wurden 110 Datensätze, entsprechend 110 Probanden, von den HNO-Experten manuell segmentiert.

2.2 Vorverarbeitungsmethoden

Die Vorverarbeitung lässt sich in drei Schritte gliedern. Das Ziel des ersten Schrittes ist das Entfernen von Rauschen in den Bildern. Hierzu wurde ein anisotroper Diffusionsfilter verwendet [1]. Danach wird eine Histogramäqulisation angewendet [1]. In Abb. 1 sind die einzelnen Schritte der Vorverarbeitung an einem Beispiel dargestellt.

Im Anschluss werden die Grauwerte der einzelnen Bilder noch normalisiert. Das heißt, es wird jeweils der Mittelwert subtrahiert und durch die Standardabweichung geteilt, sodass die Grauwerte einer Normalverteilung folgen.

2.3 Die U-Net Architektur

Die folgende Netzwerkarchitektur wurde von Ronneberger et al. vorgeschlagen [4]. Aufgrund seiner Form in dieser Darstellung wird es als U-Net bezeichnet. Hier haben wir die Architektur in der ursprünglichen Form [4] verwendet.

Ein U-Net lässt sich in die typische Encoder-Decoder-Struktur unterteilen. Im ersten Teil des Netzwerks wird die Größe der Aktivierungen immer weiter verkleinert, wobei die Anzahl der Filter der Convolutional Layer jeweils nach einem Verkleinerungsschritt verdoppelt wird.

Im zweiten Teil des Netzwerks wird mittels Up-Sampling die Größe der Aktivierungen wieder erhöht, wobei durch Halbierung der Filter die Tiefe jeweils verringert wird. Um die entgültige Segmentierungsmasken zu erhalten wird die Ausgabe des Netzwerkes noch mittels eines Thresholds binarisiert, dieser Wert wurde auf 0.5 festgesetzt.

3 Ergebnisse

Die Segmentierungen werden mit Hilfe des DICE-Koeffizienten ausgewertet, wobei die manuallen Segmentierungen von HNO Experten bereitgestellt wurden. Das Training Set besteht aus 101 MRT Datensätzen, von welchen 20% randomisiert zur Validierung verwendet wurden, um die Hyperparameter des Models zu optimieren. Das Test Set besteht aus neun Datensätzen, welche zufällig aus dem gesamten Datensatz gewählt wurden.

Dieser lässt sich mit Hilfe von True Positives TP, False Positives FP und False Negatives FN schreiben als

$$\text{DICE} = \frac{2\text{TP}}{2\text{TP} + \text{FP} + \text{FN}} \tag{1}$$

In den durchgeführten Experimenten wurden neben den Parametern für Diffusionsfilter und Datenerweiterungsmethoden auch die Netzwerkarchitektur auf verschiedene Weisen variiert. Einerseits wurden die Anzahl und Größe der Filter optimiert und andererseits die Verwendung von Dropout und Batch Normalisierung getestet. Hierbei konnte festgestellt werden, dass die Anzahl von 64 Filtern in der ersten Ebene des Netzwerkes, wie sie von der originalen U-Net-Architektur [4] verwendet wird, hier zu einer zu komplexen Architektur führte. Dies zeigte sich in starkem overfitting. Speziell die Verwendung von Batch Normalisierung war in diesem Fall nicht mehr sinnvoll, da die Batches aufgrund der gegebenen Speicherlimitierung nur noch zu wenige Beispiele enthielten [9].

Original	Anisotroper Diffusionsfilter	Histogramäqualisation
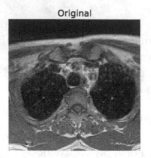	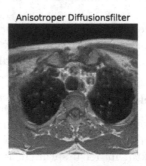	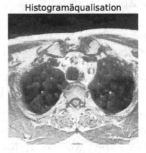

Abb. 1. Die einzelnen Vorverarbeitungsschritte am Beispiel: links das originale Bild, mittig das Bild nach der Anwendung des Diffusionsfilters, und rechts nach Histogramäqualisation.

Tabelle 1. Ergebnisse auf dem Testdatensatz für verschiedene Größen und Anzahlen an Filtern. Das Netzwerk wurde ohne Dropout trainiert.

Filteranzahl	8	8	16	16
Filtergröße	3	5	3	5
DICE [%]	93.3 ± 1.6	92.5 ± 2.8	93.9 ± 2.2	93.4 ± 2.0

Die Ergebnisse auf einem unabhängigen Testdatensatz aus 360 Bildern sind in Tab. 1 zusammengetragen. Der DICE-Koeffizient ist dabei jeweils als Mittelwert und Standardabweichung über die verschiedenen Scans angegeben. Die Verwendung von Dropout konnte nur in einem kleinen Bereich von Wahrscheinlichkeiten das overfitting vermindern (Abb. 3). Dieser Bereich lag bei etwa 0.2.

Zusätzlich sollen hier auch noch die Laufzeiten der Netzwerke untersucht werden. Diese teilen sich auf die Vorverarbeitung der Bilder und die eigentliche Segmentierung auf. Die Vorhersagen der Netzwerke wurden dabei auf einer Nvidia Titan X GPU gemacht. Als Zeit für die Vorverarbeitung ergaben sich auf einem Cluster mit 12 × Intel(R) Core(TM) i7 CPU @ 3.33 GHz 23 Gb DDR4 durchschnittlich 0.38 s. Die Segmentierungen benötigten 0.24 s bei 8 Filtern beziehungsweise 0.39 s bei 16 Filtern in der ersten Schicht des Netzwerkes. Als gesamte Laufzeit des Algorithmus ergab sich also bei der Konfiguration, welche den höchsten DICE-Koeffizienten erzielte 0.77 s.

4 Diskussion

In Abb. 2 sind exemplarisch zwei Segmentierungen, wie sie vom U-Net erzeugt wurden gezeigt. Bei der Betrachtung aller Segmentierungen fällt auf, dass im oberen, sowie im unteren Bereich der Trachea, verglichen mit den mittleren Bereichen etwas schlechtere Ergebnisse erzielt werden. Dies lässt sich einerseits dadurch begründen, dass im unteren Bereich der Scans besonders starkes Rauschen vorkommt, was die Segmentierung deutlich erschwert. Das zweite Problem, welches mehrfach zu beobachten war, liegt darin, dass Flächen auf Bildern in denen die Trachea bereits nicht mehr zu sehen war, nicht als solche erkannt wurden. Speziell im Bereich knapp oberhalb der Trachea trat dieses Problem auf.

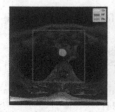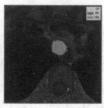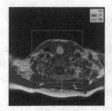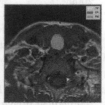

Abb. 2. Exemplarische Darstellung automatischer Segmentierungen, wobei jeweils True Positives, False Positives und False Negatives markiert wurden im unteren (links) und im oberen Bereich (rechts) der Trachea

198   Dietrich et al.

Abb. 3. Darstellung der Trainingskurven des DICE 2D -Koeffizienten (für die Trainings-Daten in blau, für die Validation-Daten in grün) in Abhängigkeit der verwendeten Dropoutrate für ein U-Net mit 16 Filtern in der ersten Ebene. Links: Dropout 0.0, Rechts: Dropout 0.2.

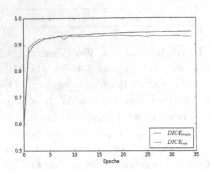 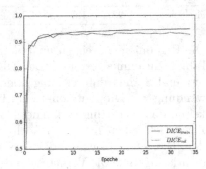

Zur Vermeidung von overfitting wurde außerdem die Verwendung von Batch Normalisierung und Dropout variiert. Hierbei konnte festgestellt werden, dass Batch Normalisierung sich dazu sehr gut eignet, sobald die Batches eine ausreichende Größe besitzen (in diesem Fall 16 Bilder). Hier wurde ein maximaler DICE-Koeffizient von $(94.4 \pm 2.1)\%$ auf den Testdaten erzielt. Jedoch ist zu erkennen, dass die Unterschiede zwischen einem Netzwerk mit Dropout (0.2) und einem Netzwerk ohne Dropout nur sehr gering sind. Zu erklären ist dies damit, dass bei der geringen Anzahl an verwendeten Filtern das overfitting nur eine sehr kleine Rolle spielt. Eine weitere Erhöhung der Dropout-Rate verschlechterte das Ergebnis wieder (Abb. 3).

Es konnte gezeigt werden, dass die Segmentierung der Trachea in MRI-Aufnahmen mittels klassischer Methoden, wie z.B. von Ivanovska et al. [5], durch CNNs deutlich verbessert (94% vs 90%) werden konnte. Die Laufzeit für eine Segmentierung konnte dabei auf unter eine Sekunde reduziert werden.

Literaturverzeichnis

1. Handels H. Segmentierung medizinischer Bilddaten. Wiesbaden: Vieweg+Teubner; 2009.
2. Simonyan K, Zisserman A. Very deep convolutional networks for large-scale image recognition. arXiv preprint arXiv:14091556. 2014.
3. Krizhevsky A, Sutskever I, Hinton GE. Imagenet classification with deep convolutional neural networks. Advances in neural information processing systems. 2012; p. 1097–1105.
4. Ronneberger O, Fischer P, Brox T; Springer. U-net: Convolutional networks for biomedical image segmentation. Proc MICCAI. 2015; p. 234–241.
5. Ivanovska T, Buttke E, Laqua R, et al. Automatic trachea segmentation and evaluation from MRI data using intensity pre-clustering and graph cuts. Proc IEEE ISPA. 2011; p. 513–518.

6. Shahid MLUR, Chitiboi T, Ivanovska T, et al. Automatic MRI segmentation of para-pharyngeal fat pads using interactive visual feature space analysis for classification. BMC Med Imag. 2017;17(1):15.
7. Seifert S, Wachter I, Dillmann R. Segmentation of intervertebral discs, trachea and spinal cord from MRI images. Proc CARS. 2006.
8. Voelzke H, Alte D, Schmidt CO, et al. Cohort profile: the study of health in Pomerania. Int J Epid. 2011;40(2):294.
9. Ioffe S. Batch renormalization: towards reducing minibatch dependence in batch-normalized models. arXiv preprint arXiv:170203275. 2017.

Abstract: Populationsbasierte 4D Bewegungsatlanten für VR Simulationen

Andre Mastmeyer, Matthias Wilms, Heinz Handels

Institut für Medizinische Informatik, Universität zu Lübeck
mastmeyer@imi.uni-luebeck.de

Atembewegte Avatare können in einem kürzlich vorgestellten visuo-haptischen Virtual Reality (VR) 4D-Simulatorkonzept modelliert [1] und GPU-basiert dargestellt [2] werden. Nadelinterventionsimulationen im hepatischen Bereich mit atmenden virtuellen Patientenkörpern sind aktuell ohne die patientenspezifische, dosisrelevante 4D-Datenerfassung nicht durchführbar. Hierbei kann ein populationsbasierter Ansatz zur Modellierung eines gemittelten, übertragbaren (4D-Atembewegungsatlas) abhelfen und die Risiken einer dosisrelevanten und teuren Erfassung eines 4D-Datensatzes mindern [3]. Diese Modelle können durch nichtlineare Registrierung auf den statischen und zu animierenden 3D-CT-Datensatz eines neuen Patienten übertragen werden [3].

Die Atmungsmodellierung mit einem linearen Vektorfeldregressionsmodell basiert auf einer Menge von 4D-CT-Datensätzen mit 3D-Atemphasenbildern und einem Spirometriesignal mit einer Hysteresesignalkomponente. Intrapatient-Interphasen-Bildregistrierungen zu einer ausgewählten patientenspezifischen Referenzphase (z.B. der maximalen Einatmung) bilden den ersten Arbeitspunkt eines Dreischritts, der in einem personalisierten Atemmodell resultiert.

Der nächste Schritt ist die Mittelung der personalisierten Atmungsmodelle. Für einen gemeinsamen Referenzrahmen wird die Atemphase bspw. der maximalen Einatmung eines Referenzpatienten ausgewählt. Dieser Rahmen ist das Ziel von Interpatientenregistrierungen der gewählten Referenzphasen. Mit den in den gleichen gemeinsamen Bezugsrahmen transformierten Bewegungsinformationen ergibt ein Mittelungsprozess das Gruppenintensitäts- und -bewegungsmodell.

Schliesslich wird das mittlere 4D-Patientenatmungsmodells durch eine personalisierende Interpatientenregistrierung auf neue 3D-Patientendaten transformiert. Diese müssen lediglich dosis- und kostensparend als 3D-CT-Datensatz in Referenzatemlage aufgenommen worden sein und können im 4D-VR-Simulator visuo-haptisch animiert [2] werden[1].

Literaturverzeichnis

1. Mastmeyer A, et al. Efficient patient modeling for visuo-haptic VR simulation using a generic patient atlas. Comp Meth Prog Biomed. 2016;132:161–175.
2. Fortmeier D, et al. Direct visuo-haptic 4D volume rendering using respiratory motion models. IEEE Trans Haptics. 2015;8(4):371–383.
3. Mastmeyer A, et al. Population-based respiratory 4D motion atlas construction and its application for VR simulations of liver punctures. Proc SPIE. 2018; p. accepted.

---

[1] VR-Simulation: 4D Intensitäts- und Atembewegungsatlas: https://goo.gl/Qog138

Abstract: Rekonstruktion der initialen Druckverteilung photoakustischer Bilder mit limitiertem Blickwinkel durch maschinelle Lernverfahren

Dominik Waibel[1,3], Janek Gröhl[1,4], Fabian Isensee[2], Klaus H. Maier-Hein[2,4], Lena Maier-Hein[1,4]

[1]Abteilung Computer-assistierte Medizinische Interventionen, Deutsches Krebsforschungszentrum (DKFZ), Heidelberg
[2]Abteilung Medizinische Bildverarbeitung, Deutsches Krebsforschungszentrum (DKFZ), Heidelberg
[3]Fakultät für Physik und Astronomie, Universität Heidelberg
[4]Medizinische Fakultät, Universität Heidelberg
d.waibel@dkfz-heidelberg.de

Die Rekonstruktion von Bildern aus unvollständigen Rohdaten ist eine fundamentale Herausforderung in der medizinischen Bildgebung. Dies gilt insbesondere auch für die Photoakustik, einer neuartigen Bildgebungstechnik, welche auf dem photoakustischen Effekt basiert, bei dem durch die Absorption von Photonen aus Laserpulsen im Gewebe Schallwellen ausgelöst werden. Durch den optischen Kontrast der Photoakustik können funktionale Parameter - wie die Blutsauerstoffsättigung - hoch aufgelöst und tief im Gewebe gemessen werden.

Anders als bei der Computer- oder Magnetresonanztomographie ist ein 360 Grad Scan in der Photoakustik aufgrund von physikalischen Limitationen außerhalb der Kleintierbildgebung nicht möglich. Stattdessen werden Bilder, ähnlich wie bei der Ultraschallbildgebung, in Abhängigkeit der Geometrie der verwendeten Sonde, aus einem eingeschränkten Winkelbereich rekonstruiert. Dies lässt keine akkurate Rekonstruktion der initialen Druckverteilung zu, da die Schallwellen nur unvollständig gemessen werden. Derzeit werden zur Bildrekonstruktion sogenannte Beamformingalgorithmen, welche für konventionelle Ultraschallsonden entwickelt wurden, auch für Photoakustiksysteme genutzt. Sie können zwar Informationen über die zugrundeliegende initiale Druckverteilung rekonstruieren, liefern jedoch keine quantitativen Resultate.

In diesem Beitrag präsentieren wir einen Ansatz zur photoakustischen Bildrekonstruktion, der ein maschinelles Lernverfahren zur Rekonstruktion der initialen Druckverteilung aus Ultraschalldaten mit einem eingeschränkten Winkelbereich nutzt. Hierzu verwenden wir eine U-Net Deep Learning Architektur, welche auf in silico Daten trainiert und mit Phantomdaten validiert wird. Die Erzeugung der Trainingsdatenbasis erfolgt durch Monte Carlo Simulationen. Erste Ergebnisse zeigen eine genauere Rekonstruktion der initialen Druckverteilung gegenüber etablierten Rekonstruktionsalgorithmen in silico und eine qualitative Verbesserung bei der Rekonstruktion von in vitro Daten.

Abstract: Erweiterung des Bildgebungsbereiches bei der Magnetpartikelbildgebung durch externe axiale Verschiebungen

Patryk Szwargulski[1,2], Nadine Gdaniec[1,2], Matthias Graeser[1,2], Martin Möddel[1,2], Florian Griese[1,2], Tobias Knopp[1,2]

[1] Abteilung für Biomedizinische Bildgebung, Universitätsklinikum Hamburg-Eppendorf
[2] Institut für Biomedizinische Bildgebung, Technische Universität Hamburg
p.szwargulski@uke.de

Die Magnetpartikelbildgebung (engl. Magnetic-Particle-Imaging, MPI) ist eine Bildgebungsmodalität, die auf der Darstellung super-paramagnetischer Nanopartikeln unter Verwendung von statischen und dynamischen Magnetfeldern basiert [1]. Das Bildgebungsverfahren weist eine hohe zeitliche Auflösung von über 40 Volumen pro Sekunde auf und ist mit einer Detektionsgrenze von 5 ng Eisen [2] ein höchst sensitives Verfahren, mit dem viele medizinische Applikationen adressiert werden können. Als Einschränkung ist der, aus Sicherheitsgründen [3] auf wenige Kubikcentimeter beschränkte, Bildgebungsbereich zu nennen. Um diese Limitierung zu umgehen, können zusätzliche Felder geschaltet und/oder das Objekt mithilfe einer externen Verschiebung durch den Bildgebungsbereich bewegt werden. Im Rahmen dieser Arbeit wurde ein Rekonstruktionsverfahren entwickelt, welches sowohl bei statischen als auch bei dynamischen Objekten genutzt werden kann und die Rohdaten in der Form bearbeitet, dass der Messfeldverschub berücksichtigt wird. Mit der entwickelten Methode konnten sowohl statische 3D Phantomdaten als auch *in-vivo* Messdaten eines dynamischen Mausexperimentes (3D+t) erfolgreich rekonstruiert werden [4].

Literaturverzeichnis

1. Gleich B, Weizenecker J. Tomographic imaging using the nonlinear response of magnetic particles. Nature. 2005;435(7046):1214 – 1217.
2. Graeser M, Knopp T, Szwargulski P, et al. Towards picogram detection of superparamagnetic iron-oxide particles using a gradiometric receive coil. Sci Rep. 2017;7:6872.
3. Saritas EU, Goodwill PW, Zhang GZ, et al. Magnetostimulation limits in magnetic particle imaging. IEEE Trans Med Imaging. 2013;32(9):1600 – 1610.
4. Szwargulski P, Gdaniec N, Graeser M, et al. Enlarging the field of view in magnetic particle imaging using a moving table approach. Proc SPIE. 2017; p. 10578–51.

Abstract: Random-Forest-basierte Segmentierung der subkutanen Fettschicht der Mäusehaut in 3D-OCT-Bilddaten

Timo Kepp[1], Christine Droigk[1], Malte Casper[2,3], Michael Evers[2,3], Nunciada Salma[3], Dieter Manstein[3], Heinz Handels[1]

[1]Institut für Medizinische Informatik, Universität zu Lübeck
[2]Institut für Biomedizinische Optik, Universität zu Lübeck
[3]Cutaneous Biology Research Center, Massachusetts General Hospital, Boston, MA
kepp@imi.uni-luebeck.de

Die Kryolipolyse ist ein nichtinvasives kosmetisches Verfahren zur lokalen Fettreduktion [1], bei der durch kontrollierte Kühlung selektiv subkutane Fettzellen zerstört werden. Für eine quantitative Evaluation des Verfahrens soll die subkutane Fettschicht in Mäusen segmentiert werden. Für eine Darstellung der Mäusehaut wurde die Optische Kohärenztomographie (OCT) als Bildmodalität genutzt, die eine detaillierte Aufnahme der subkutanen Fettschicht in Mikrometer-Auflösung ermöglicht. Aufgrund der großen Datenmenge ist eine manuelle Segmentierung der Daten nicht durchführbar. Daher präsentieren wir in diesem Beitrag einen Ansatz für die automatische Segmentierung der subkutanen Fettschicht der Mäusehaut in 3D-OCT-Bilddaten [2]. Hierzu verwenden wir einen Random Forest (RF), der auf manuell segmentierten B-Scans trainiert wird. Die für den RF ausgewählten Merkmale basieren sowohl auf Bildintensitäten sowie auf Kanteninformationen. Des Weiteren werden dem Merkmalsvektor Deskriptoren hinzugefügt, um Umgebungsinformationen zu integrieren. Die Berechnung der Merkmale wird sowohl global als auch lokal in der näheren Nachbarschaft durchgeführt. Im Anschluss an die RF-Segmentierung verwenden wir den graphenbasierten Ansatz aus [3], um die Segmentierung des RF zu optimieren. Für die Bewertung unseres Ansatzes führen wir eine Leave-One-Out-Evaluation durch. Hierbei wird ein mittlerer Dice-Koeffizient von $0.921 \pm 0.045\,\mu m$ und eine mittlere symmetrische Oberflächendistanz von $11.80 \pm 6.05\,\mu m$ erreicht. Darüber hinaus konnte gezeigt werden, dass die graphenbasierte Optimierung eine erhöhte räumliche Konsistenz und Genauigkeit gewährleistet.

Literaturverzeichnis

1. Manstein D, Laubach H, Watanabe K, et al. Selective cryolysis: a novel method of non-invasive fat removal. Laser Surg Med. 2008;40(9):595–604.
2. Kepp T, Droigk C, Casper M, et al. Segmentation of subcutaneous fat within mouse skin in 3D OCT image data using random forests. In: Proc SPIE; 2018. Accepted.
3. Li K, Wu X, Chen DZ, et al. Optimal surface segmentation in volumetric images - a graph-theoretic approach. IEEE Trans Pattern Anal Mach Intell. 2006;28(1):119–131.

Towards Whole-body CT Bone Segmentation

André Klein[1,2], Jan Warszawski[2], Jens Hillengaß[3], Klaus H. Maier-Hein[1]

[1]Division of Medical Image Computing, Deutsches Krebsforschungszentrum (DKFZ)
[2]Medical Faculty, University of Heidelberg
[3]Section Multiple Myeloma, Department of Hematology, Oncology and Rheumatology, University of Heidelberg
andre.klein@dkfz-heidelberg.de

Abstract. Bone segmentation from CT images is a task that has been worked on for decades. It is an important ingredient to several diagnostics or treatment planning approaches and relevant to various diseases. As high-quality manual and semi-automatic bone segmentation is very time-consuming, a reliable and fully automatic approach would be of great interest in many scenarios. In this publication, we propose a U-Net inspired architecture to address the task using Deep Learning. We evaluated the approach on whole-body CT scans of patients suffering from multiple myeloma. As the disease decomposes the bone, an accurate segmentation is of utmost importance for the evaluation of bone density, disease staging and localization of focal lesions. The method was evaluated on an in-house data-set of 6000 2D image slices taken from 15 whole-body CT scans, achieving a dice score of 0.96 and an IOU of 0.94.

1 Introduction

Fast and accurate automatic bone segmentation is important for analysis, staging and treatment planning of various diseases like multiple myeloma. Despite several years of research, it is still a significant challenge in some aspects [1] caused by the inhomogeneous structure and various shapes of bones and the fact that CT scans in clinical routine are often captured with a low dose which leads to inferior image quality.

Bones can be assigned to four different categories based on their shape: long bones, short bones, flat bones, and irregular bones [2]. As shown in Fig. 1 bones are composes of three different tissue types: cortical (compact) bone, cancellous (trabecular, spongy) bone and bone marrow. The cortical bone is the most dense and solid part with high Hounsfield Units (HU), surrounding the bone marrow compartment [2]. Because of the variation in density, the different types of bone have huge differences in HU. Cancellous bone and bone marrow are less dense, with HU being more similar to those of soft tissue like muscles. Pathological changes in the bone, e.g., caused by multiple myeloma can influence the density and therefore the HU of bone tissue [3].

The gold standard for bone segmentation is still semi-automated slice-by-slice hand contouring, which is very time-consuming [4]. Fully automatic bone

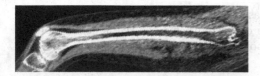

Fig. 1. CT scan of the femur. Cortical bone appears white and surrounds the less dense cancellous bone and the bone marrow.

segmentation has therefore been of great interest to research for a long time. Numerous studies can be found in literature addressing the issue, as described by Pinheiro et al. [5] and Buie et al. [5]. In the large number of studies, a lot of different approaches were proposed. Yet, bone segmentation is still considered an open problem in several aspects [1].

Some authors consider bone segmentation as a local problem, concentrating on specific bones. Krčah et al. and Younes et al. address the issue by focusing on the femur [1, 6]. Younes et al. propose primitive shape recognition and statistical shape models. A more general approach is proposed by Pinheiro et al. [5]. They regard it as a local problem, too. However, they are not focusing on a particular bone, but on a user-defined region of interest, applying a level-set based protocol. Other authors like Pérez-Carrasco et al. apply more general heuristics to whole-body scans [7], in their case continuous max-flow optimization. Furthermore, approaches are based on region growing, intensity thresholding (e.g., Buie et al. [4]), energy minimizing spline curves, edge detection or combinations of these algorithms. They often rely on expensive pre- and post-processing steps or are depending on the specific initialization [8]. While deep learning algorithms have become a methodology of choice in many areas of automatic medical image segmentation problems [9], their performance on a bone segmentation task remains to be evaluated. Some initial work can be found in the "Bone Segmenter" project by Kevin Mader of 4Quant[1].

In this paper, we present our most recent efforts towards bone segmentation on whole-body CT images, more specifically: low quality low dose CT scans that were captured as part of a PET/CT study during standard assessment for patients with multiple myeloma. We propose a network based on the U-Net architecture by Ronneberger et al. [10]. The goal of our work is to locate and segment cortical and cancellous tissue as well as bone marrow of long, short, flat and irregular bones in whole-body scans of patients with multiple myeloma.

2   Materials and methods

2.1   Data

We use an in-house data-set that consists of 15 whole-body low quality CT scans of patients diagnosed with multiple myeloma. We perform a k-fold cross-validation with k=5, thus using 9 patients for training ($\approx$3800 slices), 3 for validation ($\approx$1300 slices) and 3 for testing ($\approx$1300 slices) in each fold. Slices are 512x512 pixels, and each scan has between 380 and 450 slices. All datasets have an equal spacing of 0.98x0.98x4 mm^3. The ground truth segmentation has been

---

[1] https://github.com/4Quant/Bone-Segmenter

performed by a medical expert who was provided with segmentations generated by an intensity threshold. Slices were corrected using the segmentation plugin of the Medical Imaging Interaction Toolkit (MITK) [11].

2.2   Architecture

We adapt the U-Net architecture that was initially proposed by Ronneberger et al. [10] as shown in Fig. 2.2. The U-Net is a fully convolutional network with 18 convolutional layers. It consists of a downsampling and a symmetric upsampling path and uses skip connections to fast forward features from shallow layers to deep ones. Our model uses padded convolutions with a kernel size of 3 to keep the spatial output dimensions equal to the input. We resized the layers to match our image size of 512x512 pixels. The number of feature channels in the first convolutional channel is set to 64 as proposed in the original paper and doubled whenever the network increases in depth. We use a 2D architecture and provide the network with axial slices as input images.

2.3   Training

Data augmentation is used to more efficiently train our network given the amount of training data [10]. We make use of $\pm180°$ rotations around the axial axis, as

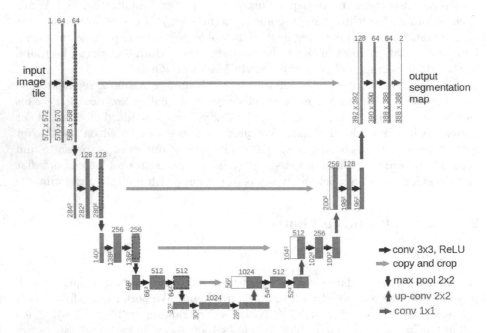

Fig. 2. U-Net architecture as proposed by Ronneberger et al. [10]. The architecture consists of a contracting path that captures semantic information and a symmetric expanding path that enables precise localization information [10].

well as randomly mirroring in x- and y-direction. We use a categorical cross-entropy loss and an adam optimizer with a learning rate of 0.0005, $\beta_1 = 0.5$, $\beta_2 = 0.999$ for our training. Our network is trained for 60 epochs with batch size 8 and 500 batches per epoch.

3   Results

The proposed segmentation algorithm achieved a dice score of 0.96 ± 0.02 and an intersection over union (IOU) of 0.94 ± 0.02. In comparison, the standard procedure, i.e. thresholding + morphological operations, achieved a dice score of 0.85 ± 0.04 and an IOU of 0.78 ± 0.06.

Both, the proposed and the standard procedure, worked well for cortical bone due to its high HU values. An example is shown in Fig. 3 for the proposed and in Fig. 4 for the standard procedure. The main issues arose when segmenting bone marrow and spongy bone. As expected, the standard approach did not segmented these structures well and also often mistook the table in the images as bony structure (Fig. 4). These issues are partly solved by our approach. However, performance on more complex body regions like the chest was still challenging as the network tends to oversegment bone like tissue such as cartilage. The most difficult task for both approaches were patients with hip or knee replacement. Segmenting bone on the according slices is a difficult task because of the artifacts that have similar HUs as cortical bone, and they are not represented sufficiently frequent in our data set for the proposed method to learn how to adequately handle such situations (Fig. 5).

The segmentation of a whole-body CT scan (512x512x400) took about 30s on an NVIDIA Titan X GPU.

4   Discussion

In this paper, we present a deep learning approach for the simultaneous segmentation of long, short, flat and irregular bones including cortical, cancellous and bone marrow structures. Our network achieved promising dice and IOU scores despite the low image quality of the applied whole-body CT scans. As expected, the segmentation of smaller bones like the ribs was more challenging, which is

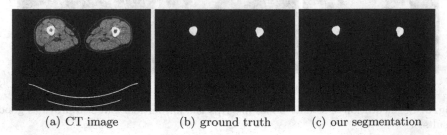

(a) CT image   (b) ground truth   (c) our segmentation

Fig. 3 The network performs best on long bones like the femur.

probably related to the fact that only small pieces of each bone are visible on

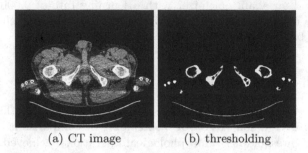

(a) CT image   (b) thresholding

Fig. 4. Segmentation created with threshold + morphological operations. The bone marrow is not segmented and the table is mistaken with bone.

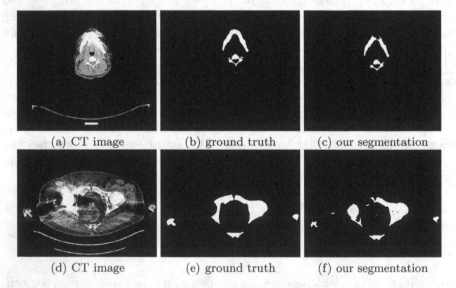

(a) CT image   (b) ground truth   (c) our segmentation

(d) CT image   (e) ground truth   (f) our segmentation

Fig. 5. Artefacts caused by tooth crowns or artificial joints lead to imperfect segmentations.

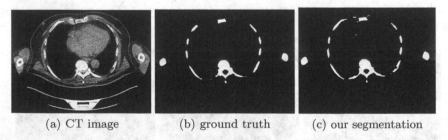

(a) CT image   (b) ground truth   (c) our segmentation

Fig. 6. Segmentation of smaller bones like rips is a harder task but still provides good results.

each slice and that tey are surrounded by more complex tissue combinations (Fig. 6).

Many different bone segmentation approaches have been published so far. It is not easy to provide a fair comparison of the different algorithms, as a lot of the work is focused on restricted problems like the segmentation of specific bony structures. To our knowledge, there do currently not exist any public benchmark datasets for the problem of general bone segmentation. Pérez-Carrasco et al. [7] presented a solution that used a continuous max-flow optimization to segment CT images. We did not reimplement the method, but on their in-house dataset the authors achieved a dice score of 0.91, requiring approx. 0.5s processing time per slice (512x512 pixels).

Our network was trained on images from a single scanner only. A larger dataset with higher heterogeneity could be established in the future to establish a more general bone segmentation method that applies to a variety of scanners and different levels of image quality. We will continue to further expand our reference dataset and plan to develop semi-supervised approaches that leverage unlabeled input data during learning.

References

1. Krčah M, Székely G, Blanc R; IEEE. Fully automatic and fast segmentation of the femur bone from 3D-CT images with no shape prior. Proc ISBI. 2011; p. 2087–2090.
2. Clarke B. Normal bone anatomy and physiology. Clin J Am Soc Nephrol. 2008;3(Supplement 3):S131–S139.
3. Hillengass J, Delorme S. Multiples Myelom: Aktuelle Empfehlungen für die Bildgebung. Der Radiologe. 2012 Apr;52(4):360–365.
4. Buie HR, Campbell GM, Klinck RJ, et al. Automatic segmentation of cortical and trabecular compartments based on a dual threshold technique for in vivo micro-CT bone analysis. Bone. 2007;41(4):505–515.
5. Pinheiro M, Alves J. A new level-set-based protocol for accurate bone segmentationfFrom CT imaging. IEEE Access. 2015;3:1894–1906.
6. Younes LB, Nakajima Y, Saito T. Fully automatic segmentation of the femur from 3D-CT images using primitive shape recognition and statistical shape models. Int J Comput Assist Rad Surg. 2014;9(2):189–196.
7. Pérez-Carrasco JA, Acha-Piñero B, Serrano C. Segmentation of bone structures in 3D CT images based on continuous max-flow optimization. Proc SPIE. 2015; p. 94133Y.
8. Malladi R, Sethian JA, Vemuri BC. Shape modeling with front propagation: A level set approach. IEEE Trans Pattern Anal Mach Intell. 1995;17(2):158–175.
9. Litjens G, Kooi T, Bejnordi BE, et al. A survey on deep learning in medical image analysis. arXiv preprint arXiv:170205747. 2017.
10. Ronneberger O, Fischer P, Brox T; Springer. U-net: Convolutional networks for biomedical image segmentation. Proc MICCAI. 2015; p. 234–241.
11. Nolden M, Zelzer S, Seitel A, et al. The medical imaging interaction toolkit: challenges and advances. Int J Comput Assist Rad Surg. 2013;8(4):607–620.

Ideal Seed Point Location Approximation for GrowCut Interactive Image Segmentation

Mario Amrehn[1], Maddalena Strumia[2], Stefan Steidl[1], Tim Horz[2],
Markus Kowarschik[2], Andreas Maier[1,3]

[1]Pattern Recognition Lab., Friedrich-Alexander University
Erlangen-Nürnberg (FAU), Germany
[2]Siemens Healthcare GmbH, Forchheim, Germany
[3]Erlangen Graduate School in Advanced Optical Technologies (SAOT), Germany
mario.amrehn@fau.de

Abstract. The C-arm CT X-ray acquisition process is a common modality in medical imaging. After image formation, anatomical structures can be extracted via segmentation. Interactive segmentation methods bear the advantage of a dynamically adjustable trade-off between time and achieved segmentation quality for the object of interest w.r.t. fully automated approaches. The segmentation's quality can be measured in terms of the Dice coefficient with the ground truth segmentation image. A user's interaction traditionally consist of drawing pictorial hints on an overlay image to the acquired image data via a graphical user interface (UI). The quality of a segmentation utilizing a set of drawn seeds varies depending on the location of the seed points in the image. In this paper, we (1) investigate the influence of seed point location on segmentation quality and (2) propose an approximation framework for ideal seed placements utilizing an extension of the well established GrowCut segmentation algorithm and (3) introduce a user interface for the utilization of the suggested seed point locations. An extensive evaluation of the predictive power of seed importance is conducted from hepatic lesion input images. As a result, our approach suggests seed points with a median of 72.5 % of the ideal seed points' associated Dice scores, which is an increase of 8.4 % points to sampling the seed location at random.

1 Introduction

The segmentation of hepatocellular carcinoma (HCC) in C-arm based computed tomography (CT) images is of vital importance for the trans-catheter arterial chemoembolization (TACE) [1] procedure. A more accurate segmentation of the tumor increases the treatment's efficacy while minimizing the toxicity for surrounding healthy tissue during treatment with chemotherapeutic agents. Contrast enhanced tumors appear as inhomogeneous hyper dense or hypo dense proliferations in the radiographic projections. A tumor represented by non-homogeneous attenuation values considerably impedes an exact distinction between cancerous cells and their surrounding healthy hepatic tissue. Due to this high variability interactive segmentation methods are superior to fully automatic segmentation approaches to obtain exact segmentations of HCC during TACE.

An interactive segmentation method may require a large amount of user interaction. The aim of this work is to reduce the user's assistance to a minimum in order to increase the efficiency of the overall segmentation process. This is realized via an automatic preselection of the seed point locations.

2   Materials and methods

2.1   Evaluation method for seed importance

Moschidis et al. [2] investigated the varying importance of sets of seed points for interactive segmentation processes incorporating pictorial hints from a user w.r.t. the resulting segmentation's quality. They concluded that seeds placed exclusively near the actual contour line of the object yield inferior segmentation results than seeds spread over the whole image space. Both alternatives are depicted in Fig. 1. Moschidis et al. exclusively analyzed seed importance by selecting seed locations sampled at random from each of the two provided categories. However, a full image of seed importance $\mathbf{D} \in \mathbb{R}^{w,h}$ with the same resolution as the 2-D input image $\mathbf{I} \in \mathbb{R}^{w,h}$ itself is desirable in order to analyze shortcomings of a given segmentation technique for each input element $\mathbf{I_x}$, where $\mathbf{x} \in \mathbb{R}^2$.

In this paper, to generate a full image of seed importance $\mathbf{D}$, at each coordinate $\mathbf{x}$ for a possible new seed point (i.e. $\mathbf{x} \notin \mathbf{X}$), this seed's location is exclusively added to the set of initial seed coordinates $\mathbf{X} \ni \{\mathbf{x}_1, \mathbf{x}_2, \ldots, \mathbf{x}_n\}$, with $n \ll w \cdot h$ for a single segmentation. The segmentation's Dice coefficient $\mathbf{D_x}$ for image coordinate $\mathbf{x}$ can be interpreted as the quality of the segmentation including seed point $\mathbf{x}$. Since the segmentation's Dice value without the current seed point (i.e. just from the initial seeds) is the same for all non-initial seed point locations $\mathbf{x} \notin \mathbf{X}$, the resulting image of Dice values can be interpreted as an image of seed location importance for the current segmentation task. Such an image transformation into the domain of a figure of merit for seed location importance

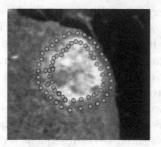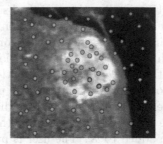

Fig. 1. Illustration of surface seeds (left) and volume seeds (right) as defined by Moschidis et al. [2]. Foreground and background seed locations are depicted in orange and green, respectively.

evaluation involves $w \cdot h - n$ separate segmentation operations for each input image. For an objective image of seed importance $\mathbf{D_{x \in X}} \lesssim \mathbf{D_{x \notin X}}$.

2.2   Seed location impact approximation

The GrowCut [3, 4] algorithm for image segmentation is based on cellular automaton theory. An automaton is defined by the tuple $(\mathbf{G_I}, \mathbf{Q}, \delta)$. $\mathbf{G_I}$ is the graph of image $\mathbf{I}$, where image elements are nodes $\mathbf{v}_e$ with associated image value $\mathbf{c}_e$. Nodes are connected by the Moore neighborhood system. The state set $\mathbf{Q}$ consists of $\mathbf{Q}_e^t = ((\mathbf{x}_e, \ell_e^t), \mathbf{\Theta}_e^t, \mathbf{c}_e, \mathbf{h}_e^t)$, where ℓ is the seed label and $\mathbf{\Theta}_e^t$ is the strength of node e at iteration t. We propose an additional variable $\mathbf{h}_e^t$ as counter for accumulated label changes of e during the GrowCut iteration, where $\mathbf{h}_e^0 = 0$. $\mathbf{\Theta}_e^0$ is 1 for initial seed locations $\mathbf{X}$, and 0 otherwise. State transitions (iterations) $\delta\left(\mathbf{Q}_e^t\right) = \mathbf{Q}_e^{t+1}$ are performed utilizing δ: start from initial seeds. Propagate labels w.r.t. local intensity features $\mathbf{c}$. every node f, at each time step t, attempts to conquer its direct neighbors. Node e is conquered if $\mathbf{\Theta}_f^t \cdot \mathrm{g}(\mathbf{c}_e, \mathbf{c}_f) > \mathbf{\Theta}_e^t$, where $\mathrm{g}(\mathbf{c}_e, \mathbf{c}_f) = 1 - \|\mathbf{c}_e - \mathbf{c}_f\|_2 / (\max_{j,k} \|\mathbf{c}_j - \mathbf{c}_k\|_2)$. If e is conquered, $\mathbf{Q}_e^{t+1} = ((\mathbf{p}_e, \ell_f^t), \mathbf{\Theta}_f^t \cdot g(c_e, c_f), \mathbf{c}_e, \mathbf{h}_e^t + 1)$, else $\mathbf{Q}_e^{t+1} = \mathbf{Q}_e^t$. The bounded node strengths are monotonously decreasing. The process is guaranteed to converge. The values of $\mathbf{h}_{\mathbf{x}}^T$, where T is the final iteration, are used to approximate the uncertainty of the segmentation method w.r.t. each seed location in input image $\mathbf{I_x}$. The index associated with the highest number of label changes $\mathrm{argmax}_{\mathbf{x}} \, \mathbf{h}_{\mathbf{x}}'^T$ is selected as most important location for an additional seed, since a minimization of the algorithms uncertainty during segmentation is synonymous with a fast convergence of the interactive segmentation's contour line outcome towards the ground truth segmentation. $\mathbf{h}'^T$ is $\mathbf{h}^T$ filtered by a Gaussian kernel with standard deviation σ. Utilizing $\mathbf{h}'^T$ instead of $\mathbf{h}^T$ reduces the importance of single high values which increases the approximation quality of the system. Using $\mathbf{h}'^T$, the area including the largest amount of label changes is preferred for seed location suggestion.

2.3   Interactive application

We utilize a UI including the described suggestion of relevant seed locations into the workflow of interactive segmentation. As depicted in Fig. 2, the UI presents two seed point locations to the user for interaction as proposed in [5]. They decide, which of the four possible variations of foreground and background labels to assign to these seed locations. Exactly one of the four represents the correct labeling. In order to assist the decision process, implicit changes to the contour line consequential to the labeling are displayed by highlighting label changing areas on the four overlay images on the right. After selection the two seed locations are added to $\mathbf{X}$. The user is presented two subsequent seed locations and interacts with the system until they are satisfied with the segmentation result. The process for determining the locations of the two seeds is an iterated version of the one described in Sec. 2.2, where after the first location suggestion $\mathbf{x}_s$, another seed is suggested with $\mathbf{X} = \mathbf{X} \cup \{\mathbf{x}_s\}$ as initial seed locations.

3   Experiments

For an evaluation the full map of seed importance $\mathbf{D}$ using the Dice score as a figure of merit is computed for 50 2-D lesion images acquired by a C-arm CT scanner. Ground truth of the tumor outlines was generated manually by medical experts. The segmentation is performed via the GrowCut method. Initial background seeds are provided along the edges of the region of interest (ROI) of fixed 100 pixels in width w and height h. At least a single initial seed is required for each class label using GrowCut. Therefore, $\mathbf{X}$ consists of these background seed locations as well as the coordinate of a single foreground seed, which is determined by the center of mass of the lesion's binary ground truth segmentation. $\sigma = 5$ is selected after initial experimentation. Subsequent to the generation of $\mathbf{D}$, which is outlined in Sec. 2.1, the approximation results utilizing the method proposed in Sec. 2.2 are evaluated with $\mathbf{D}$ as ground truth.

4   Results

The influence of a seed's location on the overall segmentation outcome is shown in Fig. 4 via the ground truth image $\mathbf{D}$ generated as described in Sec. 2.1. The evaluation of the seed location suggestion approach is depicted in Tab. 1. A detailed illustration of the achieved segmentation quality per input image is given in Fig. 3.

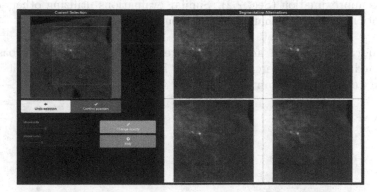

Fig. 2. The proposed application's UI for the seed point approximation method consists of four buttons to select groups of seed points generated by seed location importance approximation. The user is asked to select the correct labels for the two chosen seed locations. Background seeds are depicted in red, foreground seeds in blue. On the left, the zoomed in region and seed locations are highlighted for improved user orientation. The dotted areas illustrate the difference in each of the four possible next segmentation outlines w.r.t. the previous iteration's outline.

Table 1. Ideal seeds from **D** which provide the maximum achievable Dice score as reference for the seed location suggestion methods are depicted in the first column. Results of the proposed seed location suggestion approach are displayed in the second column. A baseline to the proposed method is provided by random sampling of seed locations as depicted in column three.

Dice score	Ideal seeds from **D** i. e. reference for 100 %	Proposed method's result relative to ideal seeds' Dice value	Random seed location sampling
Mean	0.696	68.5 % (i. e. +6.2 % points)	62.3 %
Median	0.758	72.5 % (i. e. +8.4 % points)	64.1 %
Std	0.221	24.1 % (i. e. +0.4 % points)	23.7 %

5   Discussion and outlook

As depicted in Fig. 4, Moschidis et al. [2] drastically simplified the distribution of seed location importance by implying that seeds from one of the two categories are inherently superior to the other. The proposed method for seed location suggestion yields superior results in comparison to the random sampling baseline as shown in Tab. 1 and Fig. 3. The maximum achievable Dice coefficient varies depending on the input image (Fig. 3). Further studies might investigate which patterns in the input image result in a low maximum Dice value in the seed location ground truth. Related to this, the influence of image scaling might be worth investigating to reduce the computation time during evaluation (Sec. 2.1) as well as approximation (Sec. 2.2). Similar evaluations utilizing other seeding segmentation approaches than GrowCut would be of interest.

Disclaimer. The concept and software presented in this paper are based on research and are not commercially available. Due to regulatory reasons its future availability cannot be guaranteed.

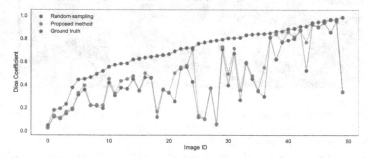

Fig. 3. Comparison of selected seed locations' influence on the Dice score. The points in red mark the maximum achievable Dice score when adding just one more seed point with coordinates **x** to an initial set of seed points **X**. The achieved Dice score by the proposed method's suggested seed location is depicted in green. A baseline suggestion is illustrated in blue. Images are sorted by their maximum achievable Dice score with one added seed point.

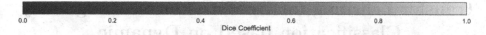

Dice Coefficient

Fig. 4. Selected results from seed location ground truth generation (Sec. 2.1) displayed as an overlay on top of each gray-valued input image. The segmentation ground truth contour line is depicted in green. The orange dot highlights the coordinate of most important / influential seed point. Dark purple indicates initial seed point locations.

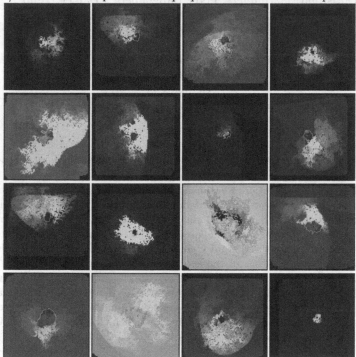

References

1. Lewandowski RJ, Geschwind JF, Liapi E, et al. Transcatheter intraarterial therapies: rationale and overview. Radiology. 2011; p. 641–657.
2. Moschidis E, Graham J. A systematic performance evaluation of interactive image segmentation methods based on simulated user interaction. Proc ISBI. 2010; p. 928–931.
3. Vezhnevets V, Konouchine V. GrowCut: interactive multi-label ND image segmentation by cellular automata. Graphicon. 2005; p. 150–156.
4. Amrehn MP, Glasbrenner J, Steidl S, et al. Comparative evaluation of interactive segmentation approaches. Procs BVM. 2016; p. 68–73.
5. Amrehn MP, Steidl S, Kortekaas R, et al.. Usability evaluation of interactive image segmentation systems; 2018.

Transfer Learning for Breast Cancer Malignancy Classification based on Dynamic Contrast-Enhanced MR Images

Christoph Haarburger[1], Peter Langenberg[1], Daniel Truhn[2],
Hannah Schneider[2], Johannes Thüring[2], Simone Schrading[2],
Christiane K. Kuhl[2], Dorit Merhof[1]

[1]Institute of Imaging and Computer Vision, RWTH Aachen University, Germany
[2]Department of Diagnostic and Interventional Radiology, University Hospital Aachen,
Germany
haarburger@lfb.rwth-aachen.de

Abstract. In clinical contexts with very limited annotated data, such as
breast cancer diagnosis, training state-of-the art deep neural networks is
not feasible. As a solution, we transfer parameters of networks pretrained
on natural RGB images to malignancy classification of breast lesions in
dynamic contrast-enhanced MR images. Since DCE-MR images comprise several contrasts and timepoints, a direct finetuning of pretrained
networks expecting three input channels is not possible. Based on the
hypothesis that a subset of the acquired image data is sufficient for a
computer-aided diagnosis, we provide an experimental comparison of all
possible subsets of MR image contrasts and determine the best combination for malignancy classification. A subset of images acquired at three
timepoints of dynamic T1-weighted images which closely corresponds to
human interpretation performs best with an AUC of 0.839.

1 Introduction

Despite decades of mammographic screening and significant advances in the field
of targeted therapies, breast cancer is still the second most prevalent cause of
cancer deaths in women [1]. Currently, dynamic contrast-enhanced magnetic
resonance imaging (DCE-MRI) is the most accurate diagnostic tool for breast
cancer diagnosis [2, 3]. With the ever expanding workload for radiologists and
lack of medical experts, the inherent risk of human error is increasing. It can
be expected that the amount of image data will increase in the future, which
will further aggravate this condition. Following the significant improvements
in image classification by deep neural networks, the transfer of such algorithms
to radiological images is a desirable goal. However, for most medical image
classification problems only a limited amount of training data is available. One
possible solution is a two-step transfer learning approach: In the first step, a
neural network is trained on a classification problem, for which a large dataset
for training is available. After that, the network is finetuned to the problem at

hand for which only a limited amount of training data is present. The potential of this approach has already been demonstrated by automated classification of RGB images of skin lesions with human-level performance [4]. However, when diagnosis is based on modalities such as CT or MRI, a different number of channels, i.e. contrasts, sequences or timepoints, may be present that is often not equal to the number of channels in the dataset the network is pretrained on (usually three). A setting that suffers from that problem is DCE-MRI of the breast: Clinical acquisition protocols usually consist of T2-weighted and DCE T1-weighted images at several timepoints constituting seven channels in total. For a transfer learning setting, this raises the question which subset of three channels is most suitable for a transfer learning classification of lesions.

In [5], Jäger et al. classified breast lesion malignancy based on diffusion weighted MR images and a custom network architecture that was trained from scratch. A comparison of transfer learning and training from scratch for medical image data was presented in [6] showing comparable results for transfer learning and training from scratch for several medical image classification problems. Transfer learning based on DCE-MRI has been demonstrated to successfully classify breast lesions into mass and non-mass types in [7] and malignant/benign in [8, 9].

Our contribution in this work is twofold: Firstly, we propose a transfer learning approach with which breast lesion malignancy can be classified with a state of the art ResNet architecture and limited amount of training data. Secondly, we provide an experimental comparison of all possible subsets of image contrasts/timepoints to determine the set that is most informative for a deep learning algorithm to classify breast lesion malignancy based on DCE-MR images.

2   Materials and methods

2.1   Dataset

Images were acquired between 2010 and 2017 at the University Hospital Aachen (Germany) utilizing a 1.5 T Scanner (Achieva; Philips Medical Systems, Best, The Netherlands). The protocol consists of the following sequences: T2-weighted turbo spin-echo sequence (acquisition matrix 512×512, spacing 0.6 mm, slice thickness 3.5 mm), coronal T1-weighted turbo spin-echo sequence and an axial two-dimensional multisection gradient-echo dynamic series (acquisition matrix 512×512, spacing 0.6 mm, slice thickness 3.5 mm). DCE T1-weighted images were acquired at 5 time points, where the first acquisition was performed before injection of 0.1 mmol of gadobutrol per kilogram of body weight (Gadovist; Bayer, Leverkusen, Germany). Subsequent postcontrast images were acquired every 90 s respectively. The first post-contrast image was subtracted from the pre-contrast image to determine a "fat-suppressed" representation of the images. This acquisition protocol leads to seven 3D images that are exemplified in Fig. 1.

All lesions were segmented manually and reviewed by a radiologist with 12 years of training using a custom software based on MeVisLab. Our dataset comprises 309 subjects and 688 lesions, where 311 lesions are malignant and 388 lesions are benign based on histology. If no histology was available, lesion malignancy was determined based on 12 month follow-up.

2.2   Preprocessing

Voxels in clinical-routine DCE-MR images are highly anisotropic with a high axial resolution and low in-plane resolution due to high slice thickness. Thus, most image information is contained in the axial plane. For this reason, we extracted axial patches based on bounding boxes around the manually annotated contours. Bounding box centers were determined by the center of mass of the segmentation mask and the patch size was set to 50×50. This approach has the advantage of incorporating the lesion context, such as enhancement of surrounding tissue, into the feature extraction. Patches that contained annotations from several lesions were removed from the dataset. The particular patch size is a tradeoff between the amount of context information that is included and the number of patches that needs to be omitted because they contain several lesions. It was not optimized in this work. Overall 1881 valid patches were extracted where 796 and 1085 patches originate from malignant and benign lesions, respectively.

MR image intensities are not necessarily on the same scale, especially if the images originate from seven years of clinical routine. To facilitate a quantitative comparison, image intensities were adjusted: First, a bias field correction was performed on all T1- and T2-weighted images using N4ITK [10]. Image intensities were then rescaled to a fixed range ensuring that the CNN can operate on the same scale across different images.

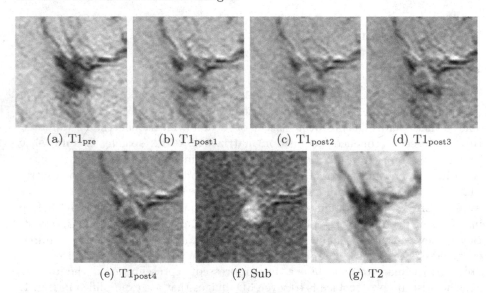

(a) $T1_{pre}$ (b) $T1_{post1}$ (c) $T1_{post2}$ (d) $T1_{post3}$

(e) $T1_{post4}$ (f) Sub   (g) T2

Fig. 1. Contrasts of an example patch depicting an invasive carcinoma.

2.3 Transfer learning

As a network architecture we chose ResNet34 [11], which we pretrained on the ImageNet [12] dataset. The key idea of the ResNet architecture are residual blocks, in which an identity connection is added parallel to stacked nonlinear layers. This improves gradient flow through the network during backpropagation allowing to train very deep models. Before feeding breast lesion patches to the network, the dataset was augmented using random rotations and flipping. Moreover, image mean and standard deviations were adjusted and dimensions were resized to 224×224 pixels to leverage the features learned during training on ImageNet. In the ResNet34 architecture, the final classification layer was adapted to our binary classification problem. During finetuning on DCE-MRI data, all layers are trained simultaneously using cross entropy loss. We employed stochastic gradient descent using a momentum of 0.9 and with a decaying learning rate starting at 0.001 and decreasing with a factor of 0.05 every 7 epochs.

3 Results

In order to determine the best set of image contrasts, all 35 combinations of three image contrasts are evaluated in a 10 fold cross validation scheme. In each fold, patches are split into training, validation and test set such that patches from a single patient are included in either training or validation or test set exclusively. All experiments were implemented using PyTorch and were executed on a workstation equipped with Intel Core i7-6400K processor and Nvidia GTX 1070 GPU.

To obtain per-lesion predictions from per-slice classifier outputs, we aggregated the subsequent predictions by taking the maximum probability of malignancy of all corresponding slices. Reported AUCs, sensitivities and specificities are based on an arbitrary cutoff of 0.5. The classification performance for the ten best performing contrast combinations in terms of AUC is given in Table 1. The best result is achieved by the set comprising $T1_{pre}$, $T1_{post3}$ and sub, which yields an AUC of 0.839.

Computation times for training a single cross validation fold based on the pretrained network was 180 seconds. Prediction for a single patch can be performed in 300 milliseconds.

4 Discussion

We presented a transfer learning approach for malignancy classification of breast lesions based on DCE-MRI and assessed the best performing combinations of contrasts. DCE-MRI is largely based on contrast agent kinetics, i.e. uptake of contrast agent and slope characteristics (persistent, plateau, washout) of the signal intensity in enhancing tissue over time [2].

Common slope characteristics are sketched in Fig. 2.

Table 1. Cross validated classification performance for ten best contrast combinations sorted by AUC.

Contrast	AUC	Sensitivity	Specificity	Accuracy
$T1_{pre}$, $T1_{post3}$, sub	0.839	0.853	0.825	0.834
$T1_{post3}$, $T1_{post4}$, sub	0.834	0.830	0.838	0.836
$T1_{pre}$, $T1_{post2}$, $T1_{post3}$	0.832	0.835	0.829	0.831
$T1_{pre}$, $T1_{post1}$, $T1_{post3}$	0.826	0.830	0.821	0.824
$T1_{pre}$, $T1_{post1}$, $T1_{post2}$	0.823	0.821	0.825	0.824
$T1_{post2}$, $T1_{post3}$, sub	0.815	0.830	0.800	0.809
$T1_{post1}$, $T1_{post4}$, sub	0.813	0.835	0.791	0.805
T2, $T1_{pre}$, sub	0.808	0.807	0.808	0.808
T2, $T1_{post4}$, sub	0.803	0.807	0.800	0.802
T2, $T1_{post2}$, sub	0.802	0.803	0.802	0.802

The top performing combinations all incorporate several timepoints of the dynamic images which is comparable to "sampling" the kinetic curve. Thus, we can conclude that the CNN extracts features that describe contrast agent kinetics. This is in line with clinical diagnostics, as contrast agent kinetics is exactly the feature that is deemed most important for malignancy classification in dynamic breast MRI by experienced radiologists [2, 3]. However, for humans not only the dynamic image stack but also the T2 image is important because it includes important structural information about masses. For the CNN on the other hand, the T2 image is less important than the set of dynamic images that capture enhancement kinetics.

When considering the results from Table 1, it is important to note that the continuous classifier output was thresholded arbitrarily at 0.5 to yield a binary prediction. The threshold is a tradeoff between sensitivity and specificity and was not tuned.

Our work has several limitations: Despite being relatively large compared to other studies related to breast cancer diagnosis, our dataset is small for a network architecture with many parameters such as ResNet. Moreover, patches containing several lesions were omitted.

A direct comparison with other works that classified breast lesion malignancy is difficult because the imaging protocols differ and the resulting accuracies depend heavily on the chosen set of malignant and benign lesions. In [5], an

Fig. 2. Contrast agent enhancement kinetics. The yellow dotted line indicates the acquisition time of the first image after bolus injection.

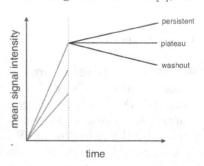

AUC > 0.9 was achieved based on diffusion weighted MR images and a custom network architecture. In future work, other approaches for representation of contrast agent kinetics in DCE-MRI will be investigated. For example, 1×1 convolutions across several timepoints may enhance exploitation of spatiotemporal properties of DCE-MRI data.

5   Conclusion

In this work, we addressed the problem of automated breast lesion malignancy classification based on DCE-MRI. Since state-of-the art deep learning algorithms require large amounts of training data, we trained our network on a large amount of RGB images and finetuned the network parameters according to our problem. In a set of experiments we showed that classification based on a subset of MR images that captures the contrast agent kinetics yields best performance.

References

1. Siegel R, Ma J, Zou Z, et al. Cancer statistics, 2014. CA Cancer J Clin. 2014;64(1):9–29.
2. Kuhl CK. The current status of breast MR imaging: part I: choice of technique, image interpretation, diagnostic accuracy, and transfer to clinical practice. Radiology. 2007;244(2):356–378.
3. Kuhl CK. Current status of breast MR imaging: part 2: clinical applications. Radiology. 2007;244(3):672–691.
4. Esteva A, Kuprel B, Novoa RA, et al. Dermatologist-level classification of skin cancer with deep neural networks. Nature. 2017 Jan;542(7639):115–118.
5. Revealing hidden potentials of the q-space signal in breast cancer. Proc MICCAI. 2017; p. 664–671.
6. Tajbakhsh N, Shin JY, Gurudu SR, et al. Convolutional neural networks for medical image analysis: full training or fine tuning? IEEE Trans Med Imaging. 2016 May;35(5):1299–1312.
7. Hadad O, Bakalo R, Ben-Ari R, et al. Classification of breast lesions using cross-modal deep learning. Proc ISBI. 2017; p. 109–112.
8. Marrone S, Piantadosi G, Fusco R, et al. An investigation of deep learning for lesions malignancy classification in breast DCE-MRI. Proc ICIAP. 2017; p. 479–489.
9. Antropova N, Huynh B, Giger M. Performance comparison of deep learning and segmentation-based radiomic methods in the task of distinguishing benign and malignant breast lesions on DCE-MRI. Proc SPIE. 2017;(10134).
10. Tustison NJ, Avants BB, Cook PA, et al. N4ITK: improved N3 bias correction. IEEE Trans Med Imaging. 2010 June;29(6):1310–1320.
11. He K, Zhang X, Ren S, et al. Deep residual learning for image recognition. Proc CVPR. 2016 June; p. 770–778.
12. Russakovsky O, Deng J, Su H, et al. ImageNet large scale visual recognition challenge. Int J Comput Vis;(3):211–252.

Traditional Machine Learning Techniques for Streak Artifact Reduction in Limited Angle Tomography

Yixing Huang[1], Yanye Lu[1], Oliver Taubmann[1,2], Guenter Lauritsch[3], Andreas Maier[1,2]

[1]Pattern Recognition Lab, Friedrich-Alexander-University Erlangen-Nuremberg
[2]Erlangen Graduate School in Advanced Optical Technologies (SAOT)
[3]Siemens Healthcare GmbH, Forchheim
yixing.yh.huang@fau.de

Abstract. In this work, the application of traditional machine learning techniques, in the form of regression models based on conventional, "hand-crafted" features, to streak reduction in limited angle tomography is investigated. Specifically, linear regression (LR), multi-layer perceptron (MLP), and reduced-error pruning tree (REPTree) are investigated. When choosing the mean-variation-median (MVM), Laplacian, and Hessian features, REPTree learns streak artifacts best and reaches the smallest root-mean-square error (RMSE) of 29 HU for the Shepp-Logan phantom. Further experiments demonstrate that the MVM and Hessian features complement each other, whereas the Laplacian feature is redundant in the presence of MVM. Preliminary experiments on clinical data suggests that further investigation of clinical applications using REPTree may be worthwhile.

1 Introduction

In computed tomography (CT), image reconstruction from data acquired in an insufficient angular range is called limited angle tomography. It arises when the gantry rotation of a CT system is restricted by other system parts or external obstacles. Because of missing data, artifacts, typically in the form of streaks, will occur in the reconstructed images.

Generally, two main approaches are utilized to deal with the limited angle problem. One is to interpolate/extrapolate the missing data in projection domain [1]. The other is to incorporate prior information into iterative algorithms. Particularly, iterative reconstruction algorithms with total variation (TV) regularization, which exploits sparsity in the image gradient domain, have achieved good performance in limited angle tomography [2, 3]. However, iterative algorithms are computationally expensive.

Recently, deep learning has outperformed the state of the art in many computer vision tasks and medical imaing processing tasks as well. The development of techniques such as convolutional neural networks (CNN), often with an encoder-decoder structure, allows to extract intrinsic features from high dimensional data and improves the learning process. Deep learning has proved effective for streak reduction in limited angle tomography [4, 5, 6]. However, the application of conventional machine learning techniques, i.e., a pixel-by-pixel prediction based on hand-crafted features, in limited angle tomography remains blank in literature. Therefore, in this paper we investigate three regression models in such a setup for limited angle tomography, namely, linear regression (LR), multi-layer perceptron (MLP), and reduced-error pruning tree (REPTree).

2   Materials and methods

2.1   Input and output

A general machine learning pipeline includes four main parts: input observations, feature extraction, a classification/regression model, and output labels. In this work, we choose the images reconstructed from the limited angle data (denoted by f_{limited}) as the input. Gu and Ye [6] point out that streak artifacts are similar to each other even though the artifact-free images are drastically different from each other. They suggest that learning the residual artifact images (denoted by f_{artifact}) is easier than learning the artifact-free images directly. Therefore, in this work we choose the residual artifact images as the output.

2.2   Feature extraction

Streak artifacts in limited angle tomography appear evidently near object boundaries. They are closely associated with object edges and have certain orientations that are determined by the acquisition geometry. Therefore, the following features are used for streak artifact prediction.

At each position (x, y), the intensity of $f_{\text{artifact}}(x, y)$ is highly related to the intensity of $f_{\text{limited}}(x, y)$. Therefore, the intensity of $f_{\text{limited}}(x, y)$ is one feature. As it is difficult to predict streak artifacts from a single pixel, the information of its neighborhood is necessary. The neighborhood, typically an image patch, can be characterized by the mean, variance, and median statistic.

The Laplacian, or the Laplace operator, is one of the most popular edge detectors. It is a second order differential operator, which is defined as,

$$\Delta f(x, y) = \nabla^2 f(x, y) = \frac{\partial^2 f(x, y)}{\partial x^2} + \frac{\partial^2 f(x, y)}{\partial y^2} \tag{1}$$

The Hessian matrix is a structure tensor constructed by second-order partial derivatives. It describes the local curvature of an image. The image $f(x, y)$ is first smoothed by a Gaussian kernel $G_s(x, y)$ with a standard deviation s, i.e., $f_s(x, y) = f(x, y) * G_s(x, y)$. The Hessian matrix is computed as,

$$H_s(x, y) = \begin{bmatrix} \frac{\partial^2 f_s(x,y)}{\partial x^2} & \frac{\partial^2 f_s(x,y)}{\partial x \partial y} \\ \frac{\partial^2 f_s(x,y)}{\partial y \partial x} & \frac{\partial^2 f_s(x,y)}{\partial y^2} \end{bmatrix} \tag{2}$$

The two eigenvalues and the orientation of the main eigenvector of $H_s(x, y)$ are chosen as the Hessian features.

2.3 Regression models

Linear regression is the most popular method in many statistical applications. It expresses the output label as a linear combination of the extracted feature attributes and the trained weights.

MLP can learn more complex, nonlinear functions than linear regression. MLP generally contains an input layer, several hidden layers, and an output layer. At hidden layers, nonlinear activation functions like the sigmoid activation function are typically used. The backpropagation method with stochastic gradient descent method is used for training.

A decision tree utilizes a tree-like structure to predict an output from the feature attributes. A tree is learnt recursively by splitting the training data set into subsets based on attribute value tests. The recursion process stops when the subset at a node has all the same value, or the tree reaches the maximum depth. Gini impurity or information gain is typically used to obtain an optimal attribute order for splitting [7]. A pruning process is employed to prevent overfitting. In this paper, we use the reduced-error pruning tree (REPTree) [8] which is a simple and fast pruning method.

2.4 Experimental set-up

To initially check the validity of different features and regression models, a 3-D standard high-contrast pixelized Shepp-Logan phantom is generated. Its image size is $512 \times 512 \times 200$. The pixel size is 0.4 mm in X and Y directions and 1.024 mm in Z direction. We pick 150 slices from the 3-D volume and one half of them are used for training, the other half for testing. We reproject these images in a parallel-beam geometry using a ray-driven method with a sampling rate of 7.5/mm. No noise is simulated. The scanned angular range is $160°$. The angular step is $0.5°$. The number of the equal-space detector pixels N_D is 1537 and the detector element size is 0.2 mm.

As preliminary experiments for clinical data, 14 patients' CT data are used, 7 patients for training and another 7 patients for testing. The selected images are reprojected in a fan-beam geometry. The scanned angular range is $170°$. The angular increment is $0.5°$. The detector has 768 pixels and the pixel size is 0.5 mm. The source to detector distance is $d = 1037$ mm and the fan angle is $20°$.

The machine learning algorithms are based on the Waikato Environment for Knowledge Analysis (Weka) [9]. MLP uses four hidden layers. The learning rate, the momentum, and the epochs are set to 0.3, 0.2 and 100, respectively. REPTree sets 1 as the minimum number of instances per leaf node and the maximum depth of the tree is set to be unlimited. The MVM features are extracted from quadratic image patches of side length 2, 4, 8 and 16. For the

Hessian features, s is set to 9. The whole implementation is based on CONRAD [10].

3   Results

The results of different machine learning algorithms using the MVM, Laplacian, and Hessian features for the Shepp-Logan phantom are displayed in Fig. 1. Figs. 1(a)-(d) show that REPTree predicts the artifacts best with only minor misclassifications. By subtracting the learnt streak artifacts, the "destreaked" images are obtained in Figs. 1(f)-(h). While streak artifacts remain in the results of LR and MLP, most of them are reduced by REPTree. The root-mean-square errors (RMSE) of the destreaked images w. r. t. the image reconstructed from full data (Fig. 1(e)) is further computed. REPTree reaches the smallest RMSE value of 29.3 HU.

To investigate the effects of different features in streak artifact classification, the results of REPTree using different combinations of features for the Shepp-Logan data are shown in Fig. 2. Figs. 2(a)-(c) indicate that using MVM only is able to predict most streak artifacts while using Laplacian or Hessian only is not sufficient. Comparing Fig. 2(d) with Fig. 2(a), the Laplacian feature is redundant in the presence of MVM since Fig. 2(d) and Fig. 2(a) have almost the same image quality. Fig. 2(e) and Fig. 1(h) also demonstrate this. Fig. 2(e) indicates that the Hessian features are beneficial, compared with Fig. 2(a).

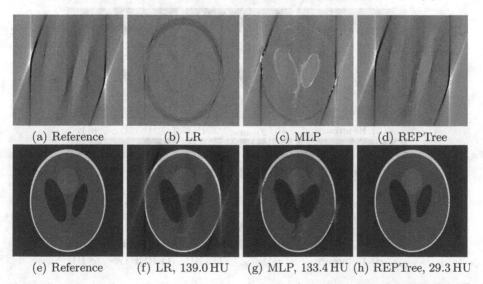

(a) Reference   (b) LR   (c) MLP   (d) REPTree

(e) Reference   (f) LR, 139.0 HU   (g) MLP, 133.4 HU   (h) REPTree, 29.3 HU

Fig. 1. Learnt streak artifacts using different machine learning algorithms and their corresponding reconstructed images in parallel-beam with a 160° trajectory. The MVM, Laplacian, and Hessian features are used. The RMSE of images learnt by LR, MLP, and REPTree are shown in the subcaptions (f)-(h). Window width for the top row: 1200 HU; window for the bottom row: [-1400, 1400] HU.

The preliminary experiments on the clinical data are displayed in Fig. 3. Figs. 3(c) and (f) demonstrate that REPTree reduces most streak artifacts well. However, it misclassifies some normal tissue as streak artifacts.

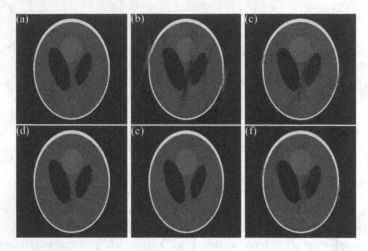

Fig. 2. The results of REPTree using different feature combinations in parallel-beam with a 160° trajectory: (a) MVM, (RMSE =) 38.4 HU; (b) Laplacian, 119.2 HU; (c) Hessian, 76.48 HU; (d) MVM and Laplacian, 38.5 HU; (e) MVM and Hessian, 28.9 HU; (f) Laplacian and Hessian, 65.0 HU. Window: [-1400, 1400] HU.

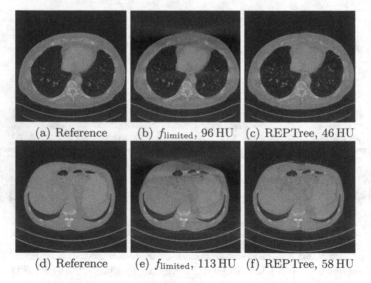

(a) Reference   (b) $f_{limited}$, 96 HU   (c) REPTree, 46 HU

(d) Reference   (e) $f_{limited}$, 113 HU   (f) REPTree, 58 HU

Fig. 3. The reference images, the limited angle reconstructions (denoted by $f_{limited}$), and the machine learning results using REPTree with the MVM and Hessian features of two clinical datasets in fan-beam with a 170° trajectory. Window: [-1150, 1300] HU.

4   Discussion

The mapping from the selected feature attributes to the streak artifacts is a complex nonlinear function. Therefore, LR fails to model that. Although a large MLP with enough hidden units can model any nonlinear functions, in our case, MLP fails to find the desired function during training. REPTree represents the mapping function well with enough nodes and it reduces the overfitting problem with pruning. Therefore, REPTree performs best in the experiments (Fig. 1).

The Laplacian feature is redundant in the presence of MVM (Fig. 2). As a potential reason, one has to consider that the Laplacian is just a linear combination of the neighboring pixels described by MVM. The Hessian features are beneficial since they stress on the strength as well as the orientation of local curvatures, which are essential properties of limited angle streak artifacts.

In summary, we investigate the application of LR, MLP, and REPTree for streak artifact reduction in limited angle tomography. The experiments on the Shepp-Logan phantom demonstrate that REPTree has the best performance on learning streak artifacts compared with LR and MLP. They also indicate that MVM and Hessian features are beneficial for streak artifact prediction while the Laplacian is redundant in the presence of MVM. The preliminary experiments on clinical data suggests that further investigation of clinical applications using REPTree may be worthwhile.

Disclaimer. The concepts and information presented in this paper are based on research and are not commercially available.

References

1. Huang Y, Huang X, Taubmann O, et al. Restoration of missing data in limited angle tomography based on Helgason-Ludwig consistency conditions. Biomed Phys Eng Express. 2017;3(3).
2. Chen Z, Jin X, Li L, et al. A limited-angle CT reconstruction method based on anisotropic TV minimization. Biomed Phys Eng Express. 2013;58(7).
3. Huang Y, Taubmann O, Huang X, et al. A new scale space total variation algorithm for limited angle tomography. Proc CT-Meeting. 2016;3(3):149–152.
4. Würfl T, Ghesu F, Christlein V, et al. Deep learning computed tomography. Proc CT-Meeting. 2016;3(3):432–440.
5. Hammernik K, Würfl T, Pock T, et al. A deep learning architecture for limited-angle computed tomography reconstruction. Proc CT-Meeting. 2017;3(3):92–97.
6. Gu J, Ye J. Multi-scale wavelet domain residual learning for limited-angle CT reconstruction. Proc CT-Meeting. 2017;3(3):443–447.
7. Loh W. Classification and regression trees. Proc CT-Meeting. 2011;1(1):14–23.
8. Quinlan J. Simplifying decision trees. Proc CT-Meeting. 1987;27(3):221–234.
9. Frank E, Hall M, Witten I. The WEKA workbench: online appendix for data mining: practical machine learning tools and techniques.. vol. 27. Int J Man Mach Stud.; 2016.
10. Maier A, Berger M, Fischer P, et al. CONRAD: a software framework for cone-beam imaging in radiology. Med Phys. 2013;40(11):111914.

Classification of Polyethylene Particles and the Local CD3+ Lymphocytosis in Histological Slices

Lara-Maria Steffes[1], Marc Aubreville[1], Stefan Sesselmann[2], Veit Krenn[3], Andreas Maier[1]

[1]Pattern Recognition Lab, Computer Sciences, Friedrich-Alexander-Universtität Erlangen-Nürnberg, Germany
[2]Professor for Innovative Concepts and Technologies in Healthcare, OTH Amberg-Weiden, Germany
[3]Center for Histopathology and Molecular Pathology, Trier, Germany
Lara.Steffes@gmx.de

Abstract. In 2014, about 400.000 endoprosthetic operations were performed in Germany [1]. Unfortunately, the lifespan is limited and already after 10 years 5 percent of the patients have primary complaints [2]. All the more important it is to clarify the causes for this failure. One main cause is an immune response to abrasion particles of the implant, an effect which is assumed to be correlated with occurrence and count of CD3+ immune/inflammatory cells [3]. For the further analysis of this effect, computer-aided classification and image analysis methods provide a high value for the medical research. Aim of this work was the development of an threshold-based algorithm for the segmentation of polyethylene abrasion particles and the CD3+ immune/inflammatory response of histological slice images.

1 Introduction

In Germany, arthroplasty, especially hip and knee endoprosthesis, is one of the most often performed surgical procedures. In 2014, about 400.000 endoprothetic operations were done [1]. For the patient, artificial endoprosthesis offers a large gain in quality of life, as pain is reduced and lost mobility is restored. Often, sporting activities can be exercised again. Unfortunately, the lifespan of endoprotheses is limited. Already after 10 years, approximately 5 percent of the patients have primary complaints, i.e. they are no longer without pain [2]. The cause of failure of endoprosthesis can be multifactorial. The main unsolved problem is the loosening of the implant from the bone and the formation of a synovial-like interface membrane (SLIM) between the implant and the bone [2]. Different abrasion materials, dependent on the used material of the sliding pair of the endoprothesis, can be found in the SLIM and are discussed to have an influence on the loosening process [3]. The occurrence and count of CD3+ immune cells, which play a central role in the immune defense, is thought of as being correlated with this deterioration process. In Fig. 1 the different forms of the polyethylene (PE) particles and the CD3+ immune/inflammatory response are shown. Micropolyethylene (MPE) particles have an expected size of less than $5\,\mu m$, macropolyethylene (MacroPE) particles between $5\,\mu m$ and $100\,\mu m$ and supramacropolyethylene (SMPE) particles above $100\,\mu m$ [4]. Because of a high time effort to count every abrasion particle (AP) and the local CD3+ immune/inflammatory response manually and the associated error susceptibility, the aim of this work is the segmentation and classification of the polyethylene APs of different sizes, and the local CD3+ immune/inflammatory response with a semi-automatic threshold-based algorithm.

2   Materials and methods

For this work, 100 labeled images of stained specimen, collected from 52 patients, were available. The 100 RGB images had a fixed width of $594\,\mu m$, corresponding to 2048 pixels. For all images the strength of the CD3+ immune/inflammatory response, the number of MacroPE/SMPE particles and the class of the MPE particles were available as reference. They were labeled semi-quantitatively by a medical expert. To avoid an optimization on the test data set the images were separated into three groups: 60 images for classifier training, while in each case 20 images were used for validation and evaluation. Two different kinds of methods, preprocessing and classification methods, were used for this work. In the preprocessing step the images were first normalized, because of color and intensity variations (Fig. 2). In literature, different approaches for the standard H&E staining of medical histological images can be found. Coloring with hematoxylin accounts for a blue-purple hue and tissue colored by eosin are visible in a bright pink color [5, 6]. The images received for this work were not colored with the

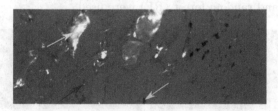

Fig. 1. Histological image with SMPE (yellow arrow), MacroPE (red arrow), MPE (blue arrow), and CD3+ immune/inflammatory response (green arrow).

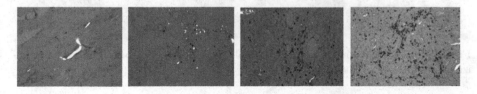

Fig. 2. Different histopathological images with a high variation in color and brightness.

usual H&E staining, because eosin would lead to a worsening of the recognition of the CD3+ cells. Nevertheless, two normalization algorithms, Macenko [7] and Reinhard [8] normalization, which were successfully used for H&E stained images, were evaluated and yielded good results (Fig. 3). Macenko et al. uses a linear per-channel normalization in optical density space [7, 9]. Reinhard et al. maps the standard deviations and means of the three channels of the original image to the corresponding channels of the target image in LAB color space [8, 9]. Both normalization algorithms are part of the stain normalization toolbox from the University of Warwick [9]. With the help of a color deconvolution (CD) [6] into the three channels corresponding to the actual stain color the visibility of the CD3+ cells and, in the most cases, the PE particles could be improved. With further preprocessing methods, simple binary thresholding, morphological operations for removing small black holes within and cracks in-between larger PE particles and a median filter for noise reduction, binary images were obtained. The PE particles, respectively the CD3+ cells, were visible as white regions on a black background. With a final blob detection method, based on the difference of Gaussian [10] and the assumption of a circular structure of the CD3+ cells, the features of the CD3+ cells were obtained. As output, the number of blobs, the area, the radii and midpoints of the blobs in the image were returned. For the purpose of classification the CD3+ immune/inflammatory response the absolute number and the total area share of these cells per image, were suitable. For finding the features of the PE particles, the number of PE particles, the areas, the perimeters and the contours, a simple contour finding algorithm provided by the OpenCV library was used. As features for separating the PE particles into MPE and MacroPE/SMPE, the perimeters and the total area occupied by PE particles per image were chosen. For classifying the MPE particles, it turned out that the number and the area of MPE particles per image were suitable. For classification the three supervised classifiers Naive Bayes (NB), support vector machine (SVM) and random forest (RF) were used.

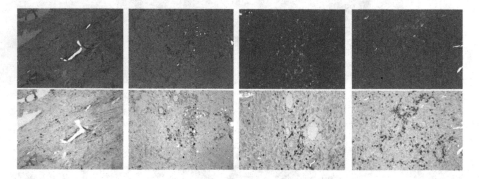

Fig. 3. Top: Macenko normalized histopatological images; Bottom: Reinhard normalized histopatological images.

3   Results

MPE particles were separated into low, moderate and high. CD3+ cells were separated into low, moderate and high immune/inflammatory response and PE particles have to be divided into MPE and MacroPE/SMPE. In Fig. 4, the normalized numbers and areas of CD3+ cells for the 60 training images, the 20 images for testing and the results of a principal component analysis (PCA) are shown top from left to right. According to the predetermined ground truth data, the red dots correspond to a low, the blue ones for a moderate and the green dots for a high CD3+ immune/inflammatory response. Although the features of the CD3+ immune/inflammatory response lie more or less on a diagonal and it can be thereby assumed that both features are correlated, a NB classifier yielded good results. An accuracy of 80 % could be reached. A PCA for dimensional reduction as well as considering just one single feature could not improve the accuracy and reached to similar results. An alternative classification algorithm (SVM, RF) yielded no significant changes in outcome, with the RF tending to overfit the training sample (Fig. 5 top). In Fig. 4, the normalized perimeters and areas of every PE particles of the PE training set (bottom left), the PE feature set of one single test image (bottom middle) and the normalized number and areas of the MPE particles for the MPE training set (bottom right) are shown, too. The NB classifier used for classification of the count of MacroPE/SMPE yielded a 55 % accurate estimation, or 90 % when a tolerated error of 1 count was introduced. For classifying the MPE particles into the three classes, a NB classifier yielded sufficient results again, revealing 80 % accuracy. In Fig. 5 the decision boundaries for the training set are shown on the respective test sets for CD3+ immune response and MPE classification. In both cases the decision

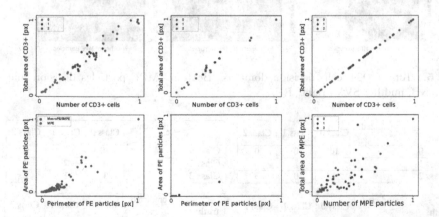

Fig. 4. Top: Ground truth labels (color coded) and CD3+-related features (number of cells, total area of cells). Left: Training set, middle: Test set, right: Training set after PCA; Bottom: PE-related features (perimeter of PE particles, area of PE particles) and MPE-related features (number of MPE particles, total area of MPE particles). Left: PE training set, middle: PE data set of a single test image, right: MPE training set.

domains are well chosen with NB. In Fig. 6 the different confusion matrices for classifier training are shown.

4 Discussion

Although the popular stain normalization methods are proven and successfully tested for the typically H&E stained colored images, it was possible to apply two of them, Macenko normalization and Reinhard normalization, to histological slice images, which were not colored with the typically H&E staining. Macenko normalization, followed by CD was suitable for the most images to improve the visibility of the available PE particles. Nevertheless sometimes smaller PE particles were not detected anymore. Generally the small image resolution and sometimes even blurred parts seemed to be problematic for the MPE particles detection. This effect accounts for some images of high MPE that were attributed to be of low MPE count and low MPE area by the feature extractor (Fig. 4 bottom right). Using the Reinhard normalization as a preprocessing step provided an

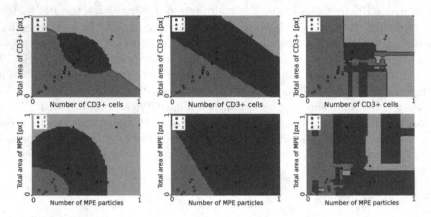

Fig. 5. Top: CD3+ cells decision domains; Bottom: MPE particles decision lines. Left: NB, middle: SVM, right: RF.

predicted: truth:	Class 0	Class 1	Class 2
Class 0	10	0	0
Class 1	3	3	0
Class 2	1	0	3

predicted: truth:	Class 0	Class 1	Class 2
Class 0	10	0	0
Class 1	4	2	0
Class 2	1	1	2

predicted: truth:	Class 0	Class 1	Class 2
Class 0	6	1	0
Class 1	1	8	2
Class 2	0	0	2

predicted: truth:	Class 0	Class 1	Class 2
Class 0	6	1	0
Class 1	1	10	0
Class 2	0	2	0

Fig. 6. Confusion matrices. Left: CD3+ classification, right: MPE classification, top: NB; Bottom: SVM.

effective means of reducing the image colouring variance significantly. After a further CD it was possible to catch the CD3+ cells with a fix threshold for all images. With the assumption of a circular structure of the CD3+ cells, it was possible to find them, although they were overlapping. Compared to the state of the art, detection of overlapping CD3+ cells was improved noticeably. Generally it can be said, that a higher number of images would have led to a better evaluation and performance of the classifiers. Nevertheless, because of the small set of very meaningful features, a classification of the cells and particles was possible and could convince with good accuracies. Especially, for the medical team it was important to gain a first indication whether the MPE correlates to the CD3+ immune/inflammatory response with a small effort. After this relationship could be confirmed, in a further step a larger study can be created, i.e. with deep learning methods [11], to verify the results and increase precision in detection.

References

1. Liebs TR. EPRD-Jahresbericht 2015. EPRD Endoprothesenregister Deutschland; 2016.
2. Hopf F. Materialabhängige CD3-Response in der SLIM bei dysfunktionalen Gelenkendoprothesen. Freie Universität Berlin; 2016.
3. Hopf F, Thomas P, Sesselmann S, et al. CD3+ lymphocytosis in the peri-implant membrane of 222 loosened joint endoprostheses depends on the tribological pairing. Acta Orthopaed. 2017; p. 1–7.
4. Krenn V, Hopf F, Thomas P, et al. Supramakropartikuläres Polyethylen bei Entzündungen periprothetischer Membranen. Der Orthopäde. 2016;45(3):256–265.
5. Magee D, Treanor D, Crellin D, et al. Colour normalisation in digital histopathology images. In: Proc MICCAI Workshop on Optical Tissue Image Analysis in Microscopy, Histopathology and Endoscopy. vol. 100. Daniel Elson; 2009.
6. Khan AM, Rajpoot N, Treanor D, et al. A nonlinear mapping approach to stain normalization in digital histopathology images using image-specific color deconvolution. IEEE Trans Biomed Eng. 2014;61(6):1729–1738.
7. Macenko M, Niethammer M, Marron J, et al. A method for normalizing histology slides for quantitative analysis. Proc ISBI. 2009; p. 1107–1110.
8. Reinhard E, Adhikhmin M, Gooch B, et al. Color transfer between images. IEEE Comp Graph App. 2001;21(5):34–41.
9. Raza SeA. Stain normalisation toolbox of warwick; 2015. [Accessed 2017-09-15]. http://www2.warwick.ac.uk/fac/sci/dcs/research/tia/software/sntoolbox/.
10. Lowe DG. Distinctive image features from scale-invariant keypoints. Int J Comput Vis. 2004;60(2):91–110.
11. Aubreville M, Knipfer C, Oetter N, et al. Automatic classification of cancerous tissue in laserendomicroscopy images of the oral cavity using deep learning. Sci Report. 2017;7(1):41598–017.

Synthetic Fundus Fluorescein Angiography using Deep Neural Networks

Florian Schiffers[1,2], Zekuan Yu[1], Steve Arguin[1], Andreas Maier[2], Qiushi Ren[1]

[1]Department of Biomedical Engineering, Peking University, China
[2]Pattern Recognition Lab, University of Erlangen-Nuremberg, Germany.
florian.schiffers@fau.de

Abstract. Fundus fluorescein angiography yields complementary image information when compared to conventional fundus imaging. Angiographic imaging, however, may pose risks of harm to the patient. The output from both types of imaging have different characteristics, but the most prominent features of the fundus are shared in both images. Thus, the question arises if conventional fundus images alone provide enough information to synthesize an angiographic image. Our research analyzes the capacity of deep neural networks to synthesize virtual angiographic images from their conventional fundus counterparts.

1 Introduction

The human retina converts incoming light into a neural signal for further processing in the brain. Because the tissue is metabolically active, early symptoms of diseases such as diabetes are detectable from retina analysis. Though fundus cameras are widely used for retinal imaging, conventional color fundus cameras are not able to image the functional state of retinal circulation [1].

Florescent angiographic methodology, in contrast, augments the capability of conventional fundus imaging. With angiographic imaging, an intravenous, fluorescent dye bounds to leukocytes, which excites the molecules when exposed to blue light. This, in turn, produces a narrow yellow-green light. The enhanced image highlights different features of the fundus. Thus, it is a routine diagnostic tool for diseases such as pseudophakic cystoid macular edema and diabetic macular edema [2]. Despite the diagnostic benefits, physicians are increasingly reluctant to use angiographic imaging technology because of its severe potential side effects [3].

Conventional color fundus imaging and fluorescence angiography are significantly different in appearance. However, many features, such as vessels or granular structures are shared between both methods. The question then emerges if an angiographic image can be efficiently estimated purely from the conventional color image. If possible, this would have the potential to further enhance diagnostic capabilities without an increase in patient risk. A successful synthetization of an angiographic image could reduce or potentially eliminate the need for actual angiographic imaging. In addition, a successful outcome in this area also serves as a potential solution to the shortage of publicly available angiographic images. Modern algorithms for image enhancement or segmentation currently cannot be efficiently trained without access to a large database of angiographic images. If these images were to be synthesized, an indefinite amount of them could be produced and therefore allow for greater research in this area.

Image synthesis and translation between different modalities has long been an area of research in the medical sciences. For example, tomographic images are a tool not only in diagnosis, but also in dose planning for cancer treatment. This method, however, often has dangerous potential side effects due to dose deposition. To circumvent this risk of harm, researchers have explored methods to generate synthetic CT images from MRI images, as MRI does not pose a risk to patients. In several studies, deep neural networks have proven to work well for typical image-translation tasks in medical imaging [4, 5].

Recently, similar image translation methods have also been applied to fundus imaging. Because access to fundus images is often restricted, Costa et al. [6] propose to synthesize fundus images from binary vessel trees in order to create large databases for other machine-learning tasks. However, to the best of our knowledge, no current algorithm exists which can estimate fundus fluorescence angiographic images from conventional color fundus images. In this work, we address this question by applying the image translation method of Zhu et al. [7] to this problem. They demonstrate image-to-image translation without the necessity of paired images from both modalities. While other methods using large databases of paired images yield superior results [8], similar-sized datasets of paired conventional and angiographic fundus images are not available. For this reason, a generative model using paired images cannot be employed.

2   Material and methods

In computer vision, generative models were long investigated to perform image synthesis. These networks were outperformed by generative adversarial networks (GANs) proposed by Goodfellow et al. [9]. Here, the generator is augmented by a discriminator, which discerns real and synthesized images. During training, the generator and the discriminator compete in a min-max game, similar to game theory. The generator network gradually refines its ability to fool the discriminator while the discriminator network gradually fine-tunes its filter to detect synthesized images. Thus, the GAN can eventually synthesize images which are indistinguishable from real images.

Recently, Zhu et al. [7] proposed a novel architecture, namely CycleGAN, translating images between two image domains A and B, without the need for tightly-coupled pairs. Unlike previous work, this setup is trained solely on the generated image quality specified by the discriminator. However, this problem is highly underdetermined and is hardly optimized. This problem is overcome by enforcing "cycle-consistency" in the sense that an image from the output domain should also translate correctly to the input domain. This backwards translation is ensured by training both a second generator and a discriminator network. Just as in standard GAN, the second generator then synthesizes from domain B to A, while the discriminator then discerns a real image B from a synthesized image B. For our problem of conventional color and angiographic fundus imaging, this architecture is visualized in Fig. 2.

2.1   Database

This study includes conventional color and angiographic fundus images from two datasets. The first provided by Hajeb et al. [10] is publicly available and contains in total 60 image pairs of 30 normal and 30 abnormal cases with a resolution of 720×576 each. The second dataset is comprised of an unpaired dataset of conventional and fluorescent images provided by the people's hospital of Jiangmen City, China. It contains 319 color and 219 fluorescent images where the resolution varies between 1380×1150 and 2800×2300.

In total, 379 color and 279 angiographic images were available in this study. From this, 365 color and 265 angiographic images are used for training, and 14 images from each group are used for testing. The test images were manually chosen to be the image pairs with the best visual alignment. Thus, the most salient image features are visible in both images.

2.2   Preprocessing

For further processing, all images were cropped to be a square with the new image center being the center of the fundus image. Subsequently, all images were downsampled to a resolution of 256×256 to keep the network from overfitting due to the lack of available training data. Color images and angiographic images are saved in the .JPG file format. Since deep learning networks require large datasets, data augmentation is a standard tool to synthetically increase the size of the dataset. In this work, each image was rotated by 90, 180, and 270 degrees, leading to a fourfold increase of training data. For further data augmentation, training samples are upscaled to 286×286 and subsequently randomly cropped to 256×256 during training.

2.3   Network architecture

This study uses the publicly available PyTorch implementation of CycleGANs provided by Zhu et al. [7]. Both generator networks are fully convolutional networks and employ the same architecture. Similarly, both discriminator networks use the same architecture. Generator networks G_C and G_F first process the image through two consecutive convolutional layers with a stride of 2. Thus, these convolutions down-sample the photo twice. The image is then subjected to six residual blocks. Subsequently, the image is brought back to its original size via two consecutive fractionally-strided convolutions with a stride of $1/2$. The discriminator networks D_C and D_F apply 70×70 PatchGANs randomly selected on the full resolution images [7]. By learning smaller patches, less parameters have to be determined, thus making the training process of the discriminator more robust. G_C takes a color image with three channels as input, then produces a grayscale image with only one channel. Vice versa, G_F inputs a grayscale image with a three channel color image as output. Respective input configurations are valid for the two discriminator networks.

The network was trained using ADAM with a batch size of 1 [7]. The learning rate was 0.0002 for the first 100 epochs, and then linearly decreased to reach 0 with epoch 200. Training with the dataset and configuration described took about 27 hours using a single GTX 1080.

3   Results

We base our evaluation on how well synthesized images resemble their ground truth counterparts. Figure 3 shows four instances taken from the test set, where an accurate registration between the image pairs were available. Each row of Fig. 3 shows from left to right the real and generated angiographic image, the input color fundus and last the backwards translated color fundus image to demonstrate the cycle consistency.

The generated images are hardly to be identified as synthetic images for a non-medically trained human. Some structures such as vessels are clearly enhanced compared to the input color image. However, there are several instances where patterns or structures in the authentic angiographic images are not synthesized correctly. For example, fine vessel structures, that are clearly visible in the real angiographic images, are unclear or not present within the synthesized images. Some local structures are located at different positions in the image, as indicated by the yellow arrow. Furthermore, the overall image brightness and contrast between ground truth and synthesized images differ.

4   Discussion

We have demonstrated that image translation between color fundus images and angiographic images is principally possible. For this, the CycleGAN architecture proposed by [7] was applied on two unpaired datasets containing conventional color and angiographic fundus images. The network was trained with downsampled and unpaired fundus images with a resolution of 256×256. A qualitative evaluation with registered image pairs independent from the training set reveals high overall resemblance with the ground truth, while some small details cannot be synthesized correctly. We are optimistic that this technique suffices to engineer robust algorithms for angiographic images by creating large synthetic databases. However, it remains unclear whether this has the potential to provide the same level of utility to a medical practitioner. This matter will be subject to a future clinical study.

Additionally, our research will focus on increasing the generated image resolution from 256×256 to state-of-the-art resolution used in medical imaging. A naive increase of the generator network's capacity to directly synthesize high-resolution data will not lead to a success, since only an insufficient amount of training samples are available. We will investigate patch-based approaches employed by similar work [6, 4] as well as more sophisticated data-augmentation methods.

References

1. Abràmoff MD, Garvin MK, Sonka M. Retinal imaging and image analysis. IEEE Rev Biomed Eng. 2010;3:169–208.
2. Shoughy SS, Kozak I. Selective and complementary use of Optical Coherence Tomography and Fluorescein Angiography in retinal practice. Eye and Vision. 2016;3(1):26.
3. Musa F, Muen W, Hancock R, et al. Adverse effects of fluorescein angiography in hypertensive and elderly patients. Acta Ophthalmologica. 2006;84(6).
4. Nie D, Cao X, Gao Y, et al.; Springer. Estimating CT image from MRI data using 3D fully convolutional networks. International Workshop on Large-Scale Annotation of Biomedical Data and Expert Label Synthesis; p. 170–178.
5. Wolterink JM, Dinkla AM, Savenije MH, et al. Deep MR to CT Synthesis using Unpaired Data. arXiv preprint arXiv:170801155.
6. Costa P, Galdran A, Meyer MI, et al. Towards adversarial retinal image synthesis. arXiv:170108974. 2017.
7. Zhu JY, Park T, Isola P, et al. Unpaired image-to-image translation using cycle-consistent adversarial networks. arXiv preprint arXiv:170310593.
8. Isola P, Zhu JY, Zhou T, et al. Image-to-image translation with conditional adversarial networks. arXiv preprint arXiv:161107004. 2016.
9. Goodfellow I, Pouget-Abadie J, Mirza M, et al. Generative adversarial nets. Adv neural Inform Process Systems; p. 2672–2680.
10. Hajeb Mohammad Alipour S, Rabbani H, Akhlaghi MR. Diabetic retinopathy grading by digital curvelet transform. Comput Math method Med. 2012;2012.

Hippocampus Segmentation and SPHARM Coefficient Selection are Decisive for MCI Detection

A. Uhl[1], M. Liedlgruber[1], K. Butz[2,3], Y. Höller[2], G. Kuchukhidze[2], A. Taylor[2], A. Thomschevski[2,3], O. Tomasi[4], E. Trinka[2,3]

[1]Department of Computer Sciences, University of Salzburg, Austria
[2]Department of Neurology, Christian Doppler Medical Centre and Centre for Cognitive Neuroscience, Paracelsus Medical University, Salzburg, Austria
[3]Spinal Cord Injury and Tissue Regeneration Centre Salzburg, Austria
[4]Department of Neurosurgery, Paracelsus Medical University, Salzburg, Austria
uhl@cosy.sbg.ac.at

Abstract. Spherical Harmonics (SPHARM), when computed from hippocampus segmentation, have been shown to be useful features for discriminating MCI affected patients from healthy controls. In this paper we assess the impact (i) of using different hippocampus segmentation techniques, among them three out-of-the-box automated segmentation tools and three human raters with different qualification, and (ii) of applying different strategies which SPHARM coefficients to submit to SVM-based two-class classification. We find that both choices are crucial for successful classification.

1 Introduction

Mild cognitive impairment (MCI) is a condition of cognitive deterioration that is difficult to classify as normal aging or as a prodromal stage to dementia. MCI needs to be treated and handled adequately, in order to prevent massive memory decline.

Neuropsychological tests alone are highly valuable but not sufficient to determine MCI or early stages thereof, since they are not sensitive enough for patients with subjective complaints and no significant and clinically detectable deficits. A reliable diagnosis is necessary for decision making in treatment of this potentially progressive condition.

Since the hippocampal formation plays a core role in memory formation and consolidation, pathological reduction in size and other structural pathologies correlate with cognitive decline. The most established application of hippocampus volumetry is the prediction of conversion from normal aging to MCI, and further to Alzheimer disease (AD). Shape-related description of hippocampi have been used as well to determine memory-related pathologies like MCI or AD [1, 2].

Segmentation of the hippocampi is of course a prerequisite for such approaches. However, several obstacles prevent from using hippocampus volumetry and (subsequent) structural characterization in standard diagnostics, among

239

them the high effort to be invested by human segmenters, which motivates the use of automated hippocampus segmentation techniques – current state-of-the-art algorithms are based on multi-atlas segmentation (MAS).

An important aspect for research efforts focusing on medical / clinical questions related to segmented hippocampi but not on segmentation techniques itself is that without proper background and significant experience, a re-implementation of proposed techniques is far from being trivial and usually requires several man-years of programming effort. Therefore, especially for research groups "only "interested in segmentation results for further analysis, available (preferably cost-free) out-of-the-box segmentation software without the need for extensive optimisation and adaption is a highly attractive (if not the only) option [3].

In this paper, we closely follow a shape-based approach to distinguish hippocampi affected by MCI from those of a healthy control group by employing spherical harmonics coefficients [2] (SPHARM) as potentially discriminating features. In this context, we investigate the impact of using different hippocampus segmentation approaches: Three cost-free and pre-compiled out-of-the-box hippocampus segmentation software packages as well as three segmentation independently conducted by human raters with different qualifications (the availability of which can be considered an extremely rare asset). Furthermore, we compare different variants of how to employ SPHARM coefficients in an SVM-based two-class (i.e. MCI vs. control group) classification.

2   Materials and methods

2.1   Spherical harmonics descriptors in structural MCI characterisation

The features used for classification are based on Spherical Harmonics (SPHARM). These are a series of functions which are used to represent functions defined on the surface of a sphere. Once a 3D object has been mapped onto a unit sphere, it is also possible to describe that object in terms of coefficients for the basis function of SPHARM. In other words, the SPHARM coefficients can be used a shape descriptors. In this work we follow the approach described in [4] in order to obtain coefficients for the hippocampi voxel volumes.

Once a voxel volume for a hippocampus has been obtained, either by automatic or manual segmentation, we first fix the topology of the voxel objects. This is necessary since to be able to map a 3D object to a sphere the respective voxel object must exhibit a spherical topology.

Based on the resampled and fixed voxel volumes, we generate 3D objects. While other implementations create objects based on triangular faces, we decided to use quadriliterals since these more naturally correspond to voxels. The 3D objects are then mapped onto a unit sphere during the initial parameterisation, which is followed by a constrained optimisation (described in more detail in [4]). The optimised parameterisation is then used to compute the SPHARM coefficients.

We are mainly interested in shape differences and thus we want to ignore orientation differences among different hippocampi. For alignment, we compute a reconstruction of the hippocampus object up to SPHARM degree 1 (based on a triangulated sphere). This results in an ellipsoid which is aligned with the main orientation of the 3D object. Using PCA we determine the principal axes of the ellipsoid and rotate the object such that all hippocampi volumes are always in the coordinate system of the principal axes (i.e. co-aligned). After the re-alignment we recompute the SPHARM coefficients up to degree 15 for each re-aligned object and use them for the subsequent classification process.

Computing SPHARM coefficients up to degree D, we obtain a total of N complex coefficients per hippocampus, where N is computed as $N = 3*(D+1)^2$. Extracting SPHARM coefficients up to degree 15 we end up with 768 coefficients per hippocampus. We have used a custom MATLAB implementation following the SPHARM-PDM code[1].

The final feature vectors F_i available for the feature selection process are composed of the absolute coefficient values for the left and right hippocampi

$$F_i = (|C_{i,1}^l|, \ldots, |C_{i,N}^l|, |C_{i,1}^r|, \ldots, |C_{i,N}^r|) \tag{1}$$

where $C_{i,n}^l$ and $C_{i,n}^r$ denote the n-th coefficient for the left and right hippocampus of subject i, respectively. These feature vectors contain 1536 coefficients in total out of which subsets can be selected for actual classification.

2.2 Experimental settings

Data In this work we use 41 T1-weighted MRI volumes, a data set that has been acquired at the Department of Neurology, Paracelsus Medical University Salzburg, including patients with mild cognitive impairment (MCI, 20 subjects) and a healthy control group (CG, 21 subjects). These data are a subset of a larger study [3]. Diagnosis / ground truth wrt. MCI was based on multimodal neurological assessment, including imaging (high resolution 3T magnetic resonance tomography, and single photon emission computed tomography with Hexamethylpropylenaminooxim), and neuropsychological testing.

Hippocampus segmentation Manual segmentation have been performed by 3 experienced raters (one senior neurosurgeon – Rater1 – and two junior neuroscientists supervised by a senior neuroradiologist – Rater2 & Rater3) on a Wacom Cintiq 22HD graphic tablet device (resolution 1920x1200) using a DTK-2200 pen and employing the 32-bit 3DSlicer software for Windows (v. 4.2.2-1 r21513) to delineate hippocampus voxels for each slice separately. The raters independently used consensus on anatomical landmarks/boarders of the hippocampus based on Henry Duvemoy's hippocampal anatomy. The procedure used was to depict the hippocampal outline in the view of all planes in the following order: sagittal – coronal – axial with subsequent cross line control through all planes.

---

[1] available at https.//www.nitrc.org/projects/spharm pdm

For automated hippocampus segmentation all three employed hippocampus segmentation software packages are already pre-compiled and available for free [3]:

FreeSurfer (FS)[2] is a popular set of tools which allow an automated labelling of subcortical structures in the brain. AHEAD (Automatic Hippocampal Estimator using Atlas-based Delineation[3]) is specifically targeted at an automated segmentation of hippocampi and employs multiple atlases and statistical learning method. Although BrainParser (BP)[4] is usually able to label various different subcortical structures, we use a version of BrainParser which is specifically tailored to hippocampus segmentation.

We also fuse the segmentation results using voxel-based majority voting (a voxel is active in the fused volume if at least two raters or segmentation tools marked that voxel as belonging to a hippocampus) and STAPLE [5]. Since for human raters there is hardly a difference between majority voting and STAPLE, the latter results are not shown.

Feature selection, classification, and evaluation protocol Features used for actual classification are selected from the feature vectors F_i according to the degree D of their coefficients. The strategy "Single$D$ "selects only coefficients of degree D for classification, while "Cumula$D$ "selects all coefficients with degree $\leq D$. Thus, for example, Single5 uses 33 coefficients of degree 5 while Cumula5 employs 108 coefficients of degrees $D = 1 \ldots 5$. In order to reduce the dimensionality of our feature vectors for large values of D, we employ sequential forward feature selection (SFFS).

For the classification of the features we use the Support Vector Machines (SVM) classifier with a linear kernel. The choice for this classifier has been made since the classifier is known to be able to cope very well with high-dimensional features.

To come up with classification accuracy estimation, we apply leave-one-out-cross-validation (LOOVC) for the feature vectors of type Single$J$ and Cumula$J$. For SFFS, in order to reduce the significant computational cost, we apply 10-fold cross validation, i.e. the hippocampi to be classified are split into 10 folds. Each fold yields a training set for which the optimal set of features is determined using SFFS, using the LOOCV accuracy of the SVM classifier as the criterion function (wrapper approach). The validation features (evaluation set) of the current fold are then classified using SVM as well. This process is repeated for all folds and from the resulting SVM predictions for the validation features the classification rates are computed.

---

[2] v. 51.0, available at http://surfer.nmr.mgh.harvard.edu

[3] v. 1.0, available at http://www.nitrc.org/projects/

[4] available at http://www.nitrc.org/projects/

Table 1. Classification Results (overall accuracy ≥ 75% in bold; AH = AHEAD; R = Rater; S = Single; C = Cumula).

	Automated Segmentation					Human Segmentation				
	STA	MV	AH	BP	FS	D.F.	M.V.	R1	R2	R3	DF
SFFS	52.50	45.24	43.18	39.53	53.49	54.28	47.62	**80.95**	50.00	71.43	62.53
S1	57.50	71.43	54.55	44.19	65.12	59.09	**80.95**	71.43	**78.57**	71.43	**85.71**
S2	**80.00**	61.90	59.09	55.81	41.86	59.09	54.76	59.52	61.90	64.29	64.29
C1	65.00	64.29	63.64	39.53	74.42	65.91	**88.10**	64.29	**78.57**	66.67	**76.19**
C2	57.50	61.90	63.64	53.49	65.12	70.45	**83.33**	**76.19**	73.81	62.29	**76.19**
C3	60.00	64.29	56.82	41.86	67.44	59.09	**78.57**	**80.95**	66.67	69.05	**80.95**
C4	60.00	66.67	59.09	48.84	60.47	54.55	**80.95**	69.05	57.14	61.90	69.05

3 Results

Tab. 1 displays the overall classification accuracy in percent for our test data set (41 T-1 MRI volumes). Results are shown up to $J = 4$ (CumulaD) and $J = 2$ (SingleD), respectively, as for higher values of J classification accuracy goes down considerably.

We have depicted results exceeding 75% in bold. The first impression of the results is that there are no bold numbers except for one outlier in the left half of the table, i.e. the employment of automated segmentation tools does not lead to any decent classification results using the considered SPHARM approach. Looking at the results of applying individual automated segmentation tools, BP results are hardly superior to random guessing, while FS and AHEAD based results are on a comparable level and clearly better than BP.

Applying Majority Voting (M.V.) or STAPLE (STA) to the individual segmentation sometimes improves the classification results as obtained when relying on a single segmentation, but not consistently so. There is no clear trend which feature selection strategy is the best one. Overall, classification accuracy obtained based on automated segmentation is too low to be useful.

The situation is different when considering the results when basing SPHARM classification on human rater segmentation. There is a clear trend that the CumulaJ feature selection strategy is superior to SingleJ selection (where only Single1 gives competitive results).

The best results are seen up to $J = 4$, and the poor results of SingleJ for $J = 2 \ldots 4$ seem to indicate that the information most important for classification is present in the low degrees $J = 0, 1$. Also, for CumulaJ, we find the Majority Voting based results as being superior to the single rater results (except for Cumula3 where a single rater is slightly better). The best result seen (88.10% accuracy with 90.91% sensitivity and 85.00% specificity) even surpasses the corresponding classification results as given in [2] for MCI vs. CG with 83%, where a bagging strategy is used for feature selection.

There is no single rater giving clearly the best results, thus, obviously the higher qualification of Rater1 does not lead to segmentation specifically well suited for subsequent SPHARM-based classification. Overall, the differences among the human raters in terms of achieved classification accuracy are considerable.

For a comparison, we have also added results from applying decision level fusion ("DF" columns in Table 1), i.e. the classification results (MCI vs. CG) of the three individual (automated or human) segmentation are combined using majority voting (instead of fusing segmentation on a voxel basis). Those results confirm the observed trends – no useful results when relying on the three employed automated tools, and reasonable results for CumulaJ, $J = 1 \ldots 3$ and Single1 for human rater segmentation.

4   Discussion

We observe that applying three out-of-the-box hippocampus segmentation software tools does not lead to satisfying classification results, even in case fusion techniques like STAPLE are applied to the three automated segmentation. For segmentation based on human raters, competitive classification results are achieved, especially when fusing three manual segmentation, since we observe high variability in the classification results when relying on single manual segmentation. Results also show that the most discriminative information resides in the lower degree SPHARM coefficients.

We may state that results published (e.g. [2]) cannot be easily reproduced with publicly available and cost-free segmentation software. availability of state-of-the-art and easy-to-use segmentation software for clinically oriented research.

Acknowledgement. This work has been partially supported by the Austrian Science Fund, project no. KLIF 00012.

References

1. Gutman B, Wang Y, et al. Disease classification with hippocampal shape invariants. Hippocampus. 2009;19(6):572–578.
2. Geradin E, Chetelat G, et al. Multidimensional classification of hippocampal shape features discriminates Alzheimer's disease and mild cognitive impairment from normal aging. Neuroimage. 2009;47(4):1476–1486.
3. Liedlgruber M, Butz K, Höller Y, et al. Variability issues in automated hippocampal segmentation: a study on out-of-the-box software and multi-rater ground truth. Proc CBMS. 2016; p. 191–196.
4. Brechühler C, Gerig G, Kübler O. Parametrization of closed surfaces for 3-D shape description. Comput Vis Image Underst. 1995;61(2):154–170.
5. Warfield SK, Zou KH, Wells WM. Simulataneous truth and performance level estimation (STAPLE): an algortihm for the validation of image segmentation. IEEE Trans Med Imaging. 2004;23(7):903–921.

Classification of Mitotic Cells
Potentials Beyond the Limits of Small Data Sets

Maximilian Krappmann[1], Marc Aubreville[1],Andereas Maier[1],
Christof Bertram[2], Robert Klopfleisch[2]

[1]Pattern Recognition Lab, Friedrich-Alexander-University Erlangen-Nuernberg,
Germany
[2]Institute of Veterinary Pathology, Freie University of Berlin, Germany
maximilian.krappmann@inveox.com

Abstract. Tumor diagnostics are based on histopathological assessments
of tissue biopsies of the suspected carcinogen region. One standard task
in histopathology is counting of mitotic cells, a task that provides great
potential to be improved in speed, accuracy and reproducability. The advent of deep learning methods brought a significant increase in precision
of algorithmic detection methods, yet it is dependent on the availability
of large amounts of data, completely capturing the natural variability
in the material. Fully segmented images are provided by the MITOS
dataset with 300 mitotic events. The ICPR2012 dataset provides 326
mitotic cells and in AMIDA2014 dataset, 550 mitotic cells for training
and 533 for testing. In contrast to these datasets, a dataset with high
number of mitotic events is missing. For this, either one of two pathologist annotated at least 10 thousand cell images for cells of the type mitosis, eosinophilic granulocyte and normal tumor cell from canine mast
cell tumor whole-slide images, exceeding all publicly available data sets
by approximately one order of magnitude. We tested performance using
a standard CNN approach and found accuracies of up to 0.93.

1 Introduction

The number of mitotic figures within a certain area is an important characteristic in tumor grading. Mitotic cell count is a valuable predictor, correlating
highly with tumor proliferation [1]. Most of the histopathological grading systems require the number of mitotic figures within a defined area (high power
field, HPF). However, this area is not defined uniquely [2]. If the number of
mitotic figures exceeds a defined limit within ten consecutive HPFs, the grading
of the tumor may change. However, this makes a clear distinction of different
grades of illness highly questionable. The consensus among different pathologists in grading was evaluated in [3], revealing an inter-oberver discordance in
50% of the cases. As a reason, the high subjectivity of the pathologists and the
flexibility in the choice of the high power fields is reported. In order to counteract these obstacles, computer-aided methods for detecting mitotic figures were
taken into account. This process can be clustered into two main tasks. First

245

of all, the detection of cells and at second, the classification of the cells found. The hosts of competitions to detect mitotic cells prepared datasets for this tasks. The ICPR2012 dataset provides 326 mitotic events in fully segmented images. In the AMIDA2014 dataset, 550 mitotic cells for training and 533 events for testing can be found. The MITOS dataset provides about 300 mitotic figures. However, it can be questioned if this amount of training data is sufficient to train accurate classifiers. It is known that mitosis can be distinguished into four different phases, each phase results in high variance in their visual representation. This work focuses on the classification task of the cells not on detection. Due to that a dataset with more than 12000 mitotic cells, 17000 tumor cells and 10000 granulocytes is provided by our dataset. These figures have been extracted by manually reviewing 100000 histological image sections of stained canine mast cell tumors. In order to prove the demand for such a dataset, a simple deep learning approach is trained and evaluated with respect to all its parameters and with respect to the modifications of the input data. To provide the correctness of the data, the cells have been annotated by pathologists.

2   Related work

In [4] a multitask learning approach is presented which is able to detect mitotic events. A deep learning architecture similar to [5] was used. This method achieved an F-score of 0.53 across 550 mitotic events in comparison to an F-score of 0.90 for 3064 lymphatic cells. The detection rate of all cells was 98%. Malon et al. [6] used the same architecture as used in this work achieved an F-score of 0.65 on the MITOS dataset. As input 72×72 cell patches were used. Handcrafted features like morphology and run length features were extracted on blue ration images. The method introduced in [7] makes use of a pixel-wise sliding window approach. Based on that, pixels were considered as true positive if a single pixel was in a specific range around a mitotic figure. Furthermore, images around the mitotic figures were cropped and the network was trained. The architecture consists of five 2×2 convolutional layers followed by 2×2 max pooling layers and two fully connected output layers. This process needs a total of 31 seconds per patch and eight minutes per HPF. The achieved F-score was 0.782. A second approach with a reduced depth of three convolutional layers resulted in an F-score of 0.758. This network was eight times faster than the original method. Albarqouini et al. [8] came up with a special type of network that is able process two types of input data. First of all, ground truth data from established datasets like ICPR2012, MITOS or AMIDA are used. The second type of data was obtained using crowd sourcing layers. These layers incorporate annotations of non-professionals. Doing this needed some sort of reliability measurement which is why an expectation maximization algorithm is used to do some weighting. The authors revealed an improvement of 0.36 in the best and 0.068 in the worst case. The best F score was 0.76. Chen et al. [9] used another deep learning approach that made use of fully convolutional networks in order to detect mitotic candidates. Therefore, a probability map of the input is obtained yielding high values for mitotic candidates. This net was trained on 94×94 input images. However, since the spatial information is preserved, the network is able to detect mitotic candidates. These candidates are then fed into a convolutional network with a fully connected output layer for classification. A F score of 0.785 was archieved by this cascaded pipeline. Moreover, the pipeline is able to predict a 2000×2000 input image within 0.49 seconds using a NVIDIA GeForce GTX Titan GPU. All current deep learning approaches made us of augmentation due to the fact that they require a comparatively large amount of training data. This is obvious since deep learning requires a comparatively large amount of training data.

3   Material and methods

3.1   Dataset

The dataset was acquired using a semi-automatic annotation GUI. Therefore, the whole slide images are processed using the openslide software [10] and manually cropped by simply clicking at cells. The position of the midpoint for a single cell was saved. In addition, the size of the cell patches can be varied if needed. As advantage, different well known deep learning models can be used without adjusting their parameters too much. The cropped candidates were forwarded to two pathologists for revision. Exemplary results of this process can be seen in Fig. 1.

3.2   Network

Using deep learning in this work was based on the feature extraction ability of this method. Since works with good features for mitosis detection could not be found, it was logical to pick a deep learning approach. The size of the cell patches was 50×50. An example of different cell types is found in Fig. 2. To classify the mitotic cells two other classes have been extracted namely tumor cells and granulocytes. Besides mitotic cells, canine mast cell tumors largely consist of those last-mentioned cell types. Moreover, the detection of other cells is required for calculating mitotic index. This index was used in [2] to increase the accordance between pathologists. The idea is to divide the mitotic cell count by the number of other cells because it is assumed that mitotic cells in sparse regions may have higher influence on the diagnosis than in studded regions. Our work will show that it is sufficient to use a simple net in order to achieve good results due to the amount of data. Therefore the LeNet architecture was chosen. To evaluate parameters that may effect the performance of the network, the deep learning pipeline is taken into account. First of all, the manipulation of the input is investigated. Afterwards, the feature extraction ability of the network must be evaluated. The standard CNN in this work consists of two 5×5 convolutional layers followed by 2×2 max pooling layer, nesterov momentum of 0.9 and a step size of 0.01 was applied. The fully connected layer consists of 256 nodes followed by a softmax activation layer. For better generalization a dropout of 0.5 was used.

Table 1. In the first part of the table methods for input manipulations are tested. At next different modifications of the CNN architecture are evaluated.

CNN	Precision	Recall	F1	support
CNN+RGB	0.91	0.91	0.91	9490
CNN+GRAY	0.92	0.92	0.92	9490
CNN+AUG	0.92	0.92	0.92	9490
CNN+RGB+AUG	0.93	0.92	0.93	9490
CNN+Moment	0.92	0.92	0.92	9490
CNN+AdaDelta	0.89	0.89	0.89	9490
CNN+AdaGrad	0.91	0.91	0.91	9490
CNN+ExtraLayer	0.89	0.88	0.88	9490

4   Results

4.1   Manipulation of the input

The augmentation of data is routinely performed to create virtually new samples. This is beneficial when the amount of data is not sufficient or the variance in

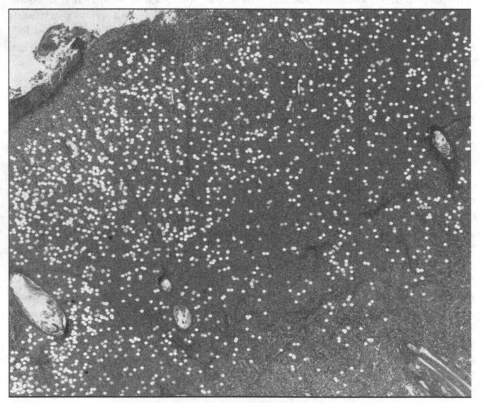

Fig. 1. Cell distribution within a partially segmented H&E slide (green: mitotic cells, blue: granulocytes, yellow: tumor cells).

Table 2. MITOS and our dataset for equal amount of mitotic and non mitotic cells.

CNN	Precision	Recall	F1	support
MITOS2014	0.66	0.65	0.65	172
OURS	0.93	0.93	0.93	4429

the test data is smaller than in real applications. To generate more varying samples, random operations like rotations, scaling, shift in colour channels or noise can be applied to achieve more robust features. If some information or small differences are missing or getting obliterated, this might also have a negative effect. Furthermore, the usage of grey scale images in contrast to RGB images is evaluated. Augmentation in combination with RGB images results in an increased performance. It is likely that the information is increased due to the usage of three channels. In addition, augmentation is used to increase the dataset and capture more variances in the images. The full impact can be seen from the first part in Table 1.

4.2   Parameters affecting the feature extraction

The feature extraction ability of a neural network is based on its adaptation of the filters. To adapt these filters a global loss function is minimized by back-propagating an error. This requires different gradient descent methods. The methods are able to overshot a global minimum or getting stuck in a local minimum. The different methods yield differnces in F-scores between 0.88 and 0.92 due to that behaviour. In addition, the depth of the network is effecting the amount and quality of the filters. If the depth is too large, the network may

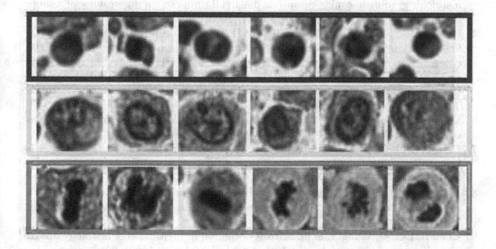

Fig. 2. Different cells of interest (green: mitotic cells, blue: granulocytes, yellow: tumor cells).

run into overfitting the training data which happened in our case. All effects are gathered in the second part in table 1.

4.3 Baseline comparison

As baseline the MITOS2014 dataset of the ICPR14 contest was used. Therefore, our dataset was translated into a two class problem. The network was trained on a $80 - 20$ split. The results in table 2 show a clear improvement on detection accuracies, as is likely induced by the increased dataset size.

5 Conclusion

Our work supports the idea that the key of boosting the classification performance is the amount of input data. The different gradient descent methods reveal their effects on the performance of network as expected. The increased depth of the network has no positive effect on the scores. The limitations of small datasets in the medical field were shown in table 2 and emphasise the need for larger datasets for pattern recognition in the medical context.

References

1. Kiupel M, Webster J, Bailey K, et al. Proposal of a 2-Tier histologic grading system for canine cutaneous mast cell tumors to more accurately predict biological behavior. Veterin Pathology. 2011;48(1):147–155.
2. Meuten D, Moore F, George J. Mitotic count and the field of view area: Time to standardize. SAGE Publications Sage CA: Los Angeles, CA; 2016.
3. Northrup N, Howerth E, Harmon B, et al. Variation among Pathologists in the histologic grading of canine cutaneous mast cell tumors with uniform use of a single grading reference. J Veterin Diagn Invest. 2005;17(6):561–564.
4. Romo-Bucheli D, Janowczyk A, Gilmore H, et al. A deep learning based strategy for identifying and associating mitotic activity with gene expression derived risk categories in estrogen receptor positive breast cancers. Cytometry A. 2017.
5. Krizhevsky A, Sutskever I, Hinton GE. Imagenet classification with deep convolutional neural networks. In: Advances in Neural Information Processing Systems; 2012. p. 1097–1105.
6. Malon CD, Cosatto E, et al. Classification of mitotic figures with convolutional neural networks and seeded blob features. J Pathol Inform. 2013;4(1):9.
7. Cireşan DC, Giusti A, Gambardella LM, et al.; Springer. Mitosis detection in breast cancer histology images with deep neural networks. Proc MICCAI. 2013; p. 411–418.
8. Albarqouni S, Baur C, Achilles F, et al. AggNet: deep learning from crowds for mitosis detection in breast cancer histology images. IEEE Trans Med Imaging. 2016;35(5):1313–1321.
9. Chen H, Dou Q, Wang X, et al. Mitosis detection in breast cancer histology images via deep cascaded networks. In: 13th AAAI Conf Artific Intell; 2016.
10. Goode A, Satyanarayanan M. A Vendor-Neutral library and viewer for whole-slide images. Computer Science Department, Carnegie Mellon University. 2008.

Markerless Coil Classification and Localization in a Routine MRI Examination Setting using an RGB-D Camera

Janani G. Nadar[1], Xia Zhong[1], Andreas Maier[1,2]

[1] Pattern Recognition Lab, Department of Computer Science,
Friedrich-Alexander-Universität Erlangen-Nürnberg
[2] Erlangen Graduate School in Advanced Optical Technologies(SAOT)
gayathri.nadar@fau.de

Abstract. In a routine MRI scan, a radio-frequency (RF) coil must be selected and placed around the region of interest (ROI). This is a crucial step in the workflow as the accurate coil placement is paramount for obtaining high-quality images. However, in the existing workflow, the position of the coil placement on the patient is estimated empirically by the medical technical assistant (MTA). This routine coil placement process has two shortcomings. On the one hand, the expertise of MTA in coil placement, taking the anatomical difference between patients into account, have a huge impact on the accuracy of the coil placement, and subsequently the image quality. On the other hand, the risk of selecting and placing the incorrect coil should be also be acknowledged. To improve the current workflow and provide feedback ahead of the MRI scans, we use an RGB-D camera to acquire extra information. Using the depth images taken before and after placing the coil, we propose a novel method to classify the coil type and localize the coil position during the coil placement process such that the MTA can place the coil correctly and accurately. We trained and evaluated our method over 100 synthetic data sets. We used two types of coils and placed and deformed them differently according to the anatomical region. The evaluation shows that we can classify the coil type without any error, and localize the coil with a mean translational error of 7.1 cm and mean rotation angle error of 0.025 rad.

1 Introduction

RF coil systems are an essential part of the MRI system, responsible for receiving the signal used for image formation. Recent receive-only flexible RF coils used in MRI provide high sensitivity in the area covered by the coil resulting in high-quality images of the organ of interest such as liver, prostate, etc. These coils can be easily wrapped or laid flat on the patient body covering all body shapes and contour. However, an accurate placement of the coil according to the planned examination is a difficult task. The MTA has to align the coil on the patient such that the coil is over the organ of interest. Even well-trained personnel

251

sometimes wrongly estimate the correct location of an organ considering different body shapes and sizes. Incorrect placement leads to increased examination time and discomfort to the patient since the positioning procedure is repeated. To improve the current workflow, an coil placement assistant system should cover two key aspects. First, a method is needed to pinpoint the target coil placement position accurately despite the difference in body shape. To this end, methods haven been proposed to fit a patient surface model using a RGB-D camera [1] and model the variation of the internal anatomy across the population [2]. Second, a method is needed to classify and localize the current coil to provide feedback to the MTA. To this end, Frohwein et al. introduce a marker-based solution for coil detection for attenuation correction for PET/MR [3]. However, the marker-based approaches are elaborate requiring accurate marker placement and additional time for their placement and removal. In this work, we assume the target coil position is given and introduce a marker-less method for the coil classification and localization method using a RGB-D camera.

2   Materials and methods

The general pipeline of our method is shown in Fig. 1. Our method consists of two main branches. First we detect the coil in the images using a trained coil detection model. Next we localize the coil through 3D feature matching and extract the 3D rigid transformation of the coil. The first step is data generation where we create a synthetic depth image dataset with two types of coil. Then we proceed to the pre-processing of the depth images. In this step, we first perform the subtraction of images with and without coil on the subject. This is followed by filtering operations for denoising and extraction of coil region from the images which is our desired ROI. Additionally, the extracted ROI is also converted into a point cloud for 3D mesh generation. Next in the pipeline, we perform a feature detection, extraction and description in the ROI images and also on the 3D meshes. In the final step, the images are divided into training and testing sets for training the SVM classifier model. The features detected in 3D meshes are used for coil localization through feature matching for 3D rigid transform estimation.

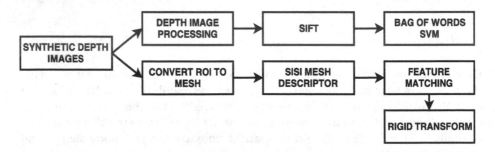

Fig. 1. An outline of our coil detection and localization pipeline.

2.1   Synthetic data generation

We start our procedure with generating synthetic depth maps. We use two types of flexible body coil meshes namely, A and B. A scene is created such that a pin-hole camera model is mounted on the ceiling directly above the scanner table looking at the patient at a distance of 300 cm from origin. We obtain 100 synthetic depth images for each type of coil by sampling mesh positions along the length and width of a human body model. We also include non-clinical coil positions to cover all possible coil locations on the subject's body. In each case, two images are obtained; one before placing the coil and one after. A ground truth file with all the transformation data such as translation, rotation, scale, and coordinates of coil position is also generated. We add a Gaussian noise distribution to the perfectly rendered depth images.

2.2   Coil ROI extraction

In the image with the coil placed on the subject's body, the coil surface is at a closer distance to the camera than the patient below. Hence, we perform a subtraction of the two images taken before and after placing the coil giving a rough outline of the coil. This is followed by thresholding such that an intensity at a pixel (x, y) above t^{MAX} is set to 0. We perform median filtering to remove noise and preserve edges.

Let the input image after denoising and filtering be S. S is a binary image in which pixels with $S(x, y) = 1$ belong to the coil and pixels with $S(x, y) = 0$ belong to the background. We detect a set of contours C such that the contours in $C = \{c_i | i = 1, 2, \ldots, N\}$ define a set of N closed borders between the foreground (1-pixels) and the background. The individual contour c_i is given by,

$$c_i = \{(x_j, y_j) | j = 1, \ldots, J \wedge x_j \in [0 \ldots w] \wedge y_j \in [0 \ldots h] \wedge x_0 = x_J \wedge y_0 = y_J\} \tag{1}$$

where w and h are width and height of the input image S respectively and J is the length of the ith contour. Next, we compute the area of all the contours and extract the one with the maximum area which gives the coil. We define a rectangular window around this area and crop the ROI. We further reconstruct the 3D world coordinates of the foreground pixels in the ROI using the camera intrinsic and extrinsic parameters. Afterwards, we apply ball-pivoting algorithm [4] to reconstruct a surface mesh from the foreground pixel point cloud.

Subsequently, we calculate the feature for both depth image and the reconstructed surface mesh using feature descriptor. In case of depth images, we use the scale-invariant feature transform (SIFT) [5] and for 3D surface meshes, we use the scale-invariant spin image (SISI) mesh descriptor [6]. For depth image S_i, we calculate a SIFT feature map $\boldsymbol{F}_i = [\boldsymbol{f}_{i,1}^T, \cdots \boldsymbol{f}_{i,N}^T]^T \in \mathbb{R}^{N \times M}$, where N denotes the number of keypoints and M denotes the dimension of the SIFT descriptor. Similarly, for each reconstructed 3D mesh $\boldsymbol{Q}_i$, we calculate a SISI feature map $\boldsymbol{F}_i' = [\boldsymbol{f}_{i,1}'^T, \cdots, \boldsymbol{f}_{i,N'}'^T]^T \in \mathbb{R}^{N' \times M'}$, where N' denotes the number of keypoints and M' denotes the dimension of the SISI descriptor.

2.3   Coil type classification

Coil type classification is performed using Bag-of-Visual-Words [7] and Support Vector Machine (SVM) [8]. Let's denote $\boldsymbol{F} = [\boldsymbol{F}_1^T, \cdots \boldsymbol{F}_K^T]^T$ as our global feature map for all K images in the dataset. We then generate a vocabulary of visual words by clustering the global feature map $\boldsymbol{F}$ with a cluster number of 100 using k-means clustering method. Using the vocabulary, the feature map in each image $\boldsymbol{F}_i$ is quantized by finding the nearest visual words for each $\boldsymbol{f}_{i,j}$ in the vocabulary to a histogram $\boldsymbol{h}_i$ showing the frequency of occurrence of visual words. Using the histogram, we train our SVM model such that,

$$\underset{\alpha_i > 0}{\text{maximize}} \quad \sum_{i=1}^{K} \alpha_i - \frac{1}{2} \sum_{i,j=1}^{K} \alpha_i \alpha_j y_i y_j k(\boldsymbol{x_i x_j})$$
$$\text{subject to} \quad \forall i : 0 < \alpha_i < C \tag{2}$$
$$\sum_{i=1}^{K} \alpha_i y_i = 0$$

where $k(\boldsymbol{x_i}, \boldsymbol{x_j})$ is the Gaussian RBF kernel, K is the number of samples, y_i is the class label such that $y_i \in \{0,1\}^K$, α_i define the weights to be learned and C is the regularization parameter. A test sample $\boldsymbol{x}$ is classified with the following decision function.

$$f(x) = \sum_i \alpha_i y_i k(\boldsymbol{x_i}, \boldsymbol{x}) + b \tag{3}$$

Here, $k(\boldsymbol{x_i}, \boldsymbol{x})$ is then the kernel function value for training sample x_i and test sample $\boldsymbol{x}$, α_i is the learned weight for training sample $\boldsymbol{x_i}$ and b is the learned bias parameter.

2.4   Coil localization

By using the features detected in the surface meshes we perform a matching with the features detected in a template mesh (Fig. 2).

The template mesh is obtained by placing the coil at origin in the defined world coordinate system (WCS) with zero translation and rotation values. Let $\mathcal{T}$ and $\mathcal{Q}$ be the template and target meshes respectively. We compute the Euclidean distance between the feature maps of $\mathcal{T}$ and $\mathcal{Q}$ and sort them in ascending order of their distance. We use the indices of first 5 nearest-neighbours and obtain a set of matched 3D vertices from $\mathcal{T}$ and $\mathcal{Q}$. We use a 3D implementation of RANSAC [9] and the Kabsch algorithm [10] to filter out the false matches or outliers. In an iterative process, 25 random points are used to compute a transformation $\mathbb{T}$ using the Kabsch algorithm. Every point from $\mathcal{T}$ is transformed with $\mathbb{T}$ and the Euclidean distance between the transformed point and the corresponding point from $\mathcal{Q}$ is computed. Points for which the resulting distance is less than a defined threshold, are selected as inliers. Using these inliers the final transformation is computed between $\mathcal{T}$ and $\mathcal{Q}$ which gives a 3×3 rotation matrix $\mathbb{R}$ depicting the rotation of Q and a 3-dimensional translation vector t. Since $\mathcal{T}$ is at origin, t gives us the the position of $\mathcal{Q}$.

3   Evaluation and Results

For coil detection, we used randomly selected 80 images and 20 images for training and testing respectively. Class 0 consists of all examples of B and Class 1 of A. Our method identifies the coils without any error with an accuracy of 1.0. For coil localization and transform estimation we compared the obtained transformations using feature matching with the ground truth. We computed the 3D rotation vector from the rotation matrix and calculated its L2-norm. For coils A and B, we get a mean error of 0.02 ± 0.01 rad and 0.03 ± 0.02 rad respectively. For translation, we computed a root-mean-squared error (RMSE) of the difference between the estimated and actual translation. We get a mean RMSE error of 6.46 ± 6.5 cm and 7.72 ± 5.19 cm for A and B respectively.

4   Discussion

We propose a novel method for markerless coil classification and localization in a routine MRI scan setting. Our method is based purely on depth images taken before and after coil placement without the need for markers. Our proposed coil classification method works efficiently achieving an accuracy of 1.0. We find that our algorithm is robust against occlusion. This is inferred by testing the algorithm on datasets where the coil is partially covered. The algorithm is able to classify the coil type correctly when the coil is half visible due to bending. Our coil localization algorithm performs well with a mean error of 0.025 radians for rotation estimation and a mean error of 7.1 cm in case of translation.

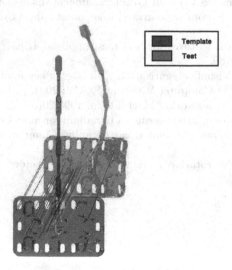

Fig. 2. An example of feature matching between template and test meshes.

For practical applicability, future work must address several current limitations. Firstly, our method assumes that the coil is already placed on the patient. In a clinical scenario, it could be beneficial to verify whether the coil is placed on the patient before coil detection and localization. Secondly, our methods can benefit from validation using real RGB-D data for e.g. from Kinect. Finally, in our study, we use depth ROI images for coil detection and the point cloud from the ROI for coil localization. A good idea would be to use point clouds for both coil detection and localization methods.

Despite current limitations, this is the first study, to our knowledge, to examine the use of depth images for MRI scan workflow optimization through coil identification and localization. An implication of these findings is that it is feasible to detect and localize RF coils using solely images mitigating the need for markers. Although our method requires further improvements for enhancing the accuracy, the results are of direct practical relevance.

Acknowledgement. We gratefully acknowledge the support of Siemens Healthineers, Erlangen, Germany. Note that the concepts and information presented in this paper are based on research, and they are not commercially available.

References

1. Singh V, Chang Y, Ma K, et al. Estimating a patient surface model for optimizing the medical scanning workflow. Proc MICCAI. 2014; p. 472–479.
2. Zhong X, Strobel N, Sanders JC, et al. Generation of Personalized Computational Phantoms Using Only Patient Metadata. Proc IEEE NSS/MIC. 2017.
3. Frohwein L, He M, Buther F, et al. Determination of position and shape of flexible mri surface coils using the Microsoft Kinect for attenuation correction in PET/MRI. Eur J Nucl Med Mol Imaging Physics. 2015;2(1):A79.
4. Bernardini F, Mittleman J, Rushmeier H, et al. The ball-pivoting algorithm for surface reconstruction. IEEE Trans Vis Comput Graphics. 1999;5(4):349–359.
5. Lowe DG. Distinctive image features from scale-invariant keypoints. Int J Comput Vision. 2004;60(2):91–110.
6. Darom T, Keller Y. Scale-invariant features for 3-D mesh models. IEEE Trans Image Process. 2012;21(5):2758–2769.
7. Csurka G, Dance C, Fan L, et al. Visual categorization with bags of keypoints. In: Workshop on Statistical Learning in Computer Vision at ECCV; 2004. p. 1–22.
8. Cortes C, Vapnik V. Support-vector networks. Mach Learn. 1995;20(3):273–297.
9. Fischler MA, Bolles RC. Random sample consensus: a paradigm for model fitting with applications to image analysis and automated cartography. Commun ACM. 1981;24(6):381–395.
10. Kabsch W. A solution for the best rotation to relate two sets of vectors. Acta Crystallogr A. 1976;32(5):922–923.

Comparative Analysis of Unsupervised Algorithms for Breast MRI Lesion Segmentation

Sulaiman Vesal[1], Nishant Ravikumar[1], Stephan Ellman[2], Andreas Maier[1]

[1]Fakultät für Pattern Recognition, FAU Erlangen-Nürnberg, Germany
[2]Radiologisches Institut, Universitätsklinikum Erlangen, Germany
sulaiman.vesal@fau.de

Abstract. Accurate segmentation of breast lesions is a crucial step in evaluating the characteristics of tumors. However, this is a challenging task, since breast lesions have sophisticated shape, topological structure, and variation in the intensity distribution. In this paper, we evaluated the performance of three unsupervised algorithms for the task of breast Magnetic Resonance (MRI) lesion segmentation, namely, Gaussian Mixture Model clustering, K-means clustering and a marker-controlled Watershed transformation based method. All methods were applied on breast MRI slices following selection of regions of interest (ROIs) by an expert radiologist and evaluated on 106 subjects' images, which include 59 malignant and 47 benign lesions. Segmentation accuracy was evaluated by comparing our results with ground truth masks, using the Dice similarity coefficient (DSC), Jaccard index (JI), Hausdorff distance and precision-recall metrics. The results indicate that the marker-controlled Watershed transformation outperformed all other algorithms investigated.

1 Introduction

Breast cancer is one of the leading causes of mortality in women [1], which can be significantly reduced through early detection and treatment. Breast lesions found during screening examinations are more likely to be smaller and still confined to the breast. There are different imaging modalities for breast cancer screening like mammograms which can find breast changes before symptom development. Ultrasound is also useful to differentiate between cysts and solid masses in women with dense breast tissues. However, in current clinical practice, Magnetic Resonance (MR) images of the breast, are assessed visually or using basic quantitative measures such as lesion diameter and apparent diffusion coefficient (from diffusion-weighted MRIs). Breast cancer diagnosis and distinguishing malignant from benign tumors is infeasible using such measures due to low precision [1]. Accurate lesion segmentation is a crucial step in evaluating tumor characteristics and addressing these limitations. This is a challenging task as, lesions boundaries are usually obscured, irregular, have low contrast and overlap with healthy tissue [2, 3].

In this study, we investigate three unsupervised methods for lesion segmentation in breast MRIs, namely, Gaussian mixture model (GMM) clustering, K-means (KM) clustering and marker-controlled Watershed transformation (MCWT), and compare their performance. The primary advantage of unsupervised methods over supervised ones is that they do not require ground truth segmentations, which are cumbersome and time-consuming to evaluate manually for radiologists. Additionally, such manual segmentations are intrinsically subjective and hence tend to vary between raters. This attribute also makes unsupervised methods uniquely suitable for automatic segmentation in real-time [4, 5].

2   Methods and materials

2.1   K-means clustering

K-means (KM) clustering is a simple unsupervised algorithm for image segmentation. The procedure follows an easy way to partition n pixels into k clusters. Each pixel is assigned to a cluster with the closest mean. The mean of each cluster is often referred to as the centroid and pixels assigned to a cluster are more similar than those assigned to other clusters. The algorithm iteratively alternates between assigning pixels to a cluster, based on their distance to cluster centroids, and refining estimates for the cluster centroids [6]. This is achieved by minimizing the mean-squared-error objective function $S(V)$ given by

$$S(V) = \sum_{i=1}^{c_i} \sum_{j=1}^{c_j} (||x_i - v_j||)^2 \tag{1}$$

where, $||x_i - v_j||$ is the Euclidean distance between pixel x_i and mean v_j, c_i is the number of pixels and c_j is the number of cluster centers. Equation 1 indicates that KM clustering is sensitive to the initial cluster assignment and the choice of the distance measure. We initialized the centroids through iterating over all pixels, find the distances between them and those with the largest distance considered as the initial centroids.

2.2   Gaussian mixture model clustering

A Gaussian Mixture Model (GMM) is a parametric probability density function represented as a weighted sum of Gaussian component densities [7]. GMM parameters are estimated from training data using the Expectation-Maximization (EM) through an iterative process. Let us consider a 2D MR image I as a vector of N pixel values $x = x_1, x_2, ..., x_N$ and assume that they are realizations of a k-component GMM. Given a class k, with parameters $\theta_k = \{\mu_k, \sigma_k\}$, the conditional probability of the ith pixel is expressed as shown in equation 2a. Assuming all pixels in an image are independent and identically distributed samples of a K component GMM, their joint probability may be expressed as shown in equation

2b. Here $\{x_i\}_{i=1...N} = X$ is a $2D$-dimensional continuous-valued image vector, $\{\theta_k\}_{k=1...K} = \Theta$ represents the set of all model parameters, $\{w_k\}_{k=1...K}$ are the mixture weights, and $\mathcal{N}(x_i|\mu_k, \sigma_k)$ are the component Gaussian densities, with mean μ_k and covariance σ_k.

$$p(x_i|\mu_k, \sigma_k) = \frac{1}{(2\pi)^{\frac{D}{2}}|\sigma_k|^{\frac{1}{2}}} \exp\{-\frac{1}{2}(x_i - \mu'_k)\Sigma_k^{-1}(x_i - \mu_k)\} \qquad (2a)$$

$$p(X|\Theta) = \prod_{i=1}^{N}\sum_{k=1}^{K} w_k \mathcal{N}(x_i|\mu_k, \sigma_k) \qquad (2b)$$

GMMs are thus parameterized by their mean vectors, covariance matrices and mixture weights of the constituent component densities. The parameters Θ are estimated using the expectation-maximization(EM) algorithm [7], which iteratively maximizes the expected complete data likelihood by alternating between the (E)xpectation and (M)aximization steps. The M-step updates for each model parameter are evaluated as follows

$$\mu_k^{(t+1)} = \frac{\sum\limits_{i=1}^{N} P_{ik}^t x_i}{\sum\limits_{i=1}^{N} P_{ik}^t} \qquad (3a)$$

$$\sigma_k^{(t+1)} = \frac{\sum\limits_{i=1}^{N}\sum\limits_{k=1}^{K} P_{ik}^t \|x_i - \mu_k^{(t+1)}\|^2}{D\sum\limits_{i=1}^{N}\sum\limits_{k=1}^{K} P_{ik}^t} \qquad (3b)$$

$$\pi_k^{(t+1)} = \frac{1}{N}\sum_{i}^{N} P_{ik}^t \qquad (3c)$$

In these equations P_{ik}^t represents the posterior probability estimated at the tth EM-iteration (Eq. 4), using the current estimates for the model parameters and D is the dimension of the data being clustered.

$$P_{ik}^t = \frac{\pi_k \mathcal{N}(x_i|\mu_k, \sigma_k)}{\sum\limits_{k=1}^{K} \pi_k \mathcal{N}(x_i|\mu_k, \sigma_k)} \qquad (4)$$

The estimated posterior probabilities, in turn, represent the cluster membership of the image pixels and are used to assign pixels to distinct clusters/classes, thereby segmenting the image.

2.3   Marker-controlled watershed transformation

In previous work [8], we proposed a robust and novel Marker-Controlled Watershed Transformation (MCWT) for the task of breast MRI lesion segmentation.

As a pre-processing step for the MCWT, we computed the morphological gradient of the image, which is the pointwise difference between a unitary dilation and erosion. The gradient image provides information about edges. Normally, there are several local minima in a gradient image due to inherent noise in the original image, and direct application of the watershed transformation generally results in over-segmentation [9]. To prevent over-segmentation, we defined markers to guide the watershed algorithm. Each marker is considered to be part of a specific watershed region and after segmentation, the boundaries of the regions are arranged to separates each object.

In MR images, tumor region is brighter and has more uniform intensity than its surroundings, which makes a good candidate for watershed segmentation. Based on this fact, we determined the internal and external markers by sorting out the pixel values in ROIs in descending order and chose n pixels with maximum intensity values as markers. To find the optimal number of markers for this dataset, we tested the algorithm by varying the number of markers between 1 and 150. We found 45 markers to be optimal based on the segmentation accuracy achieved.

2.4 Data acquisition

MR images for this study were acquired on 1.5 T scanners Magnetom Avanto and 3.0 T Magnetom Verio, Siemens Healthineers, Erlangen, Germany, with dedicated breast array coils and the patient in a prone position. The contrast media was applied into the cubital vein after the first of six dynamic acquisitions with a flow of 1.0 mL/sec chased by a 20 mL saline flush. One hundred and six lesions were identified from a representative set of 80 female patients by two expert radiologists who have more than 7 years of experience in evaluation of clinical findings. The mean patient age was 50 ± 13 and in all cases, cancer status was confirmed using histopathology. 42 of the lesions were diagnosed as benign and the remaining 64 as malignant.

2.5 Pre-processing

In this study, a 2D slice was picked from the T1-weighted subtraction MR volume manually, based on the ground truth segmentation (also in 2D) provided by radiologists. Subsequently, a regions of interest(ROI) was drawn around the lesions, ensuring that all lesions identified by the radiologist were completely covered, as in some cases there were several lesions present, scattered across the breast. Additionally, to enhance image contrast, we applied contrast-limited adaptive histogram equalization(CLAHE) [10]. The evaluation of segmentation methods described above was conducted using Dice similarity coefficient (DSC), Jaccard index (JI), Hausdorff distance (HD), precision (PR) and recall (RE) metrics [7, 11].

Table 1. DSC, JI and HD results (*mean ± std*) for the different algorithms.

Methods	DSC	JI	HD(mm)	PR	RE
K-Means	0.732±0.206	0.612±0.209	2.292±1.05	0.805±0.243	0.702±0.204
GMM	0.746±0.180	0.623±0.193	2.275±1.08	0.855±0.213	0.697±0.195
MCWT	0.786±0.172	0.679±0.217	2.265±1.24	0.866±0.199	0.752±0.250

3 Experimental results

Table 1 summarizes the segmentation accuracy achieved using each method (evaluated in terms of five metrics), for 106 lesions. Dice Coefficient, Jaccard index, Hausdorff distance, precision, and recall values were evaluated with respect to the ground truth segmentations and averaged over all cases, for each algorithm. Table 1 indicates that MCWT achieved higher segmentation accuracy compared to the rest and fewer false positives and false negative. Fig.1 shows examples of segmentation for each algorithm, along with their corresponding ground truth.

4 Discussion and conclusion

Lesion segmentation is a crucial step for the characterization of tumors in breast MR images. In this work, we presented a comparison of 3 unsupervised segmentation methods for the task of MRI breast lesions to evaluate their performance. The algorithms have been applied to 106 lesions and MCWT outperformed the other methods marginally. The results presented in Fig.1 shows that MCWT could connect those disjoint areas in the lesion better than other two methods.

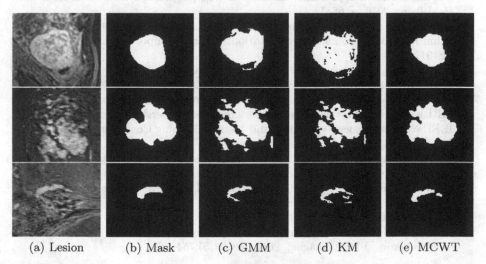

(a) Lesion   (b) Mask   (c) GMM   (d) KM   (e) MCWT

Fig. 1. Comparison of segmentation results for different methods, column one is the lesions, second is the ground truth masks and column third, fourth and fifth are the segmentation output for GMM, KM, and MCWT.

The markers in watershed transformation typically include the neighborhood pixels which has the lower intensity to a particular region. However, this method is sensitive to noise and the soft edges computed by evaluating the gradient image. KM segmentation approach could not segment some of the pixels within the lesions in comparison to the GMM, as it can be seen in the first two sample cases in Fig.1. In general, the key advantage of these unsupervised segmentation methods is that they do not require a manually-segmented reference image. A manually-created ground truth image is intrinsically subjective and creating such a reference image is a time-consuming process, particularly in the case of breast MR lesion segmentation in 3D. Future work will look to extend our proposed 2D watershed algorithm to 3D and combine it with a lesion detection technique, to establish a complete computer-aided-diagnosis system, with minimum manual intervention.

References

1. Xi X, Shi H, Han L, et al. Breast tumor segmentation with prior knowledge learning. Neurocomputing. 2017;237(Supplement C):145 – 157.
2. Jayender J, Chikarmane S, Jolesz FA, et al. Automatic segmentation of invasive breast carcinomas from dynamic contrast-enhanced MRI using time series analysis. J Mag Res Imaging. 2014;40(2):467–475.
3. Thomassin-Naggara I, Trop I, Lalonde L, et al. Tips and techniques in breast MRI. Diagnost Intervent Imaging. 2012;93(11):828 – 839.
4. Zhang H, Fritts JE, Goldman SA. Image segmentation evaluation: a survey of unsupervised methods. Comput Vis Image Understg. 2008;110(2):260 – 280.
5. Amrehn M, Glasbrenner J, Steidl S, et al. Comparative evaluation of interactive segmentation approaches. In: Bildverarbeitung für die Medizin 2016. Berlin Heidelberg; 2016. p. 68–73.
6. Moftah HM, Azar AT, Al-Shammari ET, et al. Adaptive k-means clustering algorithm for MR breast image segmentation. Neural Comput Appl. 2014 Jun;24(7-8):1917–1928.
7. Soffientini CD, De Bernardi E, Zito F, et al. Background based gaussian mixture model lesion segmentation in PET. Med Phys. 2016;43(5):2662–2675.
8. Vesal S, Diaz-Pinto A, RaviKumar N, et al. Semi-automatic algorithm for breast MRI lesion segmentation using marker-controlled watershed transformation. In: IEEE Nuclear Science Symposium and Medical Imaging Conference Record; 2017. In press.
9. Diaz A, Morales S, Naranjo V, et al. Glaucoma diagnosis by means of optic cup feature analysis in color fundus images. Proc EUSIPCO. 2016 Aug; p. 2055–2059.
10. Reza AM. Realization of the contrast limited adaptive histogram equalization (CLAHE) for real-time image enhancement. J VLSI Sign Process Syst Sign Image Vid Tech. 2004 Aug;38(1):35–44.
11. Xu S, Liu H, Song E. Marker-controlled watershed for lesion segmentation in mammograms. J Digit Imaging. 2011 Oct;24(5):754–763.

Segmentation of Fat and Fascias in Canine Ultrasound Images

Oleksiy Rybakov[1], Daniel Stromer[1], Irina Mischewski[2], Andreas Maier[1]

[1] Pattern Recognition Lab, Friedrich-Alexander-University Erlangen-Nuremberg
[2] Institut für Spezielle Zoologie und Evolutionsbiologie mit Phyletischem Museum,
Friedrich-Schiller-University Jena

oleksiy.or.rybakov@fau.de

Abstract. The connective tissue between fat and muscle termed fascia has been of interest to the recent clinical and biological research. However, in the canine and human medicine, the anatomic knowledge is still limited. To analyze the superficial fascia in canine medicine, a database with around 200 ultrasound images of one dog has been created. The superficial fascia contains fat compartments and is closely connected to the surrounding structures such as the skin's dermis and the epimysium of the muscles. This work proposes a semi-automatic and fully-automatic segmentation algorithm separating the different layers of ultrasound images of canine. Both algorithms were evaluated on a set of 24 expert-labeled images achieving high accuracy scores up to 95.9 %.

1 Introduction

Fascias play an important role for the stabilization of the body of humans or animals and when fascias get overstressed, pain can be encountered. In that case, a common modality used for diagnosis of the fascia is ultrasound imaging, which works in real-time, causes no radiation exposure and is portable and cost-efficient [1, 2]. One drawback of ultrasound imaging is that it is highly depended on the skills of the operator. Moreover, the quality of the images can be affected by the presence of various artifacts [3, 4] which might lead to edge diffusion, making clinical diagnosis and biometric measurements more challenging.

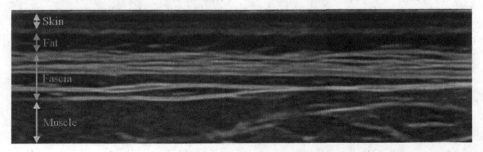

Fig. 1. An ultrasound image of a dog showing its skin, fat, fascia and muscles.

A very important task in medical image analysis is segmentation. Usually, this technique is used to locate objects and boundaries in images. Segmentation of medical ultrasound images is considered as a challenging task due to the occurring artifacts. Although there exist many segmentation approaches of ultrasound images (e. g. the method for segmentation of ultrasound images of plantar fascia proposed by Boussouar et al. [5]), the knowledge on segmentation approaches in the field of human and canine medicine is still limited. Commonly, ultrasound images of dogs contain four layers: skin, fat, fascia and muscles (Fig. 1). Our work presents two approaches – a semi-automatic and a fully-automatic algorithm – separating the four layers by subsequently segmenting the fat and the fascia layer in ultrasound images of dogs. We evaluate our proposed algorithms on a database consisting of 200 ultrasound images of one dog. The database was created by an expert measuring all body parts of the animal. We think that biologists working in the area of fascia research can highly benefit from our work as we will provide an open-source GUI. In addition, the resulting labeled images can be used for developing machine learning algorithms.

2   Materials and methods

2.1   Pre-processing

Since ultrasound images tend to suffer from speckles, noise and other artifacts, we have to pre-process the input to enhance the image quality before the actual segmentation is performed. Since fascias are rather thin, it is important that the applied filters preserve edges.

The first pre-processing step is to apply Bilateral filtering. A Bilateral filter [6] is a non-linear filter commonly used in image processing to reduce noise in an image while preserving edges. The filter replaces the intensity of each pixel with a weighted average of intensity values from close pixels. Those weights $w(x, y)$ depend on the pixels' geometric and photometric distances. To reduce the runtime, we used parallel programming techniques. We also tested Guided filtering [7], however, the results for the Bilateral filter were more accurate.

In canine ultrasound images, fascias look similar to white vessels (Fig. 1). In addition, fat can be also considered as a thick dark tubular structure. Frangi et al. [8] proposed an approach which achieved good results for vessel segmentation. First, the image is pre-smoothed with a Gaussian filter of scaling $s_i = (s_x, s_y)$. Then, the eigenvalues λ_1 and λ_2 of the Hessian $H(x, y)$ are computed at each pixel (x, y). Let us assume that the absolute value of the first eigenvalue λ_1 is larger than λ_2 and $\lambda_2 \approx 0$. Then, a good model for vessels is achieved if $R_B = \lambda_2/\lambda_1 \to 0$ and $S = \sqrt{\lambda_1^2 + \lambda_2^2}$ is high. Calculating

$$V_{ves}(x, y) = \begin{cases} 0, & \text{if } \lambda_1 \approx 0 \\ \exp\left(-\frac{R_B^2}{2\beta^2}\right)\left(1 - \exp\left(-\frac{S^2}{2c^2}\right)\right), & \text{if } \lambda_1 > 0 \end{cases} \quad (1)$$

yields to a probability for the vessel where β and c denote control parameters that depend on the gray scale ($\beta = 0.5$ and $c = 4$). The calculations are performed for different scalings s_i. The actual Vesselness is then given as the maximum over all Vesselness images for the scalings s_i. Fig. 2 shows an example ultrasound image (Left) and the output after applying the pre-processing steps (Right).

2.2 Fat segmentation

Within the semi-automatic approach, the user can decide in which region of interest (ROI) the fat layer is located. Usually, fat can be delimited using a rectangular box aligned to the x- and y-axes of the image, where the uppermost y-coordinate does not variate from the lowermost y-coordinate by a huge number. The user sets the ROI by giving both delimiting y-coordinates as arguments.

In the automatic approach, this step is performed by a customized algorithm instead. First, for each row in the Vesselness image, we compute the amount of pixels n smaller than a certain threshold ϵ_{Fat} within the row and store those values in a histogram. For the fat layer, n tends to be high. Knowing that the fat layer is usually located in the upper part of the image, we can restrict the histogram to the upper part of our image. Then, we are searching for the minima close to the global maximum inside the restricted region. This maximum corresponds to the center of the fat layer. Since the Vesselness measure gets higher at the boundary of the fat image, a good approach to find the rows delimiting the fat layer would be to search for minima close to the global maximum. In order to prevent arriving at too high minima, high local minima are deprecated. Afterwards, the Vesselness measure at each pixel within the ROI is compared to a pre-defined threshold. If the Vesselness value at a pixel within the ROI is lower than the threshold, the pixel is classified as fat, otherwise as no-fat-area.

Since the quality of the segmentation can still be corrupted by small artifacts, several post-processing steps are applied to the segmented image. The first step in this pipeline is to remove smaller artifacts by applying morphological operators like dilation and erosion [9]. Additionally, some segmented images tend to have a top layer which does not belong to the actual fat layer. Usually, if the most pixels of the upper boundary of the top layer are also located at the upper boundary of the rectangular box, the pixels can be classified as top-layer-pixels.

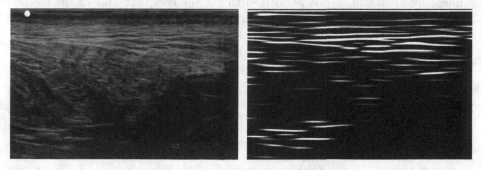

Fig. 2. (Left) Canine ultrasound image. (Right) Pre-processed image – Output after Bilateral and Vesselness filtering.

The remaining parts of the top layer can be removed by applying another dilation step. Afterwards, the image might have some gaps inside the fat layer due to occlusion. Those gaps have to be removed since the fat layer has to be homogeneous. For this purpose, each column of the image is traversed and subdivided into intervals where each pixel has been classified as fat. The remaining no-fat regions in the column apart from the uppermost and the lowermost no-fat regions are then filled with the color corresponding to the fat layer. Finally, the image is smoothed by applying median filtering.

2.3   Fascia segmentation

The semi-automatic approach for fascia segmentation is similar to our fat segmentation approach. Again, within the semi-automatic approach the user has to define a ROI where the fascia is located. Since the lower boundary of fat corresponds to the upper boundary of the fascia, only the lower boundary of the fascia has to be defined by the user. However, a rectangular box does usually not model fascias correctly. Instead, a good model to delimit the fascia is given by two intersecting straight lines (Fig. 3 (Left)). The left straight line intersects the points $(0, y_l)$ and (x_c, y_c). The right straight line intersects the points (x_c, y_c) and $(w - 1, y_r)$ where w is the width of the image. Within the semi-automatic approach, the remaining four coordinates y_l, x_c, y_c and y_r are then given to the segmentation algorithm as input parameters.

In the fully-automatic approach, this step is performed by a customized algorithm similar to the one from automatic fat segmentation. Like fascias, muscles tend to have a large Vesselness measure. However, fascias and muscles are separated by a small layer of low Vesselness measures. The boundary between fascia and muscle is then obtained by finding the rightmost local minimum within the fascia-muscle region that is small enough. Afterwards, each pixel within the resulting ROI has to be compared with the Vesselness measure at the same pixel. If, and only if, the Vesselness image at a pixel is higher than a pre-defined threshold, the pixel is classified as fascia. The resulting fascia is shown in the central image of Fig. 3. However, since fascias are usually non-homogeneous, a linear interpolation step is performed to get the complete area of the fascia. Afterwards, the image is smoothed by applying median filtering. The result is shown in Fig. 3 (Right). Finally, thresholding can be applied to the interpolated image to distinguish between fascial structures (high Vesselness measure) and fat compartments within the fascia region (low Vesselness measure).

3   Experiments and results

The proposed algorithms have been evaluated on a database with 213 ultrasound images of one single dog, where 24 images have been manually segmented by an expert. For the remaining 189 images, the semi-automatic segmentation has been selected as the ground truth image. The given problem can be reduced to a two-class task where positives are given by fat and fascia while negatives show the

Table 1. Performance measures for fully- and semi-automatic segmentation algorithm.

Measure	Accuracy	Sensitivity	Precision	Specificity	F1 score
Semi-automatic fat	98.6%	78.6%	82.6%	99.4%	80.0%
Fully-automatic fat	98.4%	79.7%	80.7%	99.2%	78.8%
Semi-automatic fascia	95.9%	92.8%	76.4%	96.0%	83.1%
Fully-automatic fascia	93.8%	74.1%	78.6%	97.6%	72.1%
Semi-automatic combined	95.9%	93.3%	83.3%	96.1%	87.8%
Fully-automatic combined	93.6%	79.6%	84.1%	97.4%	79.8%

background. Table 1 shows how our two presented algorithms performed on the manually labeled dataset with respect to commonly used accuracy measures [10]. One can see, that the semi-automatic approach shows promising results with a F1 score of 80.0 % for fat and 83.1 % for fascia segmentation whereas the fully-automatic version has a F1 score of 78.8 % for fat and 72.1 % for fascia segmentation. An example of the completed segmentation is visualized in Fig. 4.

4   Discussion and outlook

We presented a semi- and a fully-automatic segmentation algorithm for fat and fascia within ultrasound images of canines. We evaluated our developed algorithms on a expert-labeled dataset of 24 images where the F1 score of the semi-automatic approach (87.8 %) is higher than the fully-automatic's (79.8 %), however, both algorithms perform well. We think that the proposed methods can be very useful for biologists as well as computer scientists. Biologists do not need to manually segment their images anymore and are able to measure fascia and fat layers efficiently. Furthermore, the newly generated labeled data can be used as a training set for future machine learning algorithms in fascia research. As the fat and fascia layers of humans do not differ a lot from canines, the algorithms can be easily extrapolated to ultrasound images of humans. The GUI will be released with the publication of the paper.

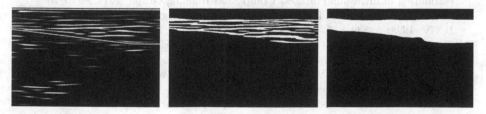

Fig. 3. (Left) A model to delimit the fascia by two straight lines (yellow). (Center) Segmented fascia structure. (Right) Interpolated area of the fascia.

Fig. 4. (Top) An expert labeled ultrasound image where the fat and fascia are delimited by the red lines. (Center) Semi-automatic resulting segmentation. (Bottom) Fully-automatic resulting segmentation. Light Grey area denotes fat, dark gray are fat compartments within the fascia and white area denotes fascia.

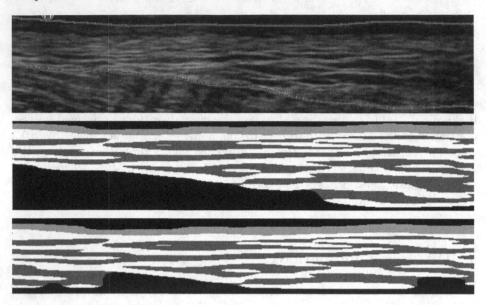

References

1. Pope JA. Medical Physics: Imaging. Heinemann; 1999.
2. Szabo TL. Diagnostic Ultrasound Imaging: Inside Out. Academic Press Series in Biomedical Engineering. Academic Press; 2013.
3. Gonzalez RC, Woods RE, Eddins SL. Digital Image Processing using MATLAB. Upper Saddle River, NJ: Prentice Hall; 2002.
4. Nelson TR, Pretorius DH, Hull A, et al. Sources and impact of artifacts on clinical three-dimensional ultrasound imaging. Ultrasound Obstetr Gyn. 2000;16(4):374–383.
5. Boussouar A, Meziane F, Crofts G. Plantar fascia segmentation and thickness estimation in ultrasound images. Comp Med Imaging Graph. 2017;56:60–73.
6. Tomasi C, Manduchi R; IEEE. Bilateral filtering for gray and color images. Proc ICCV. 1998; p. 839–846.
7. He K, Sun J, Tang X. Guided image filtering. IEEE Trans Pattern Anal Mach Intell. 2013;35(6):1397–1409.
8. Frangi AF, Niessen WJ, Vincken KL, et al. Multiscale vessel enhancement filtering. In: Proc MICCAI. Springer; 1998. p. 130–137.
9. Heijmans HJ. Connected morphological operators for binary images. Comp Vis Image Underst. 1999;73(1):99–120.
10. Goutte C, Gaussier E; Springer. A probabilistic interpretation of precision, recall and F-score, with implication for evaluation. Proc ECIR. 2005;5:345–359.

Manifold Learning-based Data Sampling for Model Training

Shuqing Chen[1], Sabrina Dorn[2], Michael Lell[3], Marc Kachelrieß[2],
Andreas Maier[1]

[1]Pattern Recognition Lab, FAU Erlangen-Nürnberg
[2]German Cancer Research Center (DKFZ), Heidelberg, Germany
[3]University Hospital Nürnberg, Paracelsus Medical University, Nürnberg, Germany
shuqing.chen@fau.de

Abstract. Training data sampling is an important task in machine
learning especially for data with small sample size and data with nonuniform sample distribution. Dividing data into different data sets randomly
can cause the problem that, the training model covers only parts of the
sampled cases and works inaccurately for weakly sampled cases. Recent
research showed the benefit of manifold learning techniques in medical
image processing. In this work, we propose a manifold learning based
approach to improve the data division and the model training. We evaluated the proposed approach using an atlas registration framework and a
deep learning framework. The final segmentation results using methods
with and without data balancing were compared. All of the final segmentations were improved after implementing the manifold learning based
approach into the frameworks. The largest improvement was 24.4%.
Thus, the proposed manifold learning based approach is effective for the
model training.

1 Introduction

To model common properties and variations from many individuals over an entire
task domain is important for many machine learning methods, such as atlas registration and deep learning. These methods can be used for varied applications,
e.g. multi-organ segmentation in the field of medical image processing. Model
training is an important part of such methods. A well-trained model works for
most cases within the domain. However, due to the limited data sample, size
and nonuniform sample distribution, problems arise in practical implementations. For many applications, the data has to be sampled into different balanced
sets before starting the modeling. With small sample size or nonuniform sample
distribution, random data selection may not work robustly.

Aljabar et al. [1] discussed the power of manifold learning in the field of
medical image processing. Using manifold learning techniques, high dimensional
medical data can be converted to lower dimensional representation while respect-
ing the intrinsic geometry [2], so that it is possible to facilitate the application of
machine learning techniques such as clustering and regression. Manifold learning

techniques can be used in the preprocessing to extract features for registration [3]. They can also improve segmentation successfully by allowing the propagation of multiple atlases to a diverse set of images [4]. Furthermore, manifold learning techniques can be used for clinical classification [1]. However, few research showed the benefit of the manifold learning to reduce the problem caused by data selection in many machine learning methods. In this paper, we proposed one manifold learning based approach to solve the data selection problem and to improve the model training.

2   Materials and methods

In order to avoid the bias due to the data selection and to keep the distribution of the data sets (i.e. training data set, test data set as well as validation data set if required) similar, three steps were employed to improve the data selection:

- *Data Representation*: Initially, the high-dimensional volumetric medical data will be projected into a low-dimensional (e.g. 2-D) visualization plane using manifold learning techniques. Each point in such visualization plane will denote a volumetric image. To improve the performance, the data should be resampled to the same image spacing before using manifold learning.
- *Data Clustering*: Afterwards, the data points can be divided into different classes using clustering techniques.
- *Data Selection*: Finally, the training data set, the validation data set and the test dataset can be built by selecting data samples from each class randomly.

To show the effectivity of this datatype-independent approach in general machine learning methods, the evaluation is designed with the multi-organ segmentation using atlas registration on computed tomography (CT) images [5] and the multi-organ segmentation using deep learning on dual-energy CT (DECT) images [6]. For our cases, the clusters are well distributed with less overlap on 2-D space. Thus, data projection on 2-D space is sufficient.

The method of the multi-organ segmentation using atlas registration is described in [5]. In this method, the data selection for the atlas modeling should focus on the inter-subject organ shape variation. Therefore, the data selection approach is applied after the step of the affine registration, in order to avoid the effect of the position variance. The atlas construction part described in [5] is improved with data selection in following steps. First of all, the data is cropped to get the region of interest (ROI) for the redundancy reduction of the atlas. Then a reference volume is selected which is the most similar to the mean volume of all samples. Subsequently, affine registration is used to reduce the variation of the rotation, the translation, the scaling and the shearing. The results after the affine registration are then split into training data set and test data set using the manifold learning based approach mentioned previously. Average volume and atlas is constructed finally after the fine alignment based on B-Spline registration as described in [5].

A 3-D cascaded fully connected network [7] was used for the multi-organ seg-mentation using deep learning technique [6]. In this network, the input training data will be augmented with more translation and rotation. Thus, unlike the atlas registration, it is not required to remove the position variation for the data selection. The data selection approach can be applied directly to the original data set without any preprocessing. Training data set, validation data set and test data set are selected using the proposed selection approach. The whole framework is kept in same as the description in [6].

3   Results

The Matlab toolbox provided by van der Maaten et al. [8] was used for manifold learning in our implementation. Dice coefficient was utilized to measure the performance of the segmentation result.

To show the effect of the data selection on atlas registration, 20 VISCERAL non-enhanced CT volumes [9] were used for the evaluation. Fig. 1 plots the

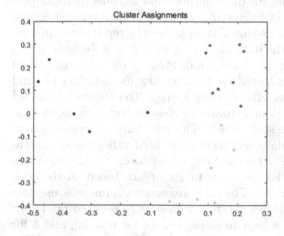

Fig. 1.   Data representation and clustering using LLE and k-Means for atlas registration data.   Colors denote classes, numbers denote volume indexes.

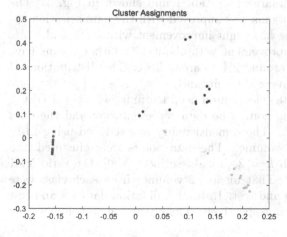

Fig. 2.   Data representation and clustering using LLE and k-Means for deep learning data. Colors denote classes, volume indexes are ignored for clarity.

Table 1. Comparison of atlas registration on CT images without and with data selection.

	Right Lung	Left Lung	Right Kidney	Left Kidney	Liver	Spleen
Without Data Selection						
Avg.	0.960	0.957	0.794	0.731	0.900	0.813
Std. Dev.	0.014	0.015	0.140	0.214	0.034	0.104
With Data Selection						
Avg.	0.965	0.960	0.834	0.821	0.912	0.842
Std. Dev.	0.009	0.010	0.080	0.121	0.024	0.051
Improvements of the average						
Diff. Avg.	0.005	0.003	0.040	0.090	0.012	0.029

20 CT volumes by characterizing the shape variation using the manifold learning approach. Each point denotes one CT volume. Locally linear embedding (LLE) [10] was chosen to reduce the dimensionality because LLE showed the best performance by experimenting the different manifold learning methods provided in the toolbox. To construct balanced training, test and validation sets, the data was clustered into k classes that should be evenly represented in each set. k-Means was used here for the data clustering with $k = 3$, because $k = 3$ is most reasonable for these volumes. This is indicated by color in Figs. 1 and 2. A 10-fold cross validation was tested for 6 target organs including left and right lung, liver, spleen, as well as left and right kidney. To construct balanced sets, one volume was selected randomly from each class as test volume, in total 3 test volumes were selected as test data set. The remaining 17 volumes were used as training data set. Test data sets were segmented using the segmentation method mentioned in [5]. For comparison, a 10-fold cross validation was tested using the 20 CT volumes for the same target organs based on the atlas construction method described in [5]. The same reference volume was used for the registrations, but training data set and test data set was selected randomly. The amount of the data sets were kept in same, i.e. 17 for training and 3 for the test. The results were summarized in Tab. 1 and shown in Fig. 3. The final segmentation of all target organs was improved with the data selection approach. Right lung and left lung has slight improvement with 0.5% and 0.3%, respectively. Liver has small improvement with about 1%. Other organs have a significant improvement from around 3% to around 9%. The distributions of the Dice coefficients are also converged significantly.

To show the effect of the data selection on deep learning, 42 clinical DECT volumes were used for the evaluation. The data representation and the data clustering is illustrated in Fig. 2. The dimensionality was reduced using LLE. Each point denotes one DECT volume. The data points were clustered into 3 classes by using k-Means with $k = 3$. Like described in [6], the ratio 5:1:1 was used for the data selection. That means, 2 volumes from each class were selected randomly for validation and test. In total, validation data set and test data set was built with 6 volumes, respectively. The remaining 30 volumes were used as training data set. The segmentation of liver, spleen, as well as left and right kidney, were evaluated. 0.9 was taken as training weight and test weight. A comparison model was experimented using same framework and same condition but with randomly generated data sets. The results were summarized in Tab. 2 and presented in Fig. 4. The data selection approach improved all final segmentation. Right kidney and left kidney has slight improvement with 0.00% and 0.7%, respectively. Liver has small improvement with about 1.5%. Spleen has significant improvement around 24.4%.

4   Discussion

We proposed a manifold learning based approach to reduce the bias of the data selection. The proposed approach was implemented into an atlas registration framework and a deep learning framework. The comparison evaluation showed the benefit of the data selection approach. Both of the machine learning methods can be improved by adding the proposed approach.

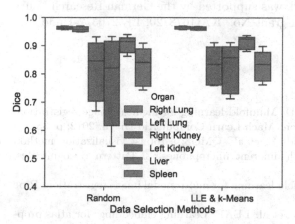

Fig. 3.   Comparision test for atlas registration with/without data selection.

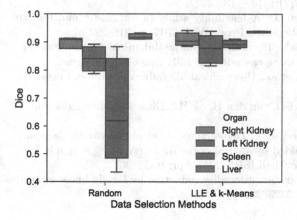

Fig. 4.   Comparison test for U-Net with/without data selection.

Table 2. Comparison of U-Net on DECT images without and with data selection.

	Right Kidney	Left Kidney	Liver	Spleen
Without Data Selection				
Avg.	0.905	0.856	0.919	0.652
Std. Dev.	0.020	0.047	0.015	0.188
With Data Selection				
Avg.	0.905	0.863	0.934	0.896
Std. Dev.	0.034	0.071	0.011	0.032
Improvements of the average				
Diff. Avg.	0.000	0.007	0.015	0.244

The approach can be tested for more machine learning methods in future. Moreover, more manifold learning techniques can be investigated further. Furthermore, other clustering techniques can be used.

Acknowledgement. This work was supported by the German Research Foundation (DFG) through research grant No. KA 1678/20, LE 2763/2-1 and MA 4898/5-1.

References

1. Aljabar P, Wolz R, Rueckert D. Manifold learning for medical image registration, segmentation, and classification. Mach Learn Comput Aid Diagn. 2012; p. 351.
2. Maier A, Schuster M, Eysholdt U, et al. QMOS: a robust visualization method for speaker dependencies with different microphones. J Pattern Recognit Res. 2009;4(1):32–51.
3. Wachinger C, Navab N. Manifold learning for multi-modal image registration. Proc BMVC. 2010 01; p. 1–12.
4. Wolz R, Aljabar P, Hajnal JV, et al. LEAP: Learning embeddings for atlas propagation. NeuroImage. 2010;49(2):1316 – 1325.
5. Chen S, Endres J, Dorn S, et al. A feasibility study of automatic multi-organ segmentation using probabilistic atlas. Proc BVM. 2017; p. 218–223.
6. Chen S, Roth H, Dorn S, et al.. Towards automatic abdominal multi-organ segmentation in dual energy CT using cascaded 3D fully convolutional network.
7. Roth HR, Oda H, Hayashi Y, et al.. Hierarchical 3D fully convolutional networks for multi-organ segmentation.
8. van der Maaten LJP, Postma EO, van den Herik HJ. Dimensionality reduction: a comparative review; 2008.
9. Jiménez-del Toro OA, Dicente Cid Y, Depeursinge A, et al. Hierarchic anatomical structure segmentation guided by spatial correlations (AnatSeg–Gspac): VISCERAL Anatomy3. Proc Visc Chall ISBI. 2015 Apr; p. 22–26.
10. Roweis ST, Saul LK. Nonlinear dimensionality reduction by locally linear embedding. Science. 2000;290(5500):2323–2326.

Computer-aided Detection of the Most Suitable MRI Sequences for Subsequent Spinal Metastasis Delineation

Georg Hille[1], Steffen Serowy[2], Klaus Tönnies[1], Sylvia Saalfeld[1]

[1]Department of Simulation and Graphics, University of Magdeburg, Germany
[2]Department of Neuroradiology, University Hospital of Magdeburg, Germany
georg.hille@ovgu.de

Abstract. Detection and segmentation of vertebral metastases is a crucial step for support of diagnosis and treatment planning, especially in minimally invasive interventions. Even though computer-assistant tools will not dispense radiologists yet, algorithmically supported detection and segmentation of spinal metastases will play a more and more important role in the near future. The usage of images, where a sufficiently good differentiation between metastases and surrounding tissue is possible, constitutes a critical requirement for successful segmentation procedures. Therefore, we proposed a pipeline, that semi-automatically sorts out unsuitable imaging sequences, as well as combinations of different images via absolute intensity difference images and returns a ranking based recommendation of which image data fits best the requirements for future segmentation tasks. We evaluated our method with 10 patient cases and matched the produced ranking with those of a segmentation field expert. With an average Spearman's ranking coefficient of 0.92 ± 0.07, our method showed promising results and could be a valueable pre-processing step to speed up clinical segmentation procedures due to omitting the time-consuming manual initialization of choosing suitable image data.

1 Introduction

Owing to the fact that cancerous diseases will be more frequently than ever and metastases located in the spine predominate while being the third most organ to metastasize [1] after lungs and liver [2], spinal metastases treatment will become invariably a more urgent task. The steadily growing amount of image data, which is acquired for diagnostical and therapeutical purposes will further increase workload of radiologists, hence the calls for assistance are getting louder. Furthermore, the detection and segmentation of vertebral metastases is a pivotal step towards diagnosis and treatment planning such as radiofrequency ablation simulation. Even though computer-assistant tools will not dispense yet the need for verification by radiologists, it gains more and more appreciation for pre-processing image data and decision support during diagnosis and therapy. Bone tumors and metastases typically replace focal bone marrow, which can

275

be visualized in magnetic resonance imaging (MRI). Dependent on the neoformation type, metastases cause characteristic signal intensities in different MR imaging sequences, arising the indispensable need for acquiring various sequences [3] during the diagnostic process to locate and assess the extent of the pathologic neoformation. For example segmentation of spinal metastases done manually is time-consuming and fatiguing considering the number of image slices and sequences acquired per patient. This leads to the importance of algorithmically assistance. Though, massive obstacles for metastasis segmentation in spine MRI are poor image contours between pathologic and healthy tissues, signal variations of the metastases and deformations due to the metastatic bone alteration. Therefore, an suitable MR sequence has to be chosen by the clinician. To simplify segmentation of anatomical structures and tissues, a sufficiently good differentiation is crucial, whether by pronounced object contours or average signal contrast towards surrounding tissues. The aim of our work is to find the most suitable MRI sequences or combination of various sequences of each patient via absolute intensity difference (AID) images for subsequent spinal metastasis segmentation procedures. Thus, our method will semi-automatically determine images with preferably high image contrast between metastases and both healthy vertebrae and discs and result in a recommendation of which image data fits best the requirements for following segmentation tasks.

2   Materials and methods

Our method starts with image fusions of all sagittal acquired MR sequences of each patient. All image volumes were isotropically up-sampled towards the in-plane resolution of the reference image (T_1-weigthed sequence) and rescaled to an 8-bit grayscale image. Related work, such as presented by Koh et al. [4] demonstrated earlier that absolute intensity difference images of variously weigthed MR sequences could pronounce tissue signals compared with native imaging sequences. Therefore, we computed all possible combinations of AID-images and included them in our study. Subsequently, we manually placed a landmark in a selectable sagittal cross-section of a single reference image in each, the diagnosed metastasis, a vertebral disk and one healthy vertebra. By cubic regions of $5 \times 5 \times 5\,$mm extent with the landmarks as center points, we could estimate local intensity features of each MR sequence and the computed AID-images. A preferably good differentiation between various tissue signals could be defined as a contrast or dissimilarity maximization problem. Hence, we searched for the MR sequence or AID-image, with the highest dissimilarity between metastasis and both vertebra and disk within joint cumulative histograms of all three tissue types (Fig. 1). As a dissimilarity measure we used correlation distance

$$d_{st} = 1 - \frac{(x_s - \bar{x}_s)(y_t - \bar{y}_t)}{\sqrt{(x_s - \bar{x}_s)(x_s - \bar{x}_s)'}\sqrt{(y_t - \bar{y}_t)(y_t - \bar{y}_t)'}} \tag{1}$$

with $\bar{x}_s = \frac{1}{n}\sum_j x_{sj}$ and $\bar{y}_t = \frac{1}{n}\sum_j y_{tj}$ and x_s and y_t as distances between both bin count vectors.

Since most metastases show hypointense signals in T_1- and partially also in T_2-weigthed images in comparison with healthy bone structures, but isointense signals towards vertebral discs, we weighted the dissimilarity between metastasis and the latter somewhat higher. Therefore, both distances were weigthed in the ratio 1 : 2 in favour of the distinction between metastasis and vertebral disk. We ranked the produced results of each patient according to the maximum correlation distances within their MR sequences or AID-images. To evaluate our method, we matched the algorithmically determined rankings with those of a segmentation field expert. It was asked, which three MR sequences or AID-images would be the most suitable for further treatment planning. We considered only to select the top three images per case due to the difficulty to subjectively rank images with hardly distinguishable tissues (where $d_{st} <$ 0.1). Our evaluation set consisted of 10 patients, who underwent radiofrequency ablations of spinal metastases, with at least three pre-interventional acquired MR sequences per case: T_1, T_2, STIR and/or contrast enhanced T_1. To check the accordance of both rankings, we modified Spearman's ranking coefficient (SRC) in order to compensate the difference in observation numbers

$$r_s = 1 - \frac{6 \sum_{i=1}^{n_E} d_i^2}{n_d (n_d^2 - 1)} \tag{2}$$

with d_i as the difference between two ranks of each observation and $n_d = n_A - n_E$ as the difference between the number of observations from our algorithmically produced ranking (n_A) and the number of observations from the expert (n_E). High SRC scores mean, our method prefers similar imaging sequences regarding to following segmentation tasks as a field expert would do.

3   Results

The overall Spearman's ranking coefficient between the algorithmically and the manually produced ranking of the suitability of certain MR sequences for further treatment planning, e.g. segmentation tasks, was 0.92 ± 0.07. The worst result was a ranking coefficient of 0.75. However, in this particular case the maximum correlation distance of the cumulative histograms of all sequences and AID-images was below half of the overall average (d_{st} of 0.15 vs. $d_{st,mean}$ of 0.32), thus, a clear differentiation between metastasis and both vertebra and disk was hardly possible. If there was no prominently suitable sequence or AID-image with a good distinction between those tissues, the chances of establishing similar rankings decreased and therefore, achieving lower ranking coefficients was expectably. Whenever there was a correlation distance above 0.25 within the joint cumulative histograms, the Spearman's ranking coefficient was above 0.90, meaning our approach found suitable images, similar to the field expert (Tab. 1). Such high accordance was achieved in two cases even though the maximum correlation distance was below 0.25 (patient case 3 and 5). Furthermore, the only two cases with a SRC score lower than 0.90 had a maximum correlation distance below 0.20 (patient case 2 and 6), meaning there is hardly any

Table 1. Spearman's ranking coefficient and the maximum correlation distance per case.

	Patient Cases									
	1	2	3	4	5	6	7	8	9	10
SRC	0.955	0.754	0.952	0.978	0.933	0.866	0.911	0.918	0.933	1
$d_{st,max}$	0.570	0.154	0.194	0.511	0.108	0.184	0.294	0.402	0.275	0.471

tissue delimitation possible. Therefore, our test set showed that high correlation distances ($d_{st} > 0.25$) guaranteed to find the most suitable sequences or AID-images, although lower distances could score a hit.

4   Discussion

Patient cases with hardly a signal emphasizing of cancerous structures in all imaging sequences mean an extremely ambitious challenge for automatically or even semi-automatically performed segmentation methods. The usage of images

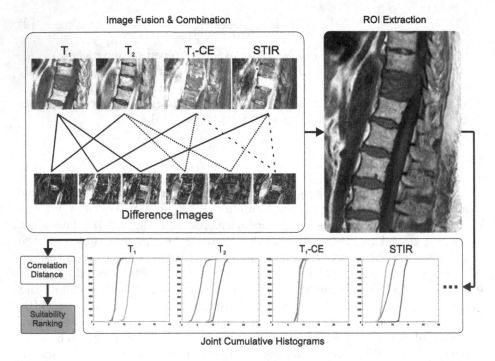

Fig. 1. The pipeline of our proposed methodology. Following image fusions of all available sagittal MRI sequences, regions of interest for each tissue were extracted. Subsequently, correlation distances of the curves were calculated in joint cumulative histograms of the metastasis (red), vertebra (green) and disk (blue) regions of each MRI sequence and their AID-images, leading to a ranking of the suitability of the images for following segmentation tasks.

that allow a sufficiently good differentiation between metastases and surrounding tissue constitutes a critical requirement for segmentation procedures. For this purpose we determined correlation distances in joint cumulative histograms of metastases, vertebrae and discs and ranked them according to their tissue discriminability. These rankings were matched with those of an expert and the SRC scores showed high accordance, which means our method prefers suitable sequences or AID-images similar to the field expert. Our evaluation showed promising results for recommending such sequences out of a bunch of diagnostically acquired images, as long as there are some that are preferable. For this purpose the user only has to place three ROIs around and within the diagnosed metastasis in a single MRI sequence instead of examining every available image. This pre-processing step could speed up semi- or fully automatic segmentation procedures due to omitting the time-consuming manual initialization of choosing reasonable images.

Acknowledgement. This work was supported by the German Ministry of Education and Research (13GW0095A) within the *STIMULATE* research campus.

References

1. Witham TF, Khavkin YA, Gallia GL, et al. Surgery insight: current management of epidural spinal cord compression from metastatic spine disease. Nature Clin Pract Neurol. 2006;2:87–94.
2. Klimo P, Schmidt MH. Surgical management of spinal metastases. The Oncologist. 2004;9:188–196.
3. Guillevin R, Vallee JN, Lafitte F, et al. Spine metastasis imaging: review of the literature. Journal of neuroradiology. 2007;34(5):311–321.
4. Koh J, Chaudhary V, Jeon EK, et al. Automatic spinal canal detection in lumbar MR images in the sagittal view using dynamic programming. Comput Med Imaging Graph. 2014;38(7):569–579.

Abstract: Deep Residual Learning for Limited Angle Artefact Correction

Alena-K. Schnurr, Khanlian Chung, Lothar R. Schad, Frank G. Zöllner

Computer Assisted Clinical Medicine, Medical Faculty Mannheim, Heidelberg University
alena-kathrin.schnurr@medma.uni-heidelberg.de

Using non-conventional scan trajectories for Cone Beam (CB) imaging promise low dose interventions and radiation protection to the personal [1]. The here investigated circular tomosynthesis yields good image quality in two preferred directions, but introduces limited angle artefacts in the third. The artefacts become more severe, the smaller the half tomo angle α gets. Han et al. have previously demonstrated the successful application of deep learning for streaking artefact correction in CT scenarios [2]. We have modified the U-Net to correct artefacts in circular tomosynthesis. 30 CBCTs and circular tomosynthesis scans of the Shepp-Logan phantom with different rotations and scalings were simulated using $\alpha \in \{25°, 35°, 45°\}$. We use 12 scans for training and 18 for validation. The network is trained using reconstructed patches as inputs and the difference between tomosynthesis and CBCT as labels. Training is performed using the Adam optimizer with mini batches. For evaluation we calculate the normalized Root Mean Squared Error ($nRMSE$) of the phantom and the reconstructed data. The CBCT reconstructions achieved a $nRMSE$ of 0.0819 ± 0.0010, while uncorrected circular tomosynthesis resulted in $nRMSE = 0.1048 \pm 0.0133$. On the training data the presented approach resulted in an average $nRMSE$ of 0.0797 ± 0.0071 which is similar to the value of the CBCTs. On the validation scans we achieved average $nRMSE$ reduction of 28% ($\alpha = 25$), 22% ($\alpha = 35$) and 12% ($\alpha = 45$) compared to the uncorrected circular tomosynthesis data. Conventional approaches such as total variation minimization become more insufficient with decreasing α which we also observed in our simulations. In conclusion our experiments have shown that deep learning can enhance circular tomosynthesis scans to a quality similar to CBCT.

References

1. Chung K, Karstensen L, Siegfarth M, et al. Investigation of scatter radiation of non-circular X-ray scan trajectories. In: Proc Int Conf 3D Image Reconstr Rad Nuc Med; 2017. p. 176–180.
2. Han Y, Yoo JJ, Ye JC. Deep residual learning for compressed sensing CT reconstruction via persistent homology analysis. CoRR. 2016;abs/1611.06391.

Abstract: AngioUnet
A Convolutional Neural Network for Vessel Segmentation in Cerebral DSA Series

Christian Neumann[1], Klaus-D. Tönnies[2], Regina Pohle-Fröhlich[1]

[1]Institut für Mustererkennung, Hochschule Niederrhein
[2]Institut für Simulation und Graphik, Universität von Magdeburg
christian.neumann@hs-niederrhein.de

Das U-net [1] ist eine vielversprechende Architektur für Segmentierungsprobleme im Bereich der Medizin. Wir zeigen, wie sich diese Architektur effektiv auf die Segmentierung von zerebralen DSA Zeitserien anwenden lässt. Durch die Erweiterung der Eingabe auf mehrere Bilder wird es möglich besser zwischen Gefäsen und Hintergrund zu unterscheiden. Die Bilder wurden so gewählt, dass sie vier vordefinierte Ausbreitungszustände des Kontrastmittels zeigen. Da Arterien und Venen nicht direkt sondern über Kapillaren verbunden sind, lassen sich so Arterien von Venen unterscheiden. Desweiteren kann das U-net auf einem kleinen Korpus trainiert werden, wenn dies mit hilfreichen Data Augmentations wie Spiegelung, Rotation und Biasing kombiniert wird. Wir verwenden alle Rotationen um 90°, deren Spiegelungen und jeweils einen Bias von ±5% des Dynamikumfangs wodurch insgesamt 24 Varianten pro Kachel entstehen. Unser Netzwerk erreicht einen Dice-Koeffizienten von 87.98% bei dieser Segmentierungsaufgabe. Wir vergleichen dies mit unterschiedlichen Konfigurationen und diskutieren den Einfluss von verschiedenen Artefakten wie sichtbaren Knochen, Kleber aus vorigen Embolisationen und die Schrauben und Marker des stereotaktischen Rahmens. Das vollständige Paper wird in den Proceedings der VISAPP 2018 erschienen sein [2].

Literaturverzeichnis

1. Ronneberger O, Fischer P, Brox T. U-Net: convolutional networks for biomedical image segmentation. arXiv preprint arXiv:150504597. 2015.
2. Neumann C, Tönnies KD, Pohle-Fröhlich R. AngioUnet: a convolutional neural network for vessel segmentation in cerebral DSA series. Proc VISIGRAPP. 2018.

Abstract: Measuring Muscle Contractions from Single Element Transducer Ultrasound Data using Machine Learning Strategies

Lukas Brausch, Holger Hewener

Fraunhofer-Institut für Biomedizinische Technik, St. Ingbert
lukas.brausch@ibmt.fraunhofer.de

Being aware of the correct execution of certain fitness exercises (e.g. squats) is important for rehabilitation and sports athletes alike. Thus, being able to non-invasively distinguish between contracted and relaxed muscle states is crucial. Measurements using optical systems (movement tracking) or kinetic approaches (muscle circumference) only provide information from the body surface with varying accuracy. Ultrasound measurements and imaging, however, can provide a more detailed view on muscle activity. In this work we present our solution using single element and array transducer ultrasound data in combination with an artificial neural net (ANN) to classify muscle contractions. The Fraunhofer Ultrasound Research Platform *DiPhAS* [1] was used to acquire ultrasound array data, while the pulser-receiver Olympus 5800PR was used with Panametrics transducers to obtain single element ultrasound A-scans serving as input data for our algorithm. Several experiments were performed on the calves of healthy volunteers. The retrieved data was used as input for our ANN and the efficiencies of different parameter choices (such as different cost functions, different minimization algorithms for the cost function, different activation functions for each neuron, etc.) were analysed. Using this approach, it is possible to distinguish between rest and knee bends with its corresponding muscle contractions. Therefore, it is shown that ultrasound measurements combined with ANNs can be used to detect certain muscle activities in the human body without relying on surrogates. The presented approach will be tested to analyse muscle activities in the forearm to control artificial hand prostheses.

References

1. Risser C, Welsch HJ, Fonfara H, et al. High channel count ultrasound beamformer system with external multiplexer support for ultrafast 3D/4D ultrasound. Proc IEEE IUS. 2016.

Abstract: Automated Segmentation of Bones for the Age Assessment in 3D MR Images using Convolutional Neural Networks

Markus Auf-der-Mauer[1], Paul-Louis Pröve[1], Eilin Jopp[2], Jochen Herrmann[3], Michael Groth[3], Michael M. Morlock[4], Ben Stanczus[1], Dennis Säring[1]

[1]Medical and Industrial Image Processing, University of Applied Sciences of Wedel
[2]Department of Legal Medicine, University Medical Center Hamburg-Eppendorf
[3]Pediatric Radiology Department, University Medical Center Hamburg-Eppendorf
[4]Institute of Biomechanics, Hamburg University of Technology
adm@fh-wedel.de

The age assessment is a complicated procedure used to determine the chronological age of an individual who lacks legal documentation. Actual studies show that the ossification degree of the growth plates in the knee joint represents a suitable indicator for the majority age. To verify this hypothesis a high number of datasets have to be analysed. Therefore, approaches which enable the detection of the bone structures are necessary. In this work a fully automatic knee segmentation in 3D MR images using convolutional neural networks is presented. A total of 76 datasets were available and divided into a training set (74%), a validation set (13%) and a test set (13%). Multiple preprocessing steps were applied to correct the images and to reduce their size. Image Augmentation was employed to virtually increase the data set size during training. The proposed architecture for the segmentation task resembles the encoder-decoder model type used for the U-Net. The trained network achieves a DSC score of 98% compared to the manual segmentations and an IoU of 96%, outperforming the results by Dam et al.[1]. The precision and recall of the model are balanced and the error has a small value of 1.2%. No overfitting was observed during training. As a proof of concept, the segmentations were used for the age estimation of a number of subjects. First results show the potential of this approach attaining a mean difference of 0.48 ± 0.32 years, which improve results from Stern et al. of 0.85 ± 0.58 years [2]. In order to fully exploit the potential of neural networks and to supply a more precise and reliable age prediction, the approach has to be tested on a larger data collective. The proposed segmentation can lead to an improvement of age estimation methods.

References

1. Dam EB, Lillholm M, Marques J, et al. Automatic segmentation of high- and low-field knee MRIs using knee image quantification with data from the osteoarthritis initiative. J Med Imaging. 2015;2(2):024001.
2. Stern D, Ebner T, Bischof H, et al. Fully automatic bone age estimation from left hand MR images. Proc MICCAI. 2014;17:220–227.

Abstract: OCT-OCTA Segmentation

A Novel Framework and an Application to Segment Bruch's Membrane in the Presence of Drusen

Julia Schottenhamml[1],[2], Eric M. Moult[1], Eduardo A. Novais[3],[4],
Martin F. Kraus[2], ByungKun Lee[1], WooJhon Choi[1], Stefan B. Ploner[2],
Lennart Husvogt[2], Chen D. Lu[1], Patrick Yiu[1], Philip J. Rosenfeld[5],
Jay S. Duker[3], Andreas K. Maier[2], Nadia Waheed[3], James G. Fujimoto[1]

[1]Research Laboratory of Electronics, Massachusetts Institute of Technology
[2]Pattern Recognition Lab, Friedrich-Alexander-University Erlangen-Nuremberg
[3]New England Eye Center, Tufts Medical Center
[4]Department of Ophthalmology, Federal University of Sao Paulo
[5]Department of Ophthalmology, University of Miami Miller School of Medicine
julia.schottenhamml@fau.de

In this work, a novel paradigm for segmenting optical coherence tomography (OCT) and optical coherence tomography angiography (OCTA) is presented [1]. Since it uses OCT and OCTA information jointly it is called "OCT-OCTA segmentation" and its usefulness is demonstrated by segmenting the Bruch's Membrane (BM) in the presence of drusen. Therefore a fully automatic graph-cut algorithm was developed and evaluated by comparing the automatic segmentation results with manual segmentation in 7 eyes (6 patients; 73.8 ± 5.7 y/o) with nascent geographic atrophy and/or drusen associated geographic atrophy. The absolute pixel-wise error between the segmentation curves were: mean: $4.5 \pm 0.89 \, \mu m$, 1st quartile: $1.9 \pm 1.35 \, \mu m$, 2nd quartile: $3.9 \pm 1.90 \, \mu m$, 3rd quartile: $6.3 \pm 2.67 \, \mu m$, which results in an absoulte mean error less than the optical axial resolution of the OCT system ($8 - 9\mu m$). The algorithm was also qualitatively assessed in healthy eyes ($n = 13$), eyes with diabetic retinopathy ($n = 21$), age-related macular degeneration (AMD) ($n = 14$), exudative AMD ($n = 5$), geographic atrophy (GA) ($n = 6$), polypoidal choroidal vasculopathy ($n = 7$) and choroidal neovascularization (CNV) ($n = 7$). The resulting segmentation contours were mostly accurate enough to form en face projections for further analysis and in cases with poorer results a correction algorithm based on outlier detection and Laplacian interpolation was applied to achieve proper results.

References

1. Schottenhamml J, Moult EM, Novais EA, et al. OCT-OCTA segmentation: a novel framework and an application to segment Bruch's membrane in the presence of drusen. Invest Ophthal Vis Sci. 2017;58(8):645–645.

Human Pose Estimation from Pressure Sensor Data

Leslie Casas[1,2], Chris Mürwald[2],Felix Achilles[1,2], Diana Mateus[1],
Dietrich Huber[2], Nassir Navab[1,2], Stefanie Demirci[1,2]

[1]Computer Aided Medical Procedures, Technische Universität München, Germany
[2]Sanvisio, Austria
[3]Computer Aided Medical Procedures, Johns Hopkins University, USA
leslie.casas@tum.de

Abstract. In-bed motion monitoring has become of great interest for
a variety of clinical applications. In this paper, we introduce a hash-
based learning method to retrieve human poses from pressure sensors
data in real time considering temporal correlation between poses. The
basis of our approach is a multimodal database describing different in-bed
activities. Database entries have been created using an array of pressure
sensors and an additional motion capture system. Our results show good
performance even in poses where the subject has minimal contact with
the sensors

1   Introduction

In today's highly digitized health care workflows, in-bed patient motion monitoring has become a crucial requirement for various aspects such as patient
positioning for precise treatment, disease and disorder diagnosis [1], detection of
bed-exit and fall events [2], and bedsore prevention [3].

Automatic monitoring systems have generally used cameras that monitor
patients in two dimensions, typically reducing a scene to a flat image. There
has been only a few attempts to monitor patient movements on a bed mattress.
An early idea presented by M. P. Toms [4], describes the use of fluid filled
cells between the patient and a support in order to detect motion via pressure
fluctuations. Alaziz et al. [5] suggest to use low-end load cells placed under
each bed leg, and classify 27 pre-defined movements by analysing the computed
forces. A similar approach has been validated by Hoque et al. [2] replacing load
cells with active RFID sensors equipped with accelerometers. Both approaches
are able to show promising results, but lack high-speed algorithmic solutions
in order to enable a real-time processing. Employing a powerful deep learning
approach, Heydarzadeh et al. [3] yield close-to-real-time in-bed patient posture
classification based on pressure data collected from a commercially available
force sensing array mat that is placed between bed mattress and linen. Despite
short processing time of the classification step, the preprocessing of pressure data
involves tedious filtering which slows down the entire speed.

In this paper we introduce a hash-based learning method to retrieve human posture poses in real time. Similar to the aforementioned approach, we retrieve pressure data from sensors that are incorporated into the patient bed mattress. Our approach is inspired by Harada et al. [6] who have proposed to solve the general computer vision pose estimation problem via a synthetic pressure distribution image generated by a surface human mesh model. This way, the pose can easily be computed by minimizing a cost function considering pressure distribution, gravity and momentum.

2 Materiales and methods

In this section, we explain the pipeline of the proposed work as depicted in Fig. 1. After presenting the acquisition and processing of the database, our encoding model learning process and the real-time estimation of the human pose are introduced.

2.1 Multimodal database

In this work, we acquired a multimodal dataset $\mathbf{D}$ using two systems. The first is an array of s pressure sensors arranged horizontally and equidistantly covering an area of 2m x 1m which delivers a pressure-based dataset $\mathbf{P} = \{\mathbf{p}_i\}$. In addition, we have employed a commercial 5-calibrated camera motion capture system, which tracks the position of a 14-joint skeleton (head, neck, shoulders, elbows, wrists, hips, knees and ankles) and delivers a 3D pose-based dataset $\mathbf{A} = \{\mathbf{a}_i\}$. The synchronization of both acquisitions has been performed offline using the time stamps of each recording and eventually setting the whole system acquisition frequency to 30Hz.

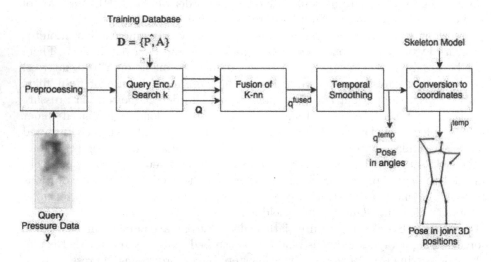

Fig. 1. Human pose estimation from a pressure distribution image.

Table 1. Description of the activities performed in the acquisition process.

Activity	Name	Description
A1	Random horizontal positions	Subject simulates sleeping positions.
A2	Fixed horizontal positions	Subject changes horizontally from left, center and right position.
A3	Rotation of joints	Keeping the trunk horizontal, subject rotates upper and lower limb joints, and head.
A4	Body stretching	Subject performs stretching positions not keeping the horizontal position.
A5	Simulated seizures	Subject performs rapid twitiching movements simulating the clonic phase of an epileptic seizure

The acquisition was performed on 6 subjects, 2 female and 4 male, performing 5 distinct activities (Tab. 1) for 1 minute each, according to an acquisition protocol inspired by work of Achilles et al. [1]. Each subject performed the activity recording lying on a mattress, which was located on top of the array of pressure sensors, and wearing motion capture sensors.

The pressure-based modality (pressure sensor array) is represented as a pressure distribution image normalized to [0,1] range per sensor. Hence, each sensor represents a stand-alone-feature in the feature space. The pose-base modality (motion capture system) is presented as joint angles describing the 14-joint skeleton in 13 segments, each segment being represented by 3 directional angles (one per axis). Therefore, each multimodal database element, which represents the acquired data in frame i, $\mathbf{D}_i = \{\mathbf{p}_i, \mathbf{a}_i\}$ consists of a tuple of the normalized pressure distribution images arranged as a vector $\mathbf{p}_i = \{p_i^1, ..., p_i^s\}$ and a vector of directional angles $\mathbf{a}_i = \{a_i^1, ..., a_i^{13 \times 3}\}$.

2.2   Hash model learning

Inspired by *Iterative Quantization* [7], we employ a similar strategy to encode the pressure distribution training data.

Let $\mathbf{X} = \{\mathbf{x}_1, \mathbf{x}_2, ..., \mathbf{x}_n\} \in \mathbb{R}^{n \times d}$ be a set of n d-dimensional, zero-centered data points. Our technique learns a binary code matrix $\mathbf{B} = sgn(\mathbf{XW}) \in \{-1, 1\}^{n \times c}$ where c is the code length and $\mathbf{W} \in \mathbb{R}^{d \times c}$ is the matrix of hyperplane coefficients.

First, an orthogonal transformation is applied to the data to reduce the dimension and obtain an initial encoding function I which maximizes the variance of each bit and provides de-correlated pairwise code bits:

$$I(\mathbf{W}) = \sum_k var(h_k(\mathbf{x})) \tag{1}$$

where $h_k(x) = sgn(x\mathbf{w}_k)$ and $\mathbf{w}_k$ are the columns of matrix $\mathbf{W}$ ($\mathbf{W}^t\mathbf{W} = 1$). When the orthogonal transformation is Principal Component Analysis (PCA),

$\mathbf{W}$ is obtained by taking the top c eigenvectors for the covariance matrix $\mathbf{X}^t\mathbf{X}$. Let $\mathbf{V} = \mathbf{XW}$ be the matrix of projected data. There exists a orthogonal transformation matrix $\mathbf{R} \in \mathbb{R}^{c \times c}$ applied to $\mathbf{V}$ such that it minimizes the quantization loss function

$$Q(\mathbf{B}, \mathbf{R}) = \|\mathbf{B} - \mathbf{VR}\|_F^2 \tag{2}$$

which measures the distance between the projected data $\mathbf{V}$ and the vertices of the hypercube $\{-1, 1\}^c$. The final encoding of $\mathbf{X}$ is $\hat{\mathbf{V}} = \mathbf{XWR}$.

Finally, using the method previously explained, let $\hat{\mathbf{P}}$ be the final encoding of our pressure based dataset $\mathbf{P}$.

2.3   Real-time pose estimation

At this stage, we employ the previously created database to realize our real-time pose estimation algorithm as online query. The huge advantage of this implementation is its speed. In the remainder of this section, we describe our algorithm according to the pipeline displayed in Fig. 1.

Step 1: Preprocessing As first step, incoming query pressure data $\mathbf{y} = \{y_1, y_2, ..., y_n\}$ is normalized to $[0, 1]$.

Step 2: Query encoding/search In this step, we apply model $\mathbf{M} = \mathbf{WR}$ learned using the initial hashing algorithm (Section 2.2) to the input pressure data vector $\mathbf{y}$ yielding an encoded representation $\hat{\mathbf{y}} = \mathbf{yM}$. Then, the search consists in finding the k closest embeddings with indexes $\{i_1, ..., i_k\}$ within the encoded pressure distribution training dataset $\hat{\mathbf{P}}$ according to Hamming distance. Finally, an array of k poses $\mathbf{Q} = \{\mathbf{a}_{i_1}, ..., \mathbf{a}_{i_k}\}$ corresponding to the k closest encoding found in the search is retrieved.

Step 3: Fusion of k poses The aim of this step is to eliminate corrupted or outlier poses within set Q in order to allow for a robust estimation. To this end, we employ median absolute deviation (MAD) to eliminate outlier poses in Q and yield an average pose set $\mathbf{q}^{fused}$.

Step 4: Temporal smoothing In order to ensure correlation between poses in subsequent frames, a computing window of $2m + 1$ frames $[t - m, t + m]$ is used to smooth the transition and avoid corrupted static poses. We also employ MAD as in Step 3 to obtain the final pose in angles $\mathbf{q}^{\text{temp}}$.

Step 5: Coordinate conversion For visualization purposes, we compute a synthetic pose in joint 3D positions $\mathbf{j}^{\text{temp}}$ from the resultant pose $\mathbf{q}^{\text{temp}}$ using a template skeleton.

Subject	MAE [deg]	MAE [m]
S1	24.223	13.379
S2	25.375	13.868
S3	22.340	10.582
S4	17.545	9.781
S5	20.283	9.762
S6	23.177	14.024

Table 2. Pose estimation mean absolute errors (MAE) using leave-one-subject-out cross validation.

Activity	MAE [deg]	MAE [cm]
A1	29.266	14.029
A2	27.954	13.871
A3	14.526	9.829
A4	33.556	21.958
A5	19.750	10.928

Table 3. Pose estimation mean absolute errors (MAE) using leave-one-activity-out cross validation.

3   Results

We have performed cross validation on our database in order to evaluate our presented approach on the subjects as well as activities. Table 2 shows the results of leave-one-subject-out cross validation. The median absolute error (MAE) in column 2 and 3, takes as reference a template skeleton to all the subjects (Step 5 in section 2.3).

Each pose estimation took 16ms in average using Matlab 2016b on a Core i7 with 2.60GHz and 12GB RAM. Table 3 shows the leave-one-subject-out cross validation results.

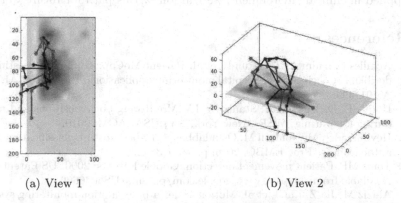

(a) View 1   (b) View 2

Fig. 2. Bad Pose Estimation: ground truth pose (black) vs. estimated pose (red).

Fig. 3. Good Pose Estimation: ground truth pose (black) vs. estimated pose (red).

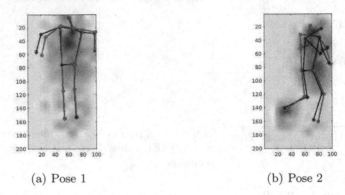

(a) Pose 1   (b) Pose 2

4 Discussion

In this paper, we have presented a simple yet effective method to yield real-time patient posture estimation from pressure sensor data.

Our experiments have revealed only a slight position error that has no severe influence on the overall posture detection. As expected, best results have been obtained when the subject is positioned flat (Fig. 3) On the other hand, poses where the subject has less contact with the surface (such as activity 4) yield the highest error (Tab. 3). However, even in those cases, the estimated pose correlates with the real patient posture (Fig. 2).

Our results further indicate that a potential inclusion of more robust learning techniques such as convolutional/recurrent neural networks (CNN/RNN) for temporal constraint, may improve the accuracy and robustness of our human pose estimation approach. In order to move forward our approach to be applied in clinical environment, we will follow this path for future work.

References

1. Achilles F, Ichim AE, Coskun H, et al. Patient MoCap: Human pose estimation under blanket occlusion for hospital monitoring applications. Proc MICCAI. 2016;Part A:491–499.
2. Hoque E, Dickerson RF, Stankovic JA. Monitoring body positions and movements during sleep using WISPs. New York, NY, USA: ACM; 2010.
3. Heydarzadeh M, Nourani M, Ostadabbas S. In-bed posture classification using deep autoencoders. Proc EMBC. 2016; p. 3839–3842.
4. Toms MP. Patient movement detection. Google Patents; 2000. US Patent 6,036,660. Available from: https://www.google.com/patents/US6036660.
5. Alaziz M, Jia Z, Liu J, et al. Motion scale: a body motion monitoring system using bed-mounted wireless load cells. Proc IEEE CHASE. 2016 June; p. 183–192.
6. Harada T, Sato T, Mori T. Pressure distribution image based human motion tracking system using skeleton and surface integration model; 2001.
7. Gong Y, Lazebnik S, Gordo A, et al.. Iterative quantization: a procrustean approach to learning binary codes for large-scale image retrieval; 2013.

Force-feedback-assisted Bone Drilling Simulation Based on CT Data

Johannes Maier[1], Michaela Huber[2], Uwe Katzky[3], Jerome Perret[4],
Thomas Wittenberg[5], Christoph Palm[1,6]

[1]Regensburg Medical Image Computing (ReMIC),
Ostbayerische Technische Hochschule Regensburg (OTH Regensburg)
[2]Department of Trauma Surgery & Emergency Department,
University Hospital Regensburg
[3]szenaris GmbH, Bremen
[4]Haption GmbH, Aachen
[5]Fraunhofer Institute for Integrated Circuits IIS, Erlangen
[6]Regensburg Center of Biomedical Engineering (RCBE),
OTH Regensburg and Regensburg University
johannes2.maier@oth-regensburg.de

Abstract. In order to fix a fracture using minimally invasive surgery approaches, surgeons are drilling complex and tiny bones with a 2 dimensional X-ray as single imaging modality in the operating room. Our novel haptic force-feedback and visual assisted training system will potentially help hand surgeons to learn the drilling procedure in a realistic visual environment. Within the simulation, the collision detection as well as the interaction between virtual drill, bone voxels and surfaces are important. In this work, the *chai3d* collision detection and force calculation algorithms are combined with a physics engine to simulate the bone drilling process. The chosen *Bullet-Physics-Engine* provides a stable simulation of rigid bodies, if the collision model of the drill and the tool holder is generated as a compound shape. Three haptic points are added to the K-wire tip for removing single voxels from the bone. For the drilling process three modes are proposed to emulate the different phases of drilling in restricting the movement of a haptic device.

1 Introduction

Fractures of the hand may lead to mechanical impairments and to a restricted flexibility of the hand. Surgeons stabilize the fracture with *K-wires* (Kirschner-wires) in the operating room [1, 2]. During the minimally invasive drilling process several structures like tendons, vessels and nerves are under risk to be damaged. This has to be prevented. Therefore, a long-term experience as well as extensive theoretical and practical training for surgeons are necessary [3]. The compact haptically and visually supported training system HaptiVisT [4], based on elements of virtual reality, haptic human-machine-interaction and gamification, will provide surgeons the possibility to train and improve their bone-drilling skills at any time in the clinic routine and on collective training courses without an incurring risk to patients [5, 6]. Within the scope of generating a realistic drilling simulation, a very complex part consists of the collision detection and the volume interaction between the virtual drill (obtained from a force-feedback haptic device) and the bones of a human hand and wrist (from pre-operative CT data) in a combined virtual three-dimensional (3D) space. On the one hand, the entire drill must be able to collide with every bone model. On the other hand, a special collision detection of the K-wire tip with the bones is required to remove individual voxels during the drilling process. For this purpose, it is necessary to find suitable simulation models for driller, K-wire tip and bones, and to combine these models in a proper way. Additionally, bone drilling with a K-wire is restricted to the forward-backward direction without the possibility to drill sideways. Consequently, in order to avoid a deviation from the drilling hole, the movement of the drill must be limited to the axial direction in order to avoid a deviation from the drilling hole. During this drilling process, it is also necessary to maintain the haptic update rate at a frequency of 1000 Hz to ensure a safe and vibration-free simulation of the calculated drilling forces [7].

2   Materials and methods

A realistic hand surgery simulation combines suitable software and hardware tools and takes the special requirements of collision detection and bone drilling into account.

2.1   Soft- and hardware tools

Generating a drilling simulation, important requirements for a programming environment have to be set. Beside a real-time simulation for haptic and graphic interfaces, stereoscopic volume as well as surface rendering in a 3D space is needed. Local coordinate systems from every integrated object have to be transferred by quaternion and matrix rotation to a common 3D space. In addition to the possibility of connecting a haptic device, collision detection between driller and bone objects is essential. The open source C++ framework chai3d (www.chai3d.org) for computer haptics fulfills these requirements. Haptical and visual rendering are separated and run parallel in a haptic and graphic thread. The haptic loop should always run with an update rate above 1000 Hz to guarantee a stable simulation of the haptic force-feedback [7]. The graphics thread with an acceptable framerate of 30 Hz is rendered using openGL (www.opengl.org) [7]. The toolkit library qt 5 (www.qt.io) provides a Graphical User Interface (GUI). To transmit the position of a drill-tip in real space to the virtual space of the computer, a haptic device (Virtuose 6D Desktop, Haption GmbH) with force-feedback is used. A real drill holder from the minimally invasive hand surgery is mounted at the end of the haptic device. Through an additional applied force-feedback to the haptic device, virtual objects, which are only visible at the computer

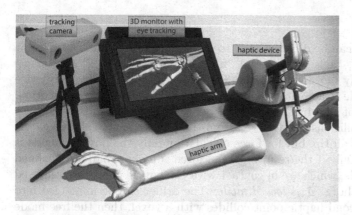

Fig. 1. HaptiVisT training system mock-up with the haptic device for haptic force-feedback and position tracking [4].

screen, become tactile. The complete mock-up can be seen in Figure 1. For more information about the training system we refer to [4].

Bones to be drilled are visualized via isosurface rendering. Real clinical hand and wrist data from a 502 layered CT with image dimensions of 512 x 512 pixels and voxel dimensions of 0.85 x 0.85 x 1.00 mm^3 are semi-automatically segmented using itksnap (www.itksnap.org). After preprocessing, resampling and upscaling a high isotropic volume resolution of 0.25 mm^3 per voxel is achieved. Each bone is cropped out of the resulting image stack, loaded into the system with setting its original position and compound together to the total hand object. With this concept, every bone can be controlled individually. For the soft tissue, the driller, the environment, and also bones, which are not yet in drilling use, a surface model rendering is sufficient to save processing power.

2.2 Collision detection

An adequate collision detection is crucial for the creation of a force-feedback-experience which realistically simulates the contact between rigid bones and a drill. Such collision detection including force calculation can be provided by a physical engine for the simulation of rigid bodies. Since bones and drill show complex surfaces, an important requirement is the support of triangle meshes. For collision between rigid objects, a dynamic collision model is generated for each object based on its surface. If the dynamic collision model of the drill collides with the bone model, the drill lingers on the bone despite continued movement of the haptic device. Due to the positional deviation between the simulated and the real drill, the strength of the transmitted force-feedback is varied. In addition to the collision model from the physics engine, a collision detection between the K-wire tip and the voxels of the bones is needed to prepare an interaction event between bone and drill to remove voxels during the drilling process. For this reason, haptic points are used, which are massless spheres with own local coordinate system and which are capable of detecting collisions with a volume voxel. These spheres are placed into the drill tip inside the physical drill collision model, because only here voxel removal induced by drilling takes place (Fig. 2b).

2.3   Bone drilling

Three drilling modes can be differentiated to emulate the basic phases for linear bone drilling: "Free", "axis locked" and "fully locked" (Fig. 2a). *Free mode:* The drill can be freely moved within the 3D space, only limited by the device conditions. This mode is activated by default at the launch of the application. By pressing the tip of the drill against the bone, force-feedback is applied to the haptic device. Collisions are detected from the physics engine as well as the haptic points in the drill tip, but for force calculation only the physics engine is taken into account. Only if the resulting axial force is higher than a predefined threshold, those voxels, which are in contact with the haptic points are removed with inclusion of the bore. *Axis locked mode:* The driller can be immerged into the bone until the second haptic point collides with a voxel, then the free mode changes to the axis locked mode. Onward, the force calculation of the physics engine is no longer active and is continued by an adapted chai3d algorithm for internal force calculation between haptic points and volume objects. The virtual proxy and goal-sphere approach for interactions with objects from chai3d is used and adjusted, allowing only an axial movement and position setting of the drill in the visualization [7]. Now, only voxels in the axial direction can be removed, but not laterally. Furthermore, the haptic device is locked in all directions and rotations, except the axial axis. Accordingly, the movement of the driller in real space is limited and only possible in the down or upward direction of the drill hole. Additional lock-forces are calculated using the lateral position deviation and the speed variation of the haptic device. The entrance point of the axis locked mode is recorded and in case of reaching this position again by pulling out the driller, the axis locked mode will be reset to the free mode. *Fully locked mode:* The fully locked mode can only be reached from the axis locked mode and is activated by deactivating the drill rotation. In this mode, all motion directions and rotations are completely locked without exception. Drill movement and voxel erosion are no longer possible. The driller remains stuck in the bone by transmitting only the restraining forces to the haptic device. This mode remains active until the bore is resumed or the drilling process is terminated by placing the K-wire in the borehole. Then, the K-wire remains in the bone while the drill can be moved freely (free mode). In order to start a new drilling operation, the next K-wire can be selected via the GUI.

3   Results

In generating a collision model for a rigid drill body, two different approaches were evaluated. In the first approach, one collision model for the K-wire and one for the drill holder were created separately and then assembled, in a way that the collision model of the K-wire can be exchanged easily. Hence during a tool change, the collision model would not have to be completely rebuilt. However, this resulted in a high instability for the K-wire collision model. The K-wire is shaped similar to a very long thin cylinder and as such its small shape it is very difficult to simulate for a physics engine. The minimum size for a moving object should not exceed 20 cm [8]. In the second approach the dynamic collision model of the physical drill is created as a compound shape including the drill tool holder and the K-wire. In case of a tool change, the collision model of the entire drill is destroyed and re-created. This resulted in an increased stability of the collision surface. For the physical simulation of rigid bodies, two engines were compared: Open-Dynamics-Engine (ODE) and Bullet-Physics-Engine (BPE). Although both models support triangular collision shapes, a stable collision detection between bone and drill is difficult with ODE, because the drill can still penetrate a bone mesh (pop through). Moreover, jitter of the moving drill model cannot completely be suppressed. With the BPE, the trembling and the pop through effect is fixed. However, the collision margin of the BPE models has to be adapted carefully to ensure a stable simulation. This collision model covers the visualized surface model of the drill. For voxel erosion three haptic points are placed within the K-wire tip. Their increasing size induce the cone-shaped K-wire tip. The size of the second and third haptic point is variable according to the size different K-wires (Fig. 2b). The three presented drill modes were tested by an experienced hand surgeon (MH). It was found, that the drilling procedure is very realistic and well covered. However, an additional fourth drilling mode is desirable, to prevent slipping effects between the sharp K-wire tip and the bone. This additional "point locked mode" will allow a smoother transition from free to axis locked mode. It will simulate the sticking effect and the restricted angular offset between the sharp tip of the driller and a bone. The update rate of the haptic thread is far above 1000 Hz with the exception of the axis locked mode. The rate temporarily falls below the required value and the simulation becomes unstable. This may be caused by the complex collision detection computation of the haptic points with numerous lateral bone voxels surrounding the bore hole. A possible solution could be a reduction of the used haptic points to a minimum.

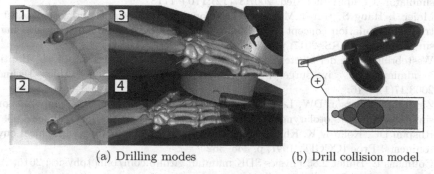

(a) Drilling modes   (b) Drill collision model

Fig. 2. (a) Visualization of the drilling modes: 1. The drill can be freely moved within the 3D world. 2. The K-wire motion is restricted to the axial direction. 3. No movement is possible during the fully locked mode. 4. The free mode is active after the K-wire has been discarded. (b) The collision model (red) superimposes the drill. Haptic points within the K-wire tip can be tool diameter dependent (grey) and independent (blue).

4   Discussion

The collision detection from the bullet engine and the chai3d voxel interaction works well with the complex triangular drill and bone models. Nevertheless, the bullet collision margins of the objects must be adapted to reduce the collision space between objects. The three haptic points should be replaced by one haptic point combined with a mathematical approach for a cone shaped K-wire hole. The presented drilling modes have to be extended by an additional point lock mode to enable a smoother transition from the free to locked axis mode. At this time only linear bone drilling is possible, but in case of K-wire bending its supposable to augment the system in enabling curved drilling. To fix the low haptic update rate a stiffness adoption during the locked axis mode may help to improve the stability of the system. The calculated force feedback has to be carefully evaluated, e.g. in using a force feedback evaluation framework [9] or in comparing it with the actual drilling force, measured by an attached load cell.

Acknowledgement. This work was supported by the German Federal Ministry of Education and Research with grant 16SV7560.

References

1. Haughton D, Jordan D, Malahias M, et al. Principles of hand fracture management. Open Orthop J. 2012;6:43–53.
2. Franssen BB, Schuurman AH, Van der Molen AM, et al. One century of Kirschner wires and Kirschner wire insertion techniques: a historical review. Acta Orthop Belg. 2010;76(1):1–6.
3. Tsai M, Hsieh M, Tsai C. Bone drilling haptic interaction for orthopedic surgical simulator. Comput Biol Med. 2007;37(12):1709–1718.
4. Maier J, Haug S, Huber M, et al. Development of a haptic and visual assisted training simulation concept for complex bone drilling in minimally invasive hand surgery. Proc CARS. 2017; p. 135–136.
5. Westebring - van der Putten EP, Goossens RHM, Jakimowicz JJ, et al. Haptics in minimally invasive surgery: a review. Minim Invasive Ther Allied Technol. 2008;17(1):3–16.
6. Zirkle M, Roberson DW, Leuwer R, et al. Using a virtual reality temporal bone simulator to assess otolaryngology trainees. Laryngoscope. 2007;117(2):258–263.
7. Ruspini DC, Kolarov K, Khatib O. The haptic display of complex graphical environments. Proc ICCGIT. 1997; p. 345–352.
8. Coumans E. Bullet 2.83 physics SDK manual. github.com/bulletphysics; 2015. Accessed: 2017-11-02.
9. Mastmeyer A, Fortmeier D, Handels H. Evaluation of direct haptic 4d volume rendering of partially segmented data for liver puncture simulation. Sci Rep. 2017;7(1):671.

Direct Volume Rendering in Virtual Reality

Ingrid Scholl, Sebastian Suder, Stefan Schiffer

Computer Graphics and Foundation of Computer Science
Mobile Autonomous Systems and Cognitive Robotics (MASCOR) Institute
FH Aachen University of Applied Sciences, Germany
scholl@fh-aachen.de

Abstract. Direct Volume Rendering (DVR) techniques are used to visualize surfaces from 3D volume data sets, without computing a 3D geometry. Several surfaces can be classified using a transfer function by assigning optical properties like color and opacity (RGBα) to the voxel data. Finding a good transfer function in order to separate specific structures from the volume data set, is in general a manual and time-consuming procedure, and requires detailed knowledge of the data and the image acquisition technique. In this paper, we present a new Virtual Reality (VR) application based on the HTC Vive headset. One-dimensional transfer functions can be designed in VR while continuously rendering the stereoscopic image pair through massively parallel GPU-based ray casting shader techniques. The usability of the VR application is evaluated.

1   Introduction

With the development of cost-efficient head-mounted displays like the Oculus Rift or the HTC Vive, the Virtual Reality (VR) market has seen an economic revival in the last years. New headsets being developed for the consumer market with a larger field of view in the range of 80° and 110° enabling a better 3D immersion for the user. VR is used as an immersive visualization tool in many fields. In medicine, visualization plays a critical role in diagnosis and therapy. VR can help the medical professional to detect and analyze complicated fractures, localize a tumor, or plan an operation from a 3D overview of the patient data. To enable this, volume data sets from CT or MRT must be loaded into the VR application and can then be visualized in 3D with volume rendering techniques.

Volume rendering in VR is a time-consuming process: a stereoscopic image pair for the left and right lense of the headset must be calculated in real-time with low latency. This implies about 90 frames per second to allow comfortable movements in the virtual scene without getting sick. Krüger et al. [1] introduced a GPU-based ray casting algorithm as direct volume rendering, to massively parallelize the ray casting process. Hadwiger et al. [2] presented the algorithm as a single-pass approach on the GPU in a CG fragment shader. Hänel et al. [3]

evaluated acceleration techniques for the visualization of volume data with immersive virtual environments (IVE). They showed that a sufficient performance for interactive volume rendering in IVEs remains a challenge.

We have realized a new VR application for real-time volume rendering using the HTC Vive headset. The user can load clinical volume data. Editing the 1D transfer function, transforming the volume and visualizing the clipping planes has been implemented and can be triggered with the HTC vive controller. We used the OpenGL rendering pipeline, and we programmed the relevant shader to parallelize the time-consuming raycasting algorithm. A user evaluation test showed that the application navigation and usability is intuitive. Users reported having a great immersion experience, and feeling as if they were inside the 3D volume.

2   Methods

The medical volume data sets are loaded into our VR application using the DICOM-Toolkit. We developed two different rendering paths which can be combined. In the next subsection we describe the underlying rendering algorithms. After that, we give a description of all user interactions and their influence on transformation and rendering parameters for the volume visualization.

2.1   VR volume and clipping plane renderer

The volume must be rendered twice, once for the left and once for the right image of the stereoscopic image pair. We integrated two methods for the volume rendering: (1) ray casting for the direct volume rendering and (2) a clipping plane rendering of the anatomical planes. Both methods are described in the following.

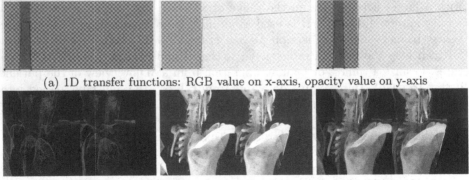

(a) 1D transfer functions: RGB value on x-axis, opacity value on y-axis

(b) Stereoscopic image pairs corresponding to the transfer functions above

Fig. 1. Transfer functions and unwarped stereoscopic rendering images.

Algorithmus 1 Pseudocode for single-pass ray casting with pre-integration.

1: Determine volume entry position
2: Compute ray line and direction
3: Apply stochastic jittering to ray start position along ray direction
4: **while** (Current ray position in volume) AND (opacity < 0.95) **do**
5:     Access scalar value at current position from volume data
6:     Classify scalar value with 2D pre-integrated transfer function
7:     Compositing of color and opacity
8:     Calculate next sample position along the ray
9: **end while**
10: Set summarized color and opacity to fragment position

Ray casting method A ray from the camera origin through each rendered image pixel is sent into the volume. A rendering integral is calculated for each ray or image pixel. The pseudocode for this sampling is shown in Algorithm 1. The basic idea of ray casting is to trace rays from the camera into the volume, computing the volume-rendering integral through sampling and compositing along these rays. We re-implemented the single-pass approach on the GPU into a fragment shader to calculate the rendering integral. Fig. 1 shows the results from the stereoscopic ray casting rendering using the corresponding 1D transfer functions from a CT data set.

Anatomical plane rendering The volume data set is stored on the GPU as a 3D texture. The sagittal, transverse and coronal anatomical planes can be extracted from the 3D texture as 2D texture coordinates. The image data are mapped on a clipping plane according to the texture coordinates. Fig. 2b shows the left image of the stereoscopic image pair which uses all anatomical planes. The ray casting result and the clipping plane are blended together.

2.2 VR interaction

Several user interactions have been implemented, allowing to pick, rotate, translate and scale the volume data in the virtual scene. Head movements, as well as

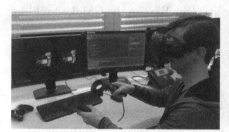
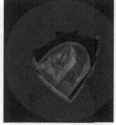

(a) Usage of the VR application   (b) Anatomical planes (c) Editing the TF in
                                    and ray casting   VR scene

Fig. 2. Interaction examples using the VR application. Only the left stereoscopic image is displayed in (b) and (c).

the HTC Vive controller movements, are connected to an event and result in a new computation of the stereoscopic rendered images. Both images are mapped to the HTC Vive displays. Fig. 2.2 summarizes the implemented events using the HTC Vive controller.

Head tracking Each motion from the headset is tracked by the HTC Vive motion capturing system. The translation and rotation parameters are translated to visualization transformations. According to this viewing transform, new stereoscopic image pairs are then rendered.

Clipping planes The anatomical plane rendering can be toggled on or off. The user can interact with each anatomical plane. A clipping plane is selected if the controller intersects the clipping plane respectively. Each plane can be moved either from front-to-back, left-to-right or top-to-bottom by picking and moving.

Volume transformations Several user interactions are implemented to pick, translate and scale the results of the volume rendering. Volume rendering can be toggled on or off. The user can pick the volume through intersection with one controller. The volume is translated through movements of the picking controller and can be scaled by movements of both controllers.

Transfer function editor We designed and integrated an editor for the 1D transfer function. The widget image from the graphical user interface is mapped on a texture and is placed in the virtual scene in 3D next to the left controller, see Fig. 1c. If the user changes the color and opacity values, a new transfer function is created and the user can see the volume visualization effect in VR in real-time. This helps to find the best classification for separating materials.

2.3 Implementation

The VR application is implemented in C++ and uses OpenGL 4.5 for the visualization, and the OpenGL shader language GLSL 4.5 for all shaders. The application is independent from the operating system. We use the CMake-building

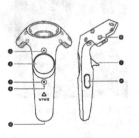

Action	Ctrl-ID	Button	Action type
Translate/rotate volume	1	Trigger	Press + move
Zoom volume	1 + 2	Grip	Press + move
Clipping plane on/off	2	Menu	Press
Translate clipping plane	2	Trigger	Press + move
TF editor on/off	2	Menu	Button press
TF left button click	1	Trigger	Pick + press
TF right button click	1	Trackpad	Pick + press

Fig. 3. Left: HTC Vive controller. Right: Table of buttons and events.

Table 1. Evaluation results of 13 users for different tasks. Values 1 to 7 correspond to a 7–step Likert scale from very difficult to very easy usability. The table shows the number of answers from the 13 test persons for every value of the Likert scale, i.e. 10 users evaluated the volume rotation and translation with a Likert scale value of 7.

Task	1	2	3	4	5	6	7	mean value	std. dev.
Volume rotation & translation	0	0	0	0	0	3	10	6.77	0.44
Volume zoom	0	0	0	1	3	2	7	6.15	1.07
Translate clipping planes	0	0	0	1	3	4	5	6.00	1.00
Toggle on/off menus	0	0	0	0	2	4	7	6.38	0.77
Edit transfer function	0	0	2	3	4	2	2	4.92	1.32

3.0.2 system and the following APIs: Qt 5.9, OpenVR 1.0.9 as interface to the HTC Vive and the DICOM-Toolkit (DCMTK) 3.6.2 as loader for the DICOM data set.

3 Evaluation

In this section we describe results of our evaluation of the performance and the usability of our VR application.

Measuring the performance of a VR application is more complex than for traditional applications. The stereoscopic image pair must be rendered for every movement of the headset and of the controller. VR applications require nearly 90 frames per second (FPS) for a good real-time feeling. Besides FPS rate, parameters like the number of dropped frames influence the VR quality. If a new rendering image is not completely computed in the current time interval, the previous rendered image can be used instead and will be displayed again. This is called dropped frames. If the number of dropped frames increases, the application starts to stutter. The SteamVR run time library uses the method of asynchronous reprojection. This allows a reprojection of an old rendered image with current tracking information. This method reduces the quality drawback effect of dropped frames.

We used the Frame Capture Analysis Tool VR (FCAT VR) of Nvidia to record and analyse the frame timing information from the headset. FCAT VR counts the number of dropped frames. Two different CT volume data sets were evaluated. The data sets differ in the image resolution and the number of slices. Data set 1 shows a human head in the dimension of $256 \times 256 \times 256$ and data set 2 a human thorax in the dimension of $512 \times 512 \times 328$. We used two different transfer functions (TFi). TF1 shows structures without transparency (bones), and TF2 uses more transparent structures. We use a fixed sample rate for the ray casting of 150 and early ray termination with an opacity value 0.95. A framerate in the range from 79.76 to 89.22 FPS could be achieved. The dropped frames percentage was under 2% with TF1 and 10.9% using TF2.

The System Usability Scale (SUS) described by John Brooke [4] provides a tool for measuring usability. It consists of a 10 item questionnaire with five positive and negative response options. A SUS score value of 100 represents a perfect score. 13 users tested the VR application, most of them with little or no VR experience. We reached a minimum, mean and maximum SUS score of 75.0, 86.65 and 92.5, respectivily. The SUS score mean value of 86.65 shows a very good usability for our application [5].

Additionally, we evaluated the user interaction through a questionnaire with five tasks listed in Tab. 1. Each task usability was rated by 13 test users on a 1 to 7 Likert scale value. 1 means very difficult and 7 means very easy. Only the usage of the transfer function editing process was experienced as difficult and must be re-engineered.

4 Discussion

The evaluation shows that our VR application provides the performance and usability required for a smooth and intuitive user experience for several reasons. First, the image refresh rate that is demanded by current VR headsets is sufficiently met and allows for a real-time stereoscopic rendering of the volume data. Second, the usability tests that we conducted, indicate that the controller interactions are in general easy to apply and intuitive, even for inexperienced users. In further development steps, we would like to improve the VR usability with regards to editing the transfer function, include illumination and other features to enhance the ray casting results.

References

1. Krüger J, Westermann R. Acceleration techniques for GPU-based volume rendering. Proc IEEE Vis. 2003; p. 38.
2. Engel K, Hadwiger M, Kniss J, et al. Real-time Volume Graphics. CRC Press; 2006.
3. Hänel C, Weyers B, Hentschel B, et al. Interactive volume rendering for immersive virtual environments. Proc IEEE 3DVis. 2014 Nov; p. 73–74.
4. Brooke J, et al. SUS-A quick and dirty usability scale. Usabil Eval Indus. 1996;189(194):4–7.
5. Albert W, Tullis T. Measuring the user experience: collecting, analyzing, and presenting usability metrics. Newnes; 2013.

Automatic Multi-modal Cervical Spine Image Atlas Segmentation
Using Adaptive Stochastic Gradient Descent

Ibraheem Al-Dhamari, Sabine Bauer, Dietrich Paulus

Medizinische Tekchnik Institut (MTI), Koblenz and Landau University
idhamari@uni-koblenz.de

1 Abstract

A personalized medicine has been advanced in different fields of medicine to combat, control and prevent a number of diseases. In personalized medicine, products are customized and only suitable for a specific patient. In spinal surgery, medical images are taken into account to implant spinal devices with the aim of minimizing the risk of insufficient implant fit. A model of the spine is generated from these images and used in biomechanic framework to simulate the effect of the customized implant on a specific patient.

To generate such a model, an efficient and practical segmentation method is needed which is proposed in this paper. The large deformation of human spine and the touching boundaries of neighboring vertebrae make the problem of spine segmentation very challenging. The classical segmentation methods e.g. thresholding or region growing fail to separate different vertebrae. The state of the art methods using shape models require a long time for training and testing. A new method for automatic multi-modal cervical spine segmentation is proposed in this paper. The proposed method requires only a few seconds to segment a specific vertebra or the whole cervical spine. It is provided as Slicer 3D plug-in which is free and open-source. The public datasets available fail to provide high quality MRI cervical spine images. Another contribution of this study is providing a high quality multi-modal cervical spine public and free dataset.

2 Introduction

In personalized medicine,"patientomized "(patient-customized) products are only suitable for the target patient and are not for other patients. Examples for patientomized therapy are the tinnitus masker, which is personalized by the manufacturer to patient tinnitus or Zenith Fenestrated AAA Endovascular Graft as an indicator for the endovascular treatment of patients with abdominal aortic or aortoiliac aneurysms having morphology [1]. In spinal surgery medical imaging are taken in to account to implant spinal devices with the aim of minimizing minimize the risk of insufficient implant fit.

Although spinal implants are available in different standardized sizes and there is the possibility of adjusting the inclination angles of the contact surfaces of the implant to the vertebral body, in some cases only an insufficient anchoring of the implant can be achieved. This can be traced back to the fact that each patient has a very individual anatomical condition. This circumstance can be responsible for insufficient anchoring of the implant or an unphysiological load distribution in the different spinal structures which could lead to pathological changes of the affected spinal structures. In some cases at least, a revision surgery is unavoidable. Therefore the aim of a patientomized spinal surgery should be to improve the surgical outcome through an exact individual adapted and adequate fitting implant to the individual anatomical needs.

A possible step to improve the patientomized spinal surgery is the integration of a biomechanical simulation in the preoperative planning. This biomechanical simulation takes the biomechanical conditions of the respective patient into account and thus spinal stress situation can be analyzed preoperative, so that a prediction of the effects of the surgical procedure can be made and the best possible surgical option can be offered. The basis of such patientomized biomechanical simulation models are surface models of each patient's vertebral body and their alignment. With the help of surface models and the knowledge of corresponding biomechanical parameters of the different patient specific spinal structures, prediction of the post-operative surgical situation can be done. For a fast surface model generation, providing an automatic segmentation of the vertebral bodies is essential. To ensure the use of patientomized simulation models in clinical daily routine, an automatic segmentation of the vertebral bodies is essential for a rapid generation of a surface model. Classical segmentation methods [2] fail to provide such accurate segmentation due to the high deformation of the spine and the touching boundaries of different vertebrae. A practical segmentation method of cervical spine is needed to achieve the goal of personalized implant.

3   Materials and methods

For the early stage of this study, 12 different clinical CT and MRI images of different patients are used. These images are anonymized to protect patient privacy. All the images have the same height and width i.e. 512x512 pixels with varied depths and resolutions. The depth ranges from 53 to 1050 slices and the resolution ranges from [0.7, 0.7, 1.0]mm to [0.9, 0.9, 2.0]mm. Sample of these images are shown in Fig. 1.

These images are part of our proposed public cervical spine dataset [1]. The number of images is small but it keeps increasing.

Atlas-based segmentation is a segmentation based on image registration [3]. The segmentation problem can be solved using this approach if an efficient image registration method is found for these images. In this study, an atlas-based

----
[1] https://mtixnat.uni-koblenz.de

segmentation method is proposed using Automatic Cochlea Image Registration (ACIR) method [4]. ACIR is an automatic multi-modal image registration method proposed for cochlea images. It uses Adaptive Stochastic Gradient Descent (ASGD)[5] to minimize Mattes's Mutual Information (MMI)[6] of a 3D rigid transform's parameters. ASGD is an optimization method for medical image registration and it is implemented as open-source in elastix toolbox[2] [7]. ACIR, ASGD and MMI are well described in the literature and available as an open source so we concentrate here on the technical details of the proposed atlas-segmentation. The reason for selected ACIR method is that it solves more challenging registration and segmentation problems successfully i.e. cochlea registration and segmentation.

To prepare the atlas model, a CT image is selected from our dataset and cropped to the cervical spine area. The cervical spine is manually segmented with different colors as in Fig. 2 left.

After that, each vertebra of the cervical spine is cropped and saved separately i.e. C1 to C7 in different files with their segmentations. These saved images will be used in the next stage as the atlas model.

To segment a new image, we locate the C2 vertebra, then the locations of other vertebrae are predicted automatically. This prediction is based on a vertical distance of 15 mm between each vertebra in the sagittal view. These location points are used for cropping each vertebra with a cube of size 90x80x60 mm. The accuracy of the predicted points is not important if a vertebra still included in the cropping cube. The previous measurements are based on our experiments and are sufficient for this purpose. Sometimes a small manual correction is needed to correct these locations which is still offered by our Slicer[3] plugin's friendly

---

[2] http://elastix.isi.uu.nl
[3] https://www.slicer.org

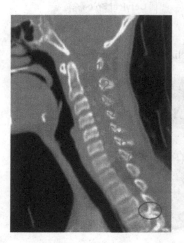 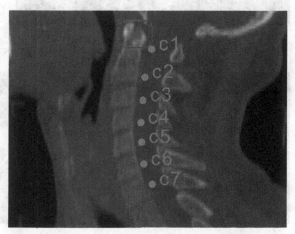

Fig. 1. Two saggital slices of cervical spine of different patients. The points of vertebrae C1-C7 and two examples of touching boundaries are shown.

user interface. We provide a video[4] tutorial to show how to use the plug-in with an example. All cervical spine vertebrae are extracted by the cropping process above and registered using ACIR to the related atlas model automatically. The result of the registrations are 3D rigid transforms' parameters. These transforms are used to transform the segmentations of the atlas model to the input image. In Fig. 2, right is a flow chart of the method steps.

4 Results

For all the tested images, the proposed method produced a visually satisfiable segmentation in a few seconds. The segmentation can be used in a model generation to be used in the simulation process later, see Fig. 3 and Fig. 4 for results samples.

The proposed method is tested against two different recent methods i.e. Fast Adaptive Gradient Descent (FASGD) [8] and Stochastic Quasi-Newton (SQN) [9] using 4 different standard measurements i.e. Dice Coefficient (DC)[10], Haus-

---

[4] https://mtixnat.uni-koblenz.de/owncloud/index.php/s/RVi3vr3JE6Q6hcF

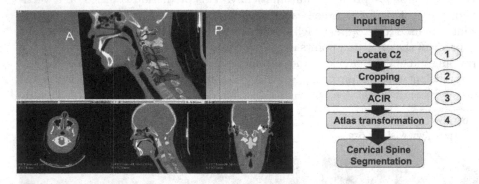

Fig. 2. Left: cervical spine atlas model. Right: flowchart of the proposed method.

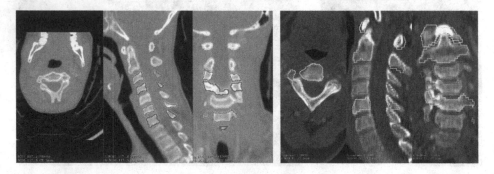

Fig. 3. Sample results: axial, sagittal and coronal slices are shown of two CT scans of two different patients. Different vertebrae are segmented and represented in different colors.

dorff (HD)[11], Matte's Mutual Information (MMI) and the Mean Squared Error(MSD). The methods are compared against the manually segmented images. In the figure, the time is represented in seconds e.g. ASGD segmented the images in 6.27 seconds. The values are rescaled to get better visualization in the chart. A sample chart of the results is provided in Fig. 5. These sample results represent the segmentation of the seventh vertebra (C7) in a CT cervical spine 3D image. The chart shows that ASGD produced faster segmentation than the other two methods. In DC, ASGD provided the largest value i.e. 0.82. In HD, MMI and MSD, ASGD produced the smallest values. FASGD and SQN were unstable and they failed to produce an output in some input images.

5 Discussion

There are two contributions in this paper. First, a public and free multi-modal cervical spine dataset. Second, using ACIR in atlas-based framework for automatic cervical spine segmentation. The idea is to deal with each vertebra separately then combine the segmentations in one final image. The proposed method handles all the segmentation issues successfully. It crops the input image into

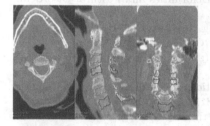 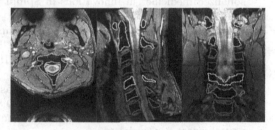

Fig. 4. Sample results: axial, sagittal and coronal slices are shown. Left: CT image, right: MRI image. Different vertebrae are segmented and represented in different colors.

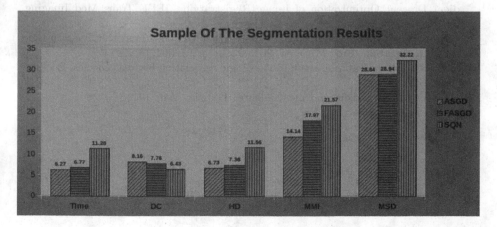

Fig. 5. Sample chart of the segmentation result.

small areas and deals with each area separately which removes all the noise and unnecessary objects and concentrates on the target object. Using ACIR without the cropping is not enough to solve the segmentation problem. This solves the low resolution and large deformation issues. It uses an atlas based model on separated vertebra which handles the issue of touching boundaries. All the steps, i.e. cropping, registration and the segmentation, are done automatically. The only human interfere is to locate C2 vertebra in the sagittal view which is quiet easy because of its long shape in addition to a few corrections if needed by moving the predicted vertebrae points to the right or the left.

There is not much difference between ASGD and FASGD in the quantitative results, see Fig. 5. The main difference is that ASGD is stable i.e. FASGD and SQN fail in some cases to produce any output. Future works include enhancing the accuracy of the proposed method by adding pre- and post-processing to correct the small segmentation errors.

References

1. Bauer S, Paulus D. Computational simulation as an innovative approach in personalized medicine. in Innovations in Spinal Deformities and Postural Disorders; 2017.
2. Gonzale R, Woods R. Digital image processing. Prentice-Hall, USA; 2006.
3. Hajnal H Hill. Medical image registration. CRC Press; 2001.
4. Al-Dhamari I, Bauer S, Paulus D, et al. ACIR: automatic cochlea image registration. Proc SPIE. 2017;10133(10):47–67.
5. Klein, Pluim, Staring, et al. Adaptive stochastic gradient descent optimisation for image registration. Int Jo Comput Vis. 2009;81(3):227–239.
6. Mattes, Haynor, Vesselle, et al. Non-rigid multimodality image registration. Proc SPIEs. 2001; p. 1609–1620.
7. Klein, Staring, Murphy, et al. elastix: a toolbox for intensity-based medical image registration. IEEE Trans Med Imaging. 2010;29(1):196–205.
8. Qiao, van Lew, Lelieveldt, et al. Fast automatic step Size Estimation for Gradient Descent Optimization of Image Registration. IEEE Trans Med Imaging. 2016;35(2):391–403.
9. Qiao Y, Sun Z, Lelieveldt B, et al. A stochastic quasi-newton method for non-rigid image registration. Proc MICCAI. 2015;9350(1):297–304.
10. Dice, R L. Measures of the amount of ecologic association between species. Ecology. 1945;26(3):297–302.
11. Hausdorff F. Grundzüge der mengenlehre. Leipzig: Veit; 1914.

SlideRunner

A Tool for Massive Cell Annotations in Whole Slide Images

Marc Aubreville[1], Christof Bertram[2], Robert Klopfleisch[2], Andreas Maier[1]

[1]Pattern Recognition Lab, Computer Sciences, Friedrich-Alexander-Universität
Erlangen-Nürnberg
[2]Institute of Veterinary Pathology, Freie Universität Berlin, Germany
marc.aubreville@fau.de

Abstract. Large-scale image data such as digital whole-slide histology
images pose a challenging task at annotation software solutions. Today,
a number of good solutions with varying scopes exist. For cell annotation, however, we find that many do not match the prerequisites for fast
annotations. Especially in the field of mitosis detection, it is assumed
that detection accuracy could significantly benefit from larger annotation databases that are currently however very troublesome to produce.
Further, multiple independent (blind) expert labels are a big asset for
such databases, yet there is currently no tool for this kind of annotation
available. To ease this tedious process of expert annotation and grading,
we introduce SlideRunner, an open source annotation and visualization
tool for digital histopathology, developed in close cooperation with two
pathologists. SlideRunner is capable of setting annotations like object
centers (for e.g. cells) as well as object boundaries (e.g. for tumor outlines). It provides single-click annotations as well as a blind mode for
multi-annotations, where the expert is directly shown the microscopy
image containing the cells that he has not yet rated.

1   Introduction

Whole-slide images enable automated image analysis in histopathology and is a
well-recognized and legally approved method for quantification of immunohisto-
chemistry in research and diagnosis. It has, beyond that, a great potential to
further support the pathologists' work in monotoneous, time-consuming tasks
such as counting rare events [1]. The availability of large amounts of data has
also paved the way for pattern recognition methods that can be used to automatically pre-annotate and analyze whole-slide images. Especially since the
advent of deep learning, the need for high-quality data annotation at a large scale
has increased significantly, but so have the prospects of high-quality detection
results.

The demand for those large-scale data sets poses two major problems to the
annotation task, that are currently unsolved for many medical image recognition
domains: The lack in quantity in data, and the lack in quality of labels. To

overcome the limitations in quantity of expert label data, Albarqouni et al. used an aggregation of expert labels and crowdsourcing with non-experts [2], showing effectively the power of an enhanced data set. However, it can be stated that expert-labelled data is generally of higher quality than non-expert labelled data.

1.1 High rating variance in expert annotations

Medical images in general, and histology images in particular, often have a high inter-observer variance in rating. As Boiesen et al. report, subjective differences in grading in breast cancer histology tumor diagnostics can lead to a significantly high variance in the tumor classification [3], which in term has implications on an individual, targeted curative treatment. This, of course, calls for computer-based assistance systems, which could significantly contribute to a highly standardized diagnosis and thus could lead to a more uniform classification.

Further, histo-pathology images are often annotated in an unsuitable way for supervised machine learning on a segmentation task (e.g. just by an arrows pointing at structures, using circles or as per-slide annotation). While this might be a suitable and sufficient annotation for a human observer, it is often too ambiguous for pattern recognition methods.

1.2 Prospects of multi label data sets

For algorithmic approaches, the quality of input data is a major bottleneck for the quality of the overall outcome. In a machine learning sense, we have to consider the labels provided by experts, usually considered as ground truth, to be noisy as well. Besides human error, also the difficulty of a certain data subset will play a role. The closer a single object is to a prototype, the easier the recognition for a human as well as for a machine learner, an effect which already successfully employed in other machine learning domains [4].

Bengio et al. suggest to exploit this difficulty in order to improve on generalization of machine learning approaches, effectively mimicking human learning, which is why they coined the term curriculum learning [5]. While there are other approaches to provide this from the confidence of machine learning approaches inherently, a very strong indicator is human error. Multi label expert data sets provide thus the possibility to differentiate prototypical from difficult samples, while at the same time supplying the learning system with a better estimate for the ground truth.

1.3 Existing software

Besides commercially available digital histopathology software, e.g. provided by the manufacturers of the scanner hardware, there is a high number of open source software solutions available for slide viewing and analysis [1], with some products supporting whole-slide images and others using standard graphics formats. Many solutions provide not only annotation capabilities, but also plug-in

Table 1. Comparison of a selection of open source software packages suited for cell annotations ([1] = bio-formats; [2] = openslide; [3] = limit at 2.1 Gigapixels).

Product	Icy [6]	Qupath [9]	Cytomine [8]	SlideRunner
Whole-Slide Image support	Yes[1]	Yes[2]	Yes[2]	Yes
Very large image support	No[3]	Yes	Yes	Yes
Multi-user Annotation	No	No	Yes	Yes
Single Click Cell Annotations	No	Yes	No	Yes
Blind Annotations	No	No	Yes	Yes
Blind Multi-labels	No	No	No	Yes
Guided Screening Process	No	No	No	Yes

systems for automated analysis or pre-processing (e.g. Icy [6] or CellProfiler [7]). As de Chaumont et al. reported, the emphasis of these projects was collaborative design and evaluation of tools and algorithms within the bioinformatics community. To extend the collaborative approach to the annotation, Marée et al. released Cytomine, an internet-based general-purpose annotation tool [8], with full integration of whole-slide images and respective on-demand loading. Since within the tool, annotations are represented in layers, it is possible to do a blind annotation with multiple experts, which is valuable for shape estimations (e.g. for tumor regions) in a blinded manner. For cell type annotations, however, multiple opinions on one cell are of great importance to judge the prototypical character of an occurrence and hence the expected difficulty.

In order to improve on current data sets, we can formulate requirements on software that would be used to aggregate data sets with multiple labels on the same cells and using big data amounts, which we do not find entirely fulfilled in state of the art solutions (Tab. 1):

- The user interface must be intuitive to use and annotations can be set with very little interactions, using one click only if possible.
- The software must be able to support blinded class labeling, where the annotated cell is displayed but the label of previous annotators is hidden.

2   Methods

SlideRunner is a GPL-licensed tool[1], written in Python 3.5 and using OpenSlide [10] as image loading backend. It provides several modes of navigation, and two major modes of operation for annotation:

- `Center annotation`: In this mode a single mouse click is needed to add an annotation in the center of an object, e.g. a cell.
- `Outline annotation`: Either using multiple clicks or click-and-drag, polygon curves can be added and annotated.

[1] available at: https://github.com/maubreville/SlideRunner

2.1   Data model

As depicted in Fig. 1(b), the major entity of our database model is the annotation. Each annotation can have multiple coordinates, with their respective x
and y coordinates, and the order they were drawn (for polygons). Further, each
annotation has a multitude of labels that were given by one person each and are
belonging to one class, respectively.

2.2   Blinded annotation

For blinded multi-annotation, it is important that the viewer is provided with a
view that does present the area or object annotations of other experts, yet hides
the information about the class the object was given but those other raters. For
this, SlideRunner provides a mode where only own annotations are provided
with (color-based) class informations in the image (Fig. 1(a)).

To leverage more gains in annotation performance, this mode is enriched by a
discovery mode, in which the user is automatically presented with a random new
image section upon completion of the currently visible view until all annotated
objects have been classified successfully. This mode is expected to considerably
reduce required time to reach for the next unclassified cells to annotate.

2.3   Guided screening

For the first annotation of the image, a guided screening mode is being provided
that guides the expert at maximum optical zoom over the complete image. This
mode will ensure that the observer will definitely examine every field of view
of the image and is therefore especially helpful if complete annotation coverage

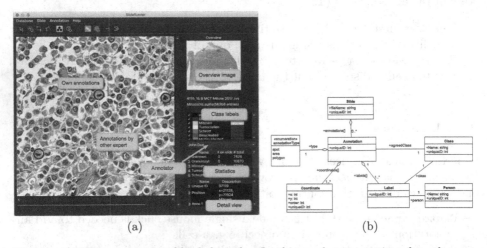

(a)   (b)

Fig. 1. a) GUI overview in blinded mode. In this mode, annotations by other experts are only visible as unknown classes (in black). b) UML diagram of database
structure. Every annotation may contain multiple labels from different persons and
multiple coordinates.

Table 2. Confusion matrix between two pathologists. Most significant disagreement was between the ambigous class and the clear classes.

	granulocytes	mitotic cells	normal tumor cells	ambiguous
granulocytes	10318	395	327	2249
mitotic cells	147	30623	202	458
normal tumor cells	27	546	18445	387
ambiguous	257	2949	1331	2420

is desired. In order to only display fields of interest containing tissue sections, white/empty areas need to be excluded from the image, which is performed by the algorithmic chain depicted in Fig. 2. After thresholding and morphologic closing, a grid is projected on the image, and non-empty slide partitions are shown to the user.

3 Results

With the means described in this text, a double-annotated database of sparsely annotated cell types from canine mast cell tumor slides was established. Histopathologically, canine cells show great similarity to human cells including the appearance and diversity of mitotic figures. As Tab. 2 shows, we found a good agreement between the raters in general, with Cohen's $\kappa = 0.815$. Most disagreement can be found between clear decisions for one of the cell classes and the ambiguous class. For a curriculum learning-based approach, this may be a good hint towards the difficulty of detection. Mean annotation times (measured as time difference between annotation events) were $6.6\,s$ and $6.3\,s$ for both raters for first annotations, and $2.0\,s$ and $2.6\,s$ for second annotations, respectively (evaluated on N=71,561 labels).

For one particular slide, one pathologist performed full annotation of mitotic figures manually, resulting in 2,252 single mitotic events distributed over the slide. For the same slide, a second pathologist performed an annotation using the guided screening mode, resulting in 4,233 mitotic events.

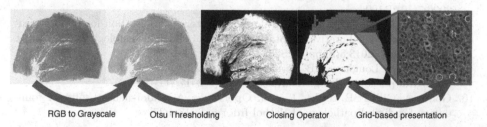

RGB to Grayscale   Otsu Thresholding   Closing Operator   Grid-based presentation

Fig. 2. Algorithmic toolchain for guided screening. Grid-based segments are presented from left to right, top to bottom.

4   Discussion

While minor differences were expected, the significant increase in mitotic figure annotations for usage of guided screening is surprising at first. Potentially, this effect can be attributed to a more thorough annotation in this mode, where the expert's attention is not focused on the center of the image. In general, statistics between both pathologists working in the same mode did not differ significantly for the whole data set.

We find that using the methods realized in SlideRunner lead to a fast annotation process of mitotic figures and other cell types. In part, however, this might also be related to a generally high mitotic count in the slides that have been labeled. In general, yet, using the tool provided means to build up a database of mitotic and other cell annotations that is unprecedented in size and could leverage precision gains provided by machine learning methods.

References

1. Bertram CA, Klopfleisch R. The pathologist 2.0: an update on digital pathology in veterinary medicine. Vet Pathol. 2017 Jun;54(5):756–766.
2. Albarqouni S, Baur C, Achilles F, et al. AggNet - deep learning from crowds for mitosis detection in breast cancer histology images. IEEE Trans Med Imaging. 2016;35(5):1313–1321.
3. Boiesen P, Bendahl PO, Anagnostaki L, et al. Histologic grading in breast cancer: reproducibility between seven pathologic departments. Acta Oncol. 2000;39(1):41–45.
4. Batliner A, Steidl S, Hacker C, et al. In: Tales of tuning: prototyping for automatic classification of emotional user states; 2005. p. 489–492.
5. Bengio Y, Louradour J, Collobert R, et al. Curriculum learning. Proc ICML. 2009; p. 41–48.
6. de Chaumont F, Dallongeville S, Chenouard N, et al. Icy: an open bioimage informatics platform for extended reproducible research. Nat Methods. 2012 Jun;9(7):690–696.
7. Carpenter AE, Jones TR, Lamprecht MR, et al. CellProfiler: image analysis software for identifying and quantifying cell phenotypes. Genome Biol. 2006;7(10):R100.
8. Marée R, Stévens B, Rollus L, et al. A rich internet application for remote visualization and collaborative annotation of digital slides in histology and cytology. Diagn Pathol. 2013;8(Suppl 1):S26.
9. Bankhead P, Loughrey MB, Fernández JA, et al. QuPath: Open source software for digital pathology image analysis. Sci Rep. 2017;7(1):16878.
10. Goode A, Gilbert B, Harkes J, et al. OpenSlide: A vendor-neutral software foundation for digital pathology. J Pathol Inform. 2013;4:27.

Automated Containerized Medical Image Processing Based on MITK and Python

A Modular System to Implement Medical Image Processing Pipelines and Visualize Meta Data

Caspar J. Goch, Jasmin Metzger, Martin Hettich, André Klein,
Tobias Norajitra, Michael Götz, Jens Petersen, Klaus H. Maier-Hein,
Marco Nolden

Medical Image Computing Group, German Cancer Research Center (DKFZ)
c.goch@dkfz.de

Modern medical image processing employs an ever widening array of tools on an ever larger pool of data. Development of the tools takes place on a variety of different platforms, determined by external circumstances, such as the availability of necessary functionality as libraries forcing the use of a specific programming language or interdependencies of third party tools requiring specific versions of specific operating systems. This problem itself is not unique to medical imaging[1] and solutions such as Docker[1] have proven themselves useful in a variety of use cases. It enables a very modularized approach to image processing where each step of a pipeline is isolated from the others. We will present a containerized pipeline of modular image processing steps, partly based on the Slicer execution model as implemented by MITK[2], partly on research software written in Python, that enables us to easily import new versions of rapidly developing tools from the developer. Managing and understanding large amounts of patient data to identify relevant patient pools for a given research question is required for efficient research. We will show equally containerized visualization tools that enable us to parse the meta data as provided by the DICOM images, make it searchable and provide a quick and easy way to interact with it using Elasticsearch[2] and Kibana[3]

References

1. Gil Y, Deelman E, Ellisman M, et al. Examining the challenges of scientific workflows. Computer;40(12):24–32.
2. Nolden M, Zelzer S, Seitel A, et al. The medical imaging interaction toolkit: challenges and advances. International Journal of Computer Assisted Radiology and Surgery. 2013;8(4):607–620.

---

[1] https://www.docker.com/
[2] https://www.elastic.co/products/elasticsearch
[3] https://www.elastic.co/products/kibana

Multi-channel Deep Transfer Learning for Nuclei Segmentation in Glioblastoma Cell Tissue Images

Thomas Wollmann[1], Julia Ivanova[1], Manuel Gunkel[2], Inn Chung[3],
Holger Erfle[2], Karsten Rippe[3], Karl Rohr[1]

[1] University of Heidelberg, BioQuant, IPMB, and DKFZ Heidelberg, Dept.
Bioinformatics and Functional Genomics, Biomedical Computer Vision Group,
[2] High-Content Analysis of the Cell (HiCell) and Advanced Biological Screening
Facility, BioQuant, University of Heidelberg, Germany
[3] Division of Chromatin Networks, DKFZ and BioQuant, Heidelberg, Germany
thomas.wollmann@bioquant.uni-heidelberg.de

Abstract. Segmentation and quantification of cell nuclei is an important task in tissue microscopy image analysis. We introduce a deep learning method leveraging atrous spatial pyramid pooling for cell segmentation. We also present two different approaches for transfer learning using datasets with a different number of channels. A quantitative comparison with previous methods was performed on challenging glioblastoma cell tissue images. We found that our transfer learning method improves the segmentation result.

1 Introduction

Segmentation of cell nuclei is a frequent and important task in quantitative microscopy image analysis and for extracting phenotypes. In this work, we consider the segmentation of nuclei from 3D tissue microscopy images of glioblastoma cells. This data is very challenging due to strong intensity variation, cell clustering, poor edge information, missing object borders, strong shape variation, and low signal-to-noise ratio (Fig. 1).

In previous work, several methods for cell segmentation were introduced (e.g., [1, 2]). Recently, deep learning methods achieved very good results [2]. When only a small dataset is available for training, it is common in video image analysis of natural scenes to pretrain a deep neural network on a large dataset like ImageNet and fine-tune the network on the considered dataset [3]. However, images of natural scenes are usually color images represented by three channels, but microscopy images generally have a varying number of channels (and often more than three channels). For a convolutional neural network, in the first layer a filter is used for each channel to extract corresponding feature maps. Hence, the number of channels is fixed in the network according to the considered data, and the pretrained network cannot directly be transferred to data with a different number of channels.

316

In this work, we introduce a novel deep neural network based on atrous spatial pyramid pooling (ASPP) for cell segmentation. We also present two transfer learning approaches which use only one channel for training and perform fine-tuning on more channels. In our application, we trained the neural network on a one-channel dataset and transfer it to a dataset with four channels. We applied our method to segment cell nuclei in challenging glioblastoma cell tissue images and performed a quantitative comparison with previous methods.

2   Methods

Our proposed deep learning method combines a U-Net [2] with batch normalization [4], residual connections [5], and atrous spatial pyramid pooling (ASPP) [6]. ASPP has the advantage that large context information can be captured at multiple image scales. We modified ASPP by using dilations of 1, 2, and 4 as well as global average pooling (pooling kernel equal to feature maps) to capture information from the whole image. After the ASPP block we employ Gaussian dropout (p=0.5). For our deep learning model we investigated PReLU [7] activation functions. Using a U-Net in conjunction with a PReLU activation function, we observed that the first layers mostly favour negative activations. However, PReLU increases the computation time. Therefore, we used PReLU only in the first layer to make use of negatively activated features, while saving computation time.

Our network was trained using cross-validation and early stopping with the Adam optimizer and a learning rate of $l_{init} = 0.001$ as well as $\beta_1 = 0.9$ and $\beta_2 = 0.999$. The dataset was always split into 50 % training, 25 % validation, and 25 % testing data. We augmented the dataset using random flipping, rotation, cropping (200×200 pixels), color shift, and elastic deformations.

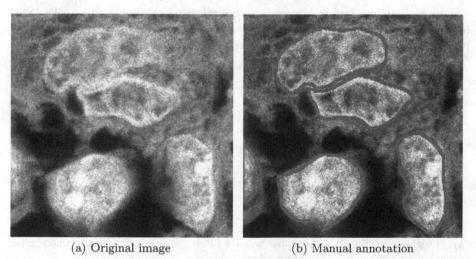

(a) Original image   (b) Manual annotation

Fig. 1. DAPI channel of original tissue image of glioblastoma cells and ground truth annotation.

For transfer learning we employed two approaches. In the first approach, we use the network trained on one channel (Fig. 2(a)) for all channels by altering the first layer of the network and using the same trained convolutional filters for all channels (Fig. 2(b)). This is motivated by the assumption that the trained filters are generic for different types of images and can therefore be applied to other channels with different stainings. In the second approach, we use the trained convolutional filters for the corresponding channel in the new dataset and initialize the filters for the other channels by MSRA initialisation [7] (Fig. 2(c)). With this approach we keep the pretrained filters for one channel and train all other filters from scratch.

2.1   Performance measures

We used four performance measures for quantitative evaluation: Object IOU, IOU, Dice, and Warping Error. The object-based intersection over union (Object IOU) measure quantifies the agreement between the segmentation result and the ground truth for each object. We matched a ground truth object to a segmented object, if the normalized overlap is more than 50 %. In addition to this object-based IOU, we also determined a pixel-based IOU. The Dice coefficient is defined as the ratio of true positive pixels and the sum of pixels in ground truth and segmentation. The Warping Error [8] is the minimum mean square error between pixels of the segmentation and pixels of the topology-preserving warped ground truth. We calculated all performance measures for each image and averaged over the whole dataset.

3   Experimental results

We applied our method to tissue microscopy images of glioblastoma cells. Segmentation of cell nuclei is important for subsequent analysis of telomeres and for patient stratification [9]. The dataset consists of five 3D images and was acquired

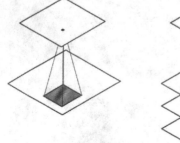 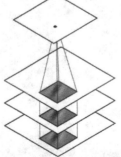 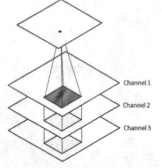

(a)   Original   filter trained on one channel

(b) Same trained filter used for all channels

(c) Individual trained filter for one channel

Fig. 2. Different approaches for transfer learning.

Table 1. Performance of different segmentation methods. Bold and underline highlights the best result, and bold indicates the second best result.

Method	Object IOU	IOU	Dice	Warp Error [10^{-4}]
Clustering & Thresholding	0.5782	**0.6520**	**0.7884**	0.093
Fast-Marching Level Set	0.5065	0.5682	0.7194	0.149
U-Net	0.6666	0.5774	0.7168	<u>0.011</u>
Proposed NN	0.7814	0.6154	0.7581	0.040
Proposed NN (transfer, same filter)	**0.7913**	0.5221	0.6709	0.045
Proposed NN (transfer, indiv. filters)	<u>0.7981</u>	**0.6426**	**0.7775**	**0.030**

by a Leica TCS SP5 point scanning confocal microscope with a 63x objective lens and a voxel size of $100 \times 100 \times 250$ nm. Four color channels were imaged sequentially: PML antibody stain (Alexa 647), FISH CY3 telomere probe, FAM labeled CENP-B PNA probe, and DAPI nuclei stain. 45 axial sections were acquired for each 3D stack. The deep learning models with transfer learning were trained on a second dataset with glioblastoma cells containing 50 images stained with DAPI nuclei stain, before training on the considered first dataset. However, the second dataset has only one channel and consists of maximum intensity projection (MIP) images. Therefore, standard transfer learning is not applicable and we need other approaches such as the two transfer learning strategies described in Section 2 above.

For a quantitative comparison, we also applied thresholding in combination with mean shift clustering. The 3D images were preprocessed using 3D Gaussian filtering ($\sigma = 2$ pixels). We used an empirically determined threshold of 160. In addition, we used an approach based on Gaussian filtering, mean shift clustering, and 3D fast-marching level sets [10]. The segmentation results were post-processed using hole filling.

All segmentation methods were evaluated on the 3D images from the first dataset, which were not used for training. We compared the segmentation results for five 3D images each containing 65 sections (in total 325 2D images per channel were used). Ground truth segmentations for all images were determined by manual annotation. Table 1 shows the results for all methods for the different evaluation metrics. It turns out that the proposed neural network combined with transferring individual filters performs best for object-based IOU and second best for IOU, Dice and Warping Error. Segmentation results for an example image are provided in Fig. 3. It can be seen that the proposed network performs best. In addition, transferring individual filters improves cell separation. The high object-based IOU and low Warping Error indicates that the proposed model is more suited to correctly merge and split objects.

4   Conclusion

We presented a deep neural network based on ASPP for cell segmentation combined with two approaches for transfer learning to transfer trained networks from one-channel data to multi-channel data. Based on a quantiative comparison using glioblastoma cell tissue images we showed that transfer learning improves the performance. Our novel deep neural network in conjunction with transfer learning and individual filters performed best for Object IOU and second best for Dice and Warping Error.

Acknowledgement. Support of the BMBF within the projects CancerTelSys (e:Med) and de.NBI (HD-HuB) is gratefully acknowledged.

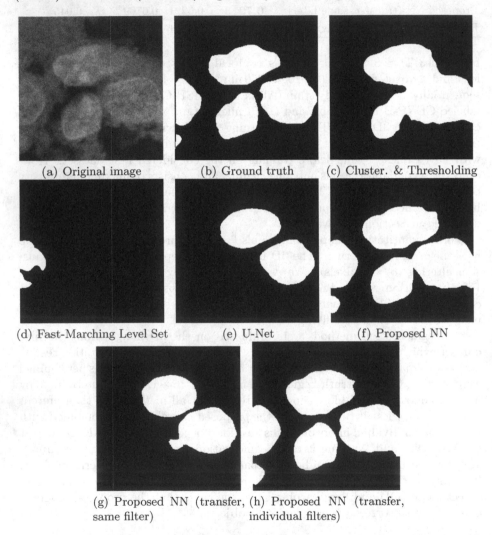

(a) Original image   (b) Ground truth   (c) Cluster. & Thresholding

(d) Fast-Marching Level Set   (e) U-Net   (f) Proposed NN

(g) Proposed NN (transfer,   (h) Proposed NN (transfer,
    same filter)   individual filters)

Fig. 3. Example tissue microscopy image of glioblastoma cells, ground truth, and segmentation results of different methods.

References

1. Dima AA, Elliott JT, Filliben JJ, et al. Comparison of segmentation algorithms for fluorescence microscopy images of cells. Cytometry Part A. 2011;79(7):545–559.
2. Ronneberger O, Fischer P, Brox T. U-Net: convolutional networks for biomedical image segmentation. Proc MICCAI. 2015; p. 234–241.
3. Huh M, Agrawal P, Efros AA. What makes ImageNet good for transfer learning?. arXiv:1608.08614; 2016.
4. Ioffe S, Szegedy C. Batch normalization: Accelerating deep network training by reducing internal covariate shift. Proc ICML. 2015; p. 448–456.
5. He K, Zhang X, Ren S, et al. Deep residual learning for image recognition. Proc CVPR. 2016; p. 770–778.
6. Chen LC, Papandreou G, Kokkinos I, et al.. Deeplab: Semantic image segmentation with deep convolutional nets, atrous convolution, and fully connected CRFs. arXiv:1606.00915; 2016.
7. He K, Zhang X, Ren S, et al. Delving deep into rectifiers: Surpassing human-level performance on imagenet classification. Proc ICCV. 2015; p. 1026–1034.
8. Jain V, Bollmann B, Richardson M, et al. Boundary learning by optimization with topological constraints. Proc CVPR. 2010; p. 2488–2495.
9. Osterwald S, Deeg KI, Chung I, et al. PML induces compaction, TRF2 depletion and DNA damage signaling at telomeres and promotes their alternative lengthening. J Cell Sci. 2015;128(10):1887–1900.
10. Sethian JA. Level Set Methods and Fast Marching Methods. vol. 3. Cambridge University Press; 1999.

Stitching Pathological Tissue Images using DOP Feature Tracking

Matthias Bergler, Maximilian Weiherer, Tobias Bergen, Malte Avenhaus,
David Rauber, Thomas Wittenberg, Christian Münzenmayer, Michaela Benz

Fraunhofer Institute for Integrated Circuits, IIS Erlangen
matthias.bergler@iis.fraunhofer.de

Abstract. This contribution introduces an approach for stitching multiple images of a histological slide to a panorama image using Differences of Paraboloids (DOP). DOP provides a novel method for the detection, description and matching of features of two overlapping images. In our context of manual whole-slide imaging (WSI), DOP extracts essential keypoints of an image and describes them with feature vectors considering the keypoint's neighborhood. The DOP feature vector of the current image is then matched against the feature vectors of all previous images. With matching correspondences, a feature based image registration is generated that estimates the translation between two overlapping images. Likewise, all images are aligned to form a whole-slide panorama. Our results reveal a superior stitching quality employing the presented DOP approach in comparison to the well-known SIFT and SURF. Our evaluation is based on the homogeneity at the artifically created edges in the panorama due to the stitching. The DOP offers a convincing solution to stitch pathological tissue.

1 Introduction

In pathology, the visual assessment and the differentiation between malign and benign tissue under a microscope is crucial. Digital representation of a histological sample needs to contain large-scale morphological structures at low magnification. Simultaneously, high optical magnification poses a key issue for the diagnosis where fine details need to be resolved. A digital panorama of the whole slide is not only useful for documentation. It also allows tele-diagnosis in cases where a second medical opinion is desired and it further enables to approach computer-aided diagnosis using computational pattern recognition. To render and provide a digital panorama of a histolocigal slide whole-slide-scanner are employed. However, still today, a pathologist routinely uses a manual microscope to investigate a histiligical sample with a series of sequential field-of-views (FoV). To him, whole-slide-scanners are expensive, time-consuming and not commonly available in his pathology department. Hence, in order to integrate scanning into his workflow we introduce a solution to stitch overlapping FoVs and to generate a panorama image on the fly. For this purpose the input data is directly captured from a video stream of a camera attached to the microscope. Using this approach, the medical staff can examine the tissue sample conventionally with his microscope while simultaneously generating a panorama for documentation purposes or a follow-up review. In this contribution we propose the new Differences of Paraboloids [1] approach for the detection, description and matching of features in order to stitch FoVs from histological slides. We tested our approach against different standard feature detection algorithms. These comprise the Scale Invariant Feature Transform (SIFT) as developed by David Lowe [2] and the Speeded-up Robust Features (SURF) by Herbert Bay [3]. Both are feature trackers, and constitute standard methods for feature based image registration. In contrast to the more general geometric registration [1] we can ignore rotation in our context since a slide under a microscope can only move along horizontal and vertical directions.

2 Material and methods

Our evaluation is based on fifteen image datasets of a gallblader tumor, a fibroma and a spindle cell sacroma. Each dataset has a different number of FoVs (Tab. 1). The images were acquired from a video stream of a USB 3.0 camera from IDS (Model UI-3260-CP-C). Through the microscope lenses a relatively large FoV was imaged on the camera sensor area of 11.3 mm×7.1 mm. We constrained on centered subimages with 1200×1200 pixel to minimize detrimental effects like imbalanced of lighting conditions or geometric distortions introduced by the microscope optics. Finally, we compared the DOP feature tracker against SIFT and SURF in order to assess the quality of our new image registration.

2.1 Feature-based image registration

The aim of image registration is to estimate the optimal transformation between two partially or fully overlapping images in order to align them in one common coordinate system. Either pixel or feature based algorithms are applicable for this task. With the DOP we address this registration problem with a feature based algorithm and generate a panorama from a series of microscopic images (FoV). The feature based approach for image registragion can generally be divided into three steps: feature detection, feature description and feature matching [4]. In our scenario of manual whole-slide imaging only the translational component needs to be determined since no rotation can occur. *Feature detection* comprises the process of detecting distinctive keypoints such as edges, corners or drop-shaped structures in the input images. A feature detector should find identical keypoints in an image even if the image was geometrically or photometrically altered [4]. In the *feature description* step a distinctive mathematical description for each keypoint is generated using the keypoint's neighborhood. The description is encoded in a feature vector. In last step, the *feature matching*, an algorithm compares the feature vectors of two or more images based on a distance measure, like the Euclidean or Hammging distance. The pair of feature vectors with a minimal distance will be used as correspondences to calculate the transformation.

2.2 DOP Filter

The design of the DOP filter [1] is based on the Laplacian of Gaussian (LoG) filter by Marr and Hildreth[5] (Fig. 1). A feature detector based on DOP registers keypoints in scale space of images at multiple levels. Normally, the scale space is generated by a convolution of the image with a gradually amplified Gaussian filter. As the computational complexity increases linearly with ascending filter size, our implementation uses an elliptical paraboloid

$$p_{\mathrm{w}}(x, y) = -a(x^2 + y^2) + b \quad \text{with} \quad a = \frac{3}{(w + 1)^2 (w^2 - w)} \quad \text{and}$$
$$b = \frac{1}{2} a w^2 \tag{1}$$

as an approximation to a Gaussian function instead for increased efficiency. In the above equation, w defines the filter size that controls the degree of smoothing. Our algorithm makes use of precalculated integral images to compute the convolution efficiently [6] independent from the filter size. Thus the result of the convolution $(I * p)(x, y)$ of an input image I at pixel position (x, y) only needs 16 look-ups [1] in the summed-area table. The fast look-up approach is beneficial to match the keypoints in real-time.

2.3 Panorama generation using DOP

Feature detection The local maxima from the filter response constitute the keypoints of the input image. The filter response is calculated as the absolute difference of two parabolic filters on different levels in scale space with the scale parameter s. Two different widths $w(s)$ and $w(s')$ [1] define the kernel size of the parabolic smoothing filter. The DOP filter response volume can now be constructed as

$$\mathcal{R}(x, y, s) = |(I * p_{\mathrm{w}(s)})(x, y) - (I * p_{\mathrm{w}(s')})(x, y)| \tag{2}$$

In the last step of the feature extraction we search for local maxima in $\mathcal{R}$ using non-maximum suppression. Each triplet (x, y, s) as the center of a 3×3×3 pixel cube with $\mathcal{R}$ above a certain threshold is tested for constituting a local maximum within this cube. A local maximum in $\mathcal{R}$ corresponds to the center of a blob feature.

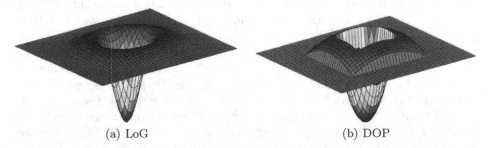

(a) LoG   (b) DOP

Fig. 1. Comparison between LoG (a) and its approximation by DOP (b).

Feature description After smoothing the image with the parabolic filter, DOP calculates binary feature vectors which are invariant to scaling and rotation. However, only a limited and relevant neighborhood of a keypoint is considered: Encoded in the elements of a feature vector are comparisons between values of the input image I at different levels and positions in scale space. For a specific selection [1] of N point-pairs $((x_i, y_i), (x_j, y_j))$ in a certain neighborhood of the regarded keypoint, every bit $k \in \{0, \ldots, N-1\}$ of the keypoint's descriptive feature vector D is given by

$$D(k) = \begin{cases} 1 & \text{if } I_{w(s_i)}(x_i, y_i) > I_{w(s_j)}(x_j, x_j) \\ 0 & \text{else} \end{cases} \tag{3}$$

with $I_{w(s)}(x, y)$ as the gray-value of I at point (x, y) for a specific level with the scale parameter s and the length of the feature vector N. Using a supervised learning algorithm N point-pairs are selected from a larger neighborhood for comparison [1]. As the stage of a microscope can only move in horizontal or vertical direction there is no necessity to treat rotation invariance.

Feature matching With the keypoint description in D we employ the Hamming-distance as a distance measure. As we intend to keep the percentage of false correspondences as low as possible, only close neighbors are considered. These are found using the nearest-neighbor distance ratio (NNDR) introduced in [2]. For feature vectors D_A, D_B and D_C with keypoint A and its two nearest neighbors B and C, the NNDR is defined as

$$\text{NNDR} = \frac{||D_A - D_B||}{||D_A - D_C||} \tag{4}$$

To decide whether or not a correspondence between A and B is acceptable, a threshold value is introduced. With an NNDR below that threshold correspondences are discarded.

2.4 Evaluation

In order to assess the quality of a generated panorama, we quantitatively describe the homogeneity of transitions between adjacent FoVs in the panorama by inspecting the smoothness of their border. This is achieved by quantify the visibility of edges by the gradient across bordering edges of the FoVs (Fig. 2). First, the sets S_X of horizontal and S_Y of vertical borders are constructed. They contain all horizontal and vertical pixel indices of adjacent FoVs execpt for adjoint background. Constrained to these sets we calculate the edge gradients E_X and E_Y of panoramas' pixel intensities $P(x, y)$ across the vertical and horizontal FoV edges as introduced by the stitching process

$$E_X := \sum_{(x,y) \in S_Y} |P(x+1, y) - P(x, y)|$$

$$E_Y := \sum_{(x,y) \in S_X} |P(x, y+1) - P(x, y)| \tag{5}$$

Table 1. Quality evaluation by gradient of stitching algorithms.

Dataset	FoVs	E DOP	SIFT	SURF
1	23	7.16	11.02	9.78
2	35	7.17	8.56	9.22
3	39	9.31	10.24	10.51
4	49	7.14	7.64	9.76
5	50	5.56	7.43	7.80
6	36	13,57	19.83	21.07
7	36	16,97	19.69	20.68
8	32	18,77	27.01	27.32
9	41	15.30	17.53	21.87
10	26	15.27	18.38	25.68
11	10	21.41	22.22	22.62
12	10	6.48	7.18	7.20
13	19	15.91	16.05	16.33
14	12	17.81	18.03	18.59
15	14	8.80	8.81	8.84

A smaller edge gradient value corresponds to smoother transition between adjacent FoVs and a better stitching quality. The real-time capability was approved by pathologists.

3   Results

To obtain a single figure of merit E we normalize E_X and E_Y by their respectively accumulated length of edges $|S_X|$ and $|S_Y|$. A smaller value of E correlates with an overall a smoother stitching appearance. With E from panoramas generated with SIFT, SURF and DOP we determinate their respective stitching accuracy. The core idea of introducing the edge gradient E is that smoother edges result in a more homogeneous image and therefore generate a better registration result with enhanced visual appearance. We maintained identical parametrization across all dataset to test the robustness and quality of the algorithms on a variety of samples. The best results were obtained with the DOP feature tracker followed by SIFT and then SURF (Tab. 1).

4   Discussion

With our experiments we demonstrate DOP as a feature tracker is suitable to generate a digital panorama representation of a slide and enables a smooth image registration for pathological tissue samples and outperforms SIFT and SURF in this context. We account this effect to the DOP feature descriptor which was

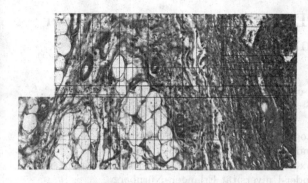

Fig. 2. Panorama of Dataset 5 generated by DOP with edges in black.

specifically designed to cope with images depicting various types of medical tissue obtained with optical sensors [1]. For all three algorithms minor stitching artefacts were noticeable with the human eye at the highest zoom level. Based on the requirements of stitching the panorama in real-time for the microscope operator moving the slide and, while maintaining high usability and quality, pixel-perfect registration is not crucial. One possible solution would be an additional post-registration step after the live-stitching process. In general, quality and speed of our presented method render the DOP a promising approach to stitch medical images.

References

1. Bergen T. Real-time Endoscopic Image Stitching for Cystoscopy; 2017. PhD-thesis, University Koblenz-Landau, in press.
2. Lowe DG. Distinctive image features from scale-invariant keypoints. Int J Comput Vis. 2004;60(2):91–110.
3. Bay H, Tuytelaars T, Van Gool L. SURF: Speeded up robust features. Proc ECCV. 2006; p. 404–417.
4. Hassaballah M, Abdelmgeid AA, Alshazly HA. Image features detection, description and matching. In: Image Feature Detectors and Descriptors. Springer; 2016. p. 11–45.
5. Marr D, Hildreth E. Theory of edge detection. Proc R Soc Lond B Biol Sci. 1980;207(1167):187–217.
6. Viola P, Jones M. Rapid object detection using a boosted cascade of simple features. Proc CVPR. 2001;1:511–518.

Motion Artifact Detection in Confocal Laser Endomicroscopy Images

Maike Stoeve[1], Marc Aubreville[1], Nicolai Oetter[2,3], Christian Knipfer[4,3], Helmut Neumann[5,3], Florian Stelzle[2,3], Andreas Maier[1,3]

[1]Pattern Recognition Lab, Computer Science,
Friedrich-Alexander-Universität Erlangen-Nürnberg
[2]Department of Oral and Maxillofacial Surgery, University Hospital Erlangen,
Friedrich-Alexander-Universität Erlangen-Nürnberg
[3]Erlangen Graduate School in Advanced Optical Technologies (SAOT),
Friedrich-Alexander-Universität Erlangen-Nürnberg
[4]Department of Oral and Maxillofacial Surgery,
University Medical Center Hamburg-Eppendorf
[5]First Department of Internal Medicine, University Hospital Mainz,
Johannes Gutenberg-Universität Mainz
maike.stoeve@fau.de

Abstract. Confocal Laser Endomicroscopy (CLE), an optical imaging technique allowing non-invasive examination of the mucosa on a (sub)-cellular level, has proven to be a valuable diagnostic tool in gastroenterology and shows promising results in various anatomical regions including the oral cavity. Recently, the feasibility of automatic carcinoma detection for CLE images of sufficient quality was shown. However, in real world data sets a high amount of CLE images is corrupted by artifacts. Amongst the most prevalent artifact types are motion-induced image deteriorations. In the scope of this work, algorithmic approaches for the automatic detection of motion artifact-tainted image regions were developed. Hence, this work provides an important step towards clinical applicability of automatic carcinoma detection. Both, conventional machine learning and novel, deep learning-based approaches were assessed. The deep learning-based approach outperforms the conventional approaches, attaining an AUC of 0.90.

1 Introduction

With over 500,000 diagnosed cases each year, head and neck squamous cell carcinoma (HNSCC) is considered the sixth most common cancer type worldwide [1]. For diagnosis of HNSCC, invasive biopsy and subsequent histopathological examination is applied as gold standard method [2]. As alternative, non-invasive optical imaging technologies as narrow-band imaging, autofluorescence imaging and confocal laser endomicroscopy (CLE) are gaining interest in research [3]. Among those technologies, CLE has already proven to be a valuable diagnostic tool in gastroenterology and has been successfully applied to examine lesions in the oral cavity [4]. Both, the interpretation of CLE images and the histopatho-logical examination of tissue samples require experience and proficiency and entail a subjective component [5]. Thus, promising approaches using machine learning techniques for automatic carcinoma detection based on CLE images were developed [6].

As the accuracy of these algorithms is highly affected by the occurrence of artifacts, artifact-tainted images were excluded manually prior to training in a time-consuming manual labeling step in all known approaches. In the scope of this work, an automatic motion artifact detection pipeline was developed and evaluated. Hence, this work provides the basis to integrate a fully automatic motion artifact detection into existing carcinoma detection frameworks, an im-portant step towards clinical applicability.

1.1 Motion artifacts

A frequent cause of image impairment are motion artifacts. They can either be caused by movements of the investigated anatomical structures or motion induced by the physician. The proportion of motion artifact images compared to good quality images is highly dependent on the experience of the physician [7]. As shown in Fig. 1, two different manifestations can be observed. The first manifestation is characterized by streaky patterns originating from the repeated acquisition of the same, shifted image line. This pattern can be observed, when the sum of the velocities of probe, organ and scanning is approximately equal to zero. This requires an organ movement in the same direction as the sam-pling pattern or a probe motion in the correspondingly opposite direction. If a significant relative motion results from organ or probe motion, the cells are stretched or blurred. This second manifestation is hard to detect, as distinction between elongated cells is difficult without the observation of adjacent frames. Finally, motion artifacts can impair the whole image leading to a total loss of information or only influence parts of the image still allowing a diagnosis based on untainted regions [7]. Due to the meander-shaped optical sampling pattern, only whole image rows are affected by motion artifacts.

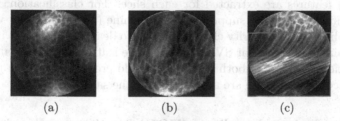

(a)   (b)   (c)

Fig. 1. CLE images containing (a) no artifacts or motion artifacts manifesting in (b) stretched cells or (c) stripe patterns (region marked in red).

2   Materials and methods

For the present work, 116 CLE sequences comprising 11,234 images from 12 patients and 4 sites within the oral cavity, namely the upper alveolar ridge, the lower inner labium, the palatal region and the lesion site itself were utilized. The CLE sequences were recorded at the department of Oral and Maxillofacial Surgery of the University Hospital Erlangen by a standalone probe-based CLE system (Cellvizio, Mauna Kea Technologies, Paris, France). The obtained images are approximately of size 576×578 pixels. The overall image quality was assessed by an expert and artifact regions were annotated manually within each image. Details on the data can be found in [6].

In the scope of this work, two different methodical approaches were established for the detection of motion artifact-tainted CLE image regions. The first approach uses conventional pattern recognition methods extracting characteristic image features, whereas the second approach applies deep learning strategies. For both approaches, images with low signal-to-noise ratio are excluded. The remaining CLE images are converted to 8-bit integer values after a quantile-based dynamic range compression following Aubreville et al. [6] was performed.

2.1   Feature-based motion artifact detection

The feature-based approach consists of three steps: pre-processing, feature extraction and classification. The pre-processing step is required due to the unusual round shape of CLE images complicating the feature extraction process. Jaremenko et al. circumvented this problem by dividing the image in overlapping, square patches and concatenating the information of all patches for the classification of the whole image [8]. As motion artifacts always cover the whole width of an image, slices with a width of the maximum extent of the CLE image in x-direction, a fixed height of 128 pixels and an overlap of 30 % (HOG) or 50 % (corrAngle) are extracted. To allow the detection of motion artifact-tainted slices of an image and differentiate them from untainted slices of the same image, either Histogram of Oriented Gradient (HOG) or angle of maximum correlation (corrAngle) features are extracted for each slice. For classification, a random forest classifier (RF) and a support vector machine (SVM) classifier were used. Undersampling of the majority class is applied to deal with the class imbalance. Prior to training of the linear SVM classifier, the feature vector is standardized. For evaluation purposes of both classifiers, 5-fold cross-validation is used. The different slices of one image are all assigned to the same fold.

Histogram of oriented gradients (HOG) The Histogram of Oriented Gradient (HOG) feature descriptor of Dalal and Triggs is frequently used in the field of object recognition [9]. Basically, the occurrence of gradient directions is computed in a local image region characterizing the local shape of an object. In contrast to the original pipeline, no gamma and color normalization is used. A cell size of 32×32 and block size of 64×64 resulted in the best classification performance. Due to the varying length of CLE image slices, the obtained HOG feature vectors are of varying length. Hence, mean, standard deviation, skewness and kurtosis are computed over all 9 bins of the feature vector individually. The statistical properties for all bins are subsequently concatenated to form a feature vector of a fixed length of 36.

Angle of maximum correlation (corrAngle) The angle of maximum correlation feature (corrAngle) is designed under consideration of the origin of the streaky patterns visible in most motion artifact-tainted images. The direction of the relative motion accounts for the angle θ characterizing the direction of the stripe pattern. To create a feature vector describing the presence or absence of motion artifact patterns in an image slice with length L, a centered reference segment of row i of the CLE image slice is extracted. For a set of angles equally distributed between $\frac{\pi}{8}$ and $\frac{7}{8}\pi$ and a fixed radius R, comparative segments are extracted with center at $(\frac{L}{2} + R\sin(\theta), j + R + R\cos(\theta))$ using bilinear interpolation. Then, the correlation coefficient of the reference segment and each comparative segment is computed as measurement of similarity. The angle responsible for the highest correlation coefficient is saved. This procedure is repeated for each row despite the first and last R rows. Finally, all approximated motion angles are concatenated to form the final feature vector. For a motion artifact-tainted image slice, the approximated angle is constant (stripe pattern). In contrast, CLE image slices without motion artifacts show high variations of the approximated motion angle over image rows.

2.2 Deep learning-based motion artifact detection (artiNet)

Building on the Inception v3 architecture of Szegedy [10] pretrained on ImageNet, the deep learning-based detector of motion artifact-tainted CLE image areas (artiNet) is build by inserting a 2d 1×1 convolutional layer after the eighth inception block followed by a column fusion and a softmax layer as depicted in Fig. 2.2. Thus, the input representation for the new layers still entails spatial information. The convolutional layer is used to map the 17×17×768 dimensional input to the two output classes motion artifact and good quality. The result is a 17×17 grid of predictions. To obtain predictions of motion artifact regions covering the whole image width comparable to the slices of the conventional approach, a column fusion layer extracts the maximum over the image width resulting in a 17×2 representation fed to the final softmax layer.

Prior to training the grayscale images are transformed to RGB color representation. Then, a centered image patch of 400×400 pixels is extracted and resized to 299×299 pixels. Due to the slice-wise detection of motion artifacts and available corresponding labels effectively representing a fully convolutional approach with a network capacity according to one with smaller patches, data augmentation seems less important. Within the TensorFlow framework, the Inception network was fine-tuned in 2000 training steps using the Adam optimizer with an initial learning rate of $5 \cdot 10^{-6}$. For the training of the new layers, a learning rate of $5 \cdot 10^{-5}$ was used. In each training step, a minibatch consisting of 25 randomly selected instances of both classes is processed to deal with the class imbalance of the data set. For evaluation, a leave-one-patient-out cross-validation was performed.

3   Results

The top result is obtained by the artiNet, where an AUC of 0.90 is achieved. The best performance following the conventional pattern recognition pipeline is achieved by the corrAngle feature and RF classification. For this combination, an AUC of 0.85 is reached. The corrAngle-based motion detection with RF performs significantly better than the RF and SVM predictors trained on HOG, where approximately equal ROC curves with AUC values of 0.73 and 0.74 are achieved. In contrast to the RF classification performance, the results of the SVM classifier trained on the corrAngle features are poor. For additional insight into the performance of the artiNet, the comparison of predictions for single image slices and respective labels is visualized in Fig. 3.

4   Discussion

Due to the included patch extraction step of the artiNet, the image borders are discarded. For motion artifact detection, the center of the slice is representative as a motion induced deterioration covers the whole extent in x-direction. Still, the information at the top and bottom of the image is removed. Thus, motion artifacts only deteriorating the rejected areas can not be detected. An improved performance is to be expected if the whole image is used. As the manifestation of stretched cells is underrepresented in the data set, a performance gap between the two possible manifestations of motion artifacts, stripe patterns and stretched cells might occur. Moreover, the performance of the proposed methods was only

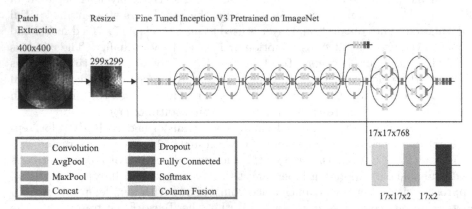

Fig. 2. Visualization of the artiNet for motion artifact detection in CLE images based on an Inception v3 network [10] pre-trained on ImageNet.

Fig. 3. Results of motion artifact detection in CLE images. a) ROC curves visualizing the average cross-validation performance of the motion artifact detection; b) Example images showing slicewise predictions of the artiNet compared to class labels.

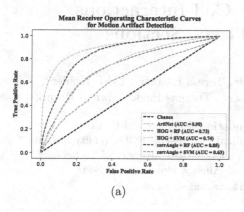

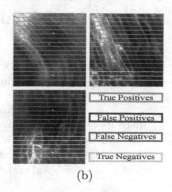

(a)   (b)

assessed on data of one clinical team. Hence, additional training instances are required to obtain a robust artifact detector.

References

1. Blaszczak W, Barczak W, Wegner A, et al. Clinical value of monoclonal antibodies and tyrosine kinase inhibitors in the treatment of head and neck squamous cell carcinoma. Med Oncol. 2017;34(4):60.
2. Oetter N, Knipfer C, Rohde M, et al. Development and validation of a classification and scoring system for the diagnosis of oral squamous cell carcinomas through confocal laser endomicroscopy. J Transl Med. 2016;14(1):159.
3. Nathan CAO, Kaskas NM, Ma X, et al. Confocal laser endomicroscopy in the detection of head and neck precancerous lesions. J Otolaryngol Head Neck Surg. 2014;151(1):73–80.
4. Thong PS, Tandjung SS, Movania MM, et al. Toward real-time virtual biopsy of oral lesions using confocal laser endomicroscopy interfaced with embedded computing. J Biomed Opt. 2012;17(5):0560091–05600910.
5. Neumann H, Vieth M, Atreya R, et al. Prospective evaluation of the learning curve of confocal laser endomicroscopy in patients with IBD. Histol Histopathol. 2011;26(7):867.
6. Aubreville M, Knipfer C, Oetter N, et al. Automatic classification of cancerous tissue in laserendomicroscopy images of the oral cavity using deep learning. Sci Rep. 2017;20(7):11979.
7. Sharman M, Bacci B, Whittem T, et al. In vivo confocal endomicroscopy of small intestinal mucosal morphology in dogs. J Vet Intern Med. 2013;27(6):1372–1378.
8. Jaremenko C, Maier A, Steidl S, et al. Classification of confocal laser endomicroscopic images of the oral cavity to distinguish pathological from healthy tissue. Proc BVM. 2015; p. 479–485.
9. Dalal N, Triggs B, et al.; IEEE. Histograms of oriented gradients for human detection. Proc CVPR. 2005;1:886–893.
10. Szegedy C, Vanhoucke V, Ioffe S, et al. Rethinking the inception architecture for computer vision. Proc VCPR. 2016; p. 2818–2826.

Variational Networks for
Joint Image Reconstruction and Classification
of Tumor Immune Cell Interactions
in Melanoma Tissue Sections

Alexander Effland[1], Michael Hölzel[2], Teresa Klatzer[3], Erich Kobler[3],
Jennifer Landsberg[4], Leonie Neuhäuser[1], Thomas Pock[3], Martin Rumpf[1]

[1]Institute for Numerical Simulation, University of Bonn
[2]Institute of Clinical Chemistry and Clinical Pharmacology, University of Bonn
[3]Institute of Computer Graphics and Vision, Graz University of Technology
[4]Department of Dermatology and Allergy, University of Bonn
alexander.effland@ins.uni-bonn.de

Abstract. Immunotherapy is currently revolutionizing the treatment of
cancer. Detailed analyses of tumor immune cell interaction in the tumor
microenvironment will facilitate an accurate prediction of a patient's
clinical response. The automatic and reliable pre-screening of histological tissue sections for tumor infiltrating immune cells (TILs) will support the development of TIL-based predictive biomarkers for checkpoint
immunotherapy. In this paper, a learning approach for image classification is presented, which allows various pattern inquires for different
types of tissue section images. The underlying trainable reaction diffusion model combines classification and denoising. The model is trained
using a stochastic generation of training data. The effectiveness of this
approach is demonstrated for immunofluorescent and for Hematoxylin
and Eosin (H&E) stained melanoma section images. A particular focus
is on the classification of TILs in the proximity to melanoma cells in an
experimental melanoma mouse model and in human melanoma. This
new learning approach for images of melanoma tissue sections will refine
the strategy for the practical clinical application of biomarker research.

1 Introduction

The clinical success of immune checkpoint inhibitors has proven the importance
of immune surveillance of tumors for the survival of patients with a variety of ma-
lignancies, particular with melanoma. However, primary and acquired resistance
to immunotherapy limit the therapeutic efficacy for many cancer patients. Thus,
there is a growing need to identify predictive biomarkers and to enhance our understanding of the complex interactions between the immune system and tumor
cells. Using melanoma tissue sections, it has been shown that tumor infiltrating
CD8+ immune cells and their distribution within the tumor microenvironment
are promising predictive biomarkers [1, 2].

This paper deals with a variational network learning approach for the detection of these biomarkers. There are diverse deep learning approaches for the automatic detection and classification of cell markers in the context of computer-aided cancer diagnosis. E.g. in [3], Sirinukunwattana et al. employed a spatially constrained convolutional neural network for the detection of relevant cell nuclei using a neighboring ensemble predictor to incorporate the spatial structure of the cells. In [4], a classification of epithelial and stromal cells based on a deep convolutional neural network is performed, where the quality of the outcome is compared to handcraft feature extracted datasets. For a recent overview of deep learning methods for classification and segmentation tasks in digital pathology we refer to [5].

In this paper, we take into account the trainable nonlinear reaction diffusion model (TNRD) [6] from image denoising, where the parameters in each time step are degrees of freedom. We minimize an L^2 loss functional over these degrees of freedom. The acquisition of training data from real histological sections is out of reach, since for each section a substantial amount of user interaction of an experienced pathologist would be needed and a robust loss function decay requires large sample sizes of such tissue sections. Hence, we train the proposed model with training data generated via a stochastic cell distribution algorithm, mimicking structure, color distribution and noise of real histological sections of cancer tissues.

2   Materials and Methods

In what follows, we will present the learning approach, the generator of training data and the image acquisition.

2.1   A "deeper" variational network

Assume, we have given a blurry and noisy $N_1 \times N_2$ color image $\mathbf{u}_0^{rgb} \in \mathcal{U}_{rgb} = ([0,1]^3)^{N_1 \times N_2}$ together with an initial segmentation mask $u_0^m \in [0,1]^{N_1 \times N_2}$. Our aim is to compute a combined color- and segmentation image $\mathbf{u} = (\mathbf{u}^{rgb}, u^m) \in \mathcal{U}_{rgbm} = ([0,1]^4)^{N_1 \times N_2}$ by using a "deeper" extension of the TNRD model. The proposed model performs N_t projected gradient steps of the form

$$\mathbf{u}_{t+1} = \mathrm{proj}_{\mathcal{U}_{rgbm}}(\mathbf{u}_t - \nabla E_t(\mathbf{u}_t)) \quad \text{for } t \in \{0, \dots, N_t - 1\}, \qquad (1)$$

where the projection operator $\mathrm{proj}_{\mathcal{U}_{rgbm}}$ refers to a simple pointwise truncation to the interval $[0,1]$. Observe that the effective step size of the gradient descent will be defined by means of the parameters of the learned model. Since this model evolves the gradient of a time-dependent variational model E_t, it is also referred to as "variational network" [7]. In this paper we propose to use the following variational model:

$$E_t(\mathbf{u}) = \sum_{\mathcal{F}_2} \phi_t^2(K_t^2 \phi_t^1(K_t^1 \mathbf{u})) + \tfrac{\lambda_t}{2}\|R\mathbf{u} - \mathbf{u}_0^{rgb}\|_2^2. \qquad (2)$$

The first term is a smoothness term, which is based on a composition of convolution operators and pointwise non-linear functions. The learned convolution operator $K_t^1 = (K_t^{1,1}, \ldots, K_t^{1,N_{f_1}}) : \mathcal{U}_{rgbm} \mapsto \mathcal{F}_1$ implements a set of N_{f_1} 2D convolutions to compute the feature space $\mathcal{F}_1 = \mathbb{R}^{N_1 \times N_2 \times N_{f_1}}$. Next, learned non-linear functions $\phi_t^1 : \mathcal{F}_1 \mapsto \mathcal{F}_1$ are applied in a pointwise manner in order to apply a non-linear transformation to the feature space $\mathcal{F}_1$. This feature space is then again filtered by a second set of convolution operators $K_t^2 = (K_t^{2,1}, \ldots, K_t^{2,N_{f_2}}) : \mathcal{F}_1 \mapsto \mathcal{F}_2$ which implement N_{f_2} learned convolution operators. This gives the second feature space $\mathcal{F}_2 = \mathbb{R}^{N_1 \times N_2 \times N_{f_2}}$ which is once more transformed by applying learned non-linear functions $\phi_t^2 : \mathcal{F}_2 \mapsto \mathcal{F}_2$. The final regularization term is then given by taking the sum over all elements of $\mathcal{F}_2$.

The second term is a data fidelity term, which is given by the squared L^2-norm between the current image $\mathbf{u}$ and the initial image $\mathbf{u}_0$. The linear operator $R : \mathcal{U}_{rgbm} \mapsto \mathcal{U}_{rgb}$ is used to restrict the norm to the RGB channels of $\mathbf{u}$.

In our iterative scheme (1), we evolve the gradient of the variational model (2). By virtue of the chain rule, the gradient is given by

$$\nabla E_t(\mathbf{u}) = (K_t^1)^\top \phi_t^{1'}(K_t^1 \mathbf{u})(K_t^2)^\top \phi_t^{2'}(K_t^2 \phi_t^1(K_t^1 \mathbf{u})) + \lambda_t R^\top(R\mathbf{u} - \mathbf{u}_0^{rgb}), \quad (3)$$

where $\phi_t^{1'}$ and $\phi_t^{2'}$ denote the derivatives of the pointwise non-linear functions.

Similar to the TNRD model [6], the functions ϕ_t^i are parameterized using Gaussian radial basis functions with weights $w_t^i \in \mathbb{R}^J$ and the convolution operators K_t^1 and K_t^2 are given by small convolution kernels. Thus, the overall parameters for the model that have to be learned are $\theta = (K_t^1, w_t^1, K_t^2, w_t^2, \lambda_t)_{t=1}^{N_t}$. As initial data for the denoising and classification we consider $\mathbf{u}_0$ with $\mathbf{u}_0^{RGB}$ being the actual tissue section image and u_0^m as uniformly distributed noise.

Let us now briefly describe our learning procedure. Given a set of sample pairs $((\mathbf{u}_0^{rgb}, u_0^m)_s, (\mathbf{g}^{rgb}, g^m)_s)_{s=1}^S$, the training problem is defined as

$$\min_{\theta \in \mathcal{T}} \sum_{s=1}^S \frac{1}{6} \|(\mathbf{u}_T^{rgb})_s - (\mathbf{g}^{rgb})_s\|_2^2 + \frac{1}{2} \|(u_T^m)_s - (g^m)_s\|_2^2, \quad (4)$$

where $\mathbf{g}^{rgb}$ and g^m define the target images and masks, respectively. The set $\mathcal{T} = \{(K_t^1, w_t^1, K_t^2, w_t^2, \lambda_t) : \|K_t^{1,i}\|_2 \leq 1, \|K_t^{2,j}\|_2 \leq 1, \lambda_t \geq 0, i = 1...N_{f_1}, j = 1...N_{f_2}, t = 1...N_t\}$ is the set of admissible model parameters. Observe that these constraints are essential to avoid a scaling problems between the filter and the corresponding non-linear functions. The coefficients in (4) ensure a balance of the loss between image reconstruction and cell detection. To solve this variational problem, the Adam optimizer [8] is employed, where a projection of θ onto $\mathcal{T}$ is performed after each gradient step.

2.2   Stochastic generator of training data

Our training data for the two prototypic scenarios considered here is based on a comparably simply structural description: ellipsoidal shapes for the different cell

Table 1. Cell specific data of all scenarios.

	category	mean color	semi axes (pixels)	number/placement
(1)	tumor cell	green	20 – 35	60 cells, random placement
	tumor nucleus	light blue	8 – 12	only 60% visible
	immune cell	red	8 – 20	40 cells, random placement, no overlapping
	immune cell nucleus	blue	7 – 8	only 60% visible
	stroma/ dediff. melanoma	blue	5 – 15	40 cells, random placement, no overlapping
(2)	tumor cell	light purple	15 – 25	5 of 7 Voronoi regions filled, no overlapping
	tumor nucleus	purple	3 – 10	only 60% visible
	immune cell	violet	4 – 8	2 of 7 Voronoi regions filled, no overlapping

components, a stochastic placement of these primitives, and an additive noise generation for the cells and background color. We consider two different tissue section image classes:

The aim of scenario 1 is the detection of the direct contact of immune cells with melanoma cells in immunofluorescent stained melanoma sections. Scenario 2 analyzes the pattern/invasion of tumor infiltrating immune cells in H&E stained melanoma sections.

The essential guidelines for the data generation are (for details see Table 1):

- All cells and cell nuclei are modeled as ellipses, where both the length of the semi axes and the inclination are drawn from a uniform distribution.
- The cells are placed randomly or in cells of a precomputed random Voronoi tessellation.
- Overlapping of cells or the location of cell midpoints inside other cells can be excluded for certain cell types.
- The colors of cells/nuclei are drawn from a multivariate normal distribution with expectation/variance extracted from a small sample of real images.
- Realistic noise is added in the composition of the geometric primitives, with covariance matrices estimated via a covariance analysis of the above sample.
- Finally, background noise is added with average color and variance again extracted from this sample.

Examples of the training data for the two problem classes are shown in Fig. 2.

Our method classifies certain types of immune cells, depending on a fluorescence marking and their local cell environment. Depending on the scenario, immune cells are marked as classified if they are located in a proximity of tumor cells (scenario 1) or if the concentration of immune cells in a neighborhood is sufficiently large (scenario 2). Local cell concentrations are computed based on the volumetric measure of cells in circular neighborhoods. A classified immune cell is indicated with a value 1.0 in the marking channel at all underlying pixels on a 0 background, i.e. for a circular cell concentration beyond a threshold 0.4 (scenario 1) or 0.2 (scenario 2). Since this measure is prone to small perturbations of the cell structures, we could improve the stability of the classification in scenario 1 by assigning to all pixels in the ground truth mask the value 0.5 if the cell concentration is in the range $[0.2, 0.4]$.

2.3   Acquisition of histological sections

To analyze immune cell and melanoma cell interactions, we used ten representative immunofluorescent stains for the immune cell marker CD45 in red, the melanocytic marker gp100 in green and the nuclei DAPI in blue of murine melanomas (staining protocol has been described previously in [9]) and ten H&E stained human melanoma metastases of the Skin Cancer Center Bonn of the University Hospital in Bonn. H&E stains were performed according to standard protocols. Stained sections were examined with a Leica DMBL immunofluorescence microscope, all images were acquired with a JVC digital camera KY-75FU.

3   Results

We consider $N_t = 10$ steps in the TNRD model and 200 random 500×500 training images. In each step, $N_{f_1} = 24$ different filters of size $11 \times 11 \times 4$ and $N_{f_2} = 24$ filters of size $5 \times 5 \times 24$, and for the activation function $J = 31$ Gaussian radial basis functions in the interval $[-1.2, 1.2]$ were used. Following [8], we performed 20000 iterations of the Adam optimizer with step size 0.001 using a batch size of 2 and the exponential decay rate parameters $\beta_1 = 0.9$ and $\beta_2 = 0.999$. The plots of the associated loss function and the peak signal-to-noise ratio (PSNR) for the RGB and the masking channel are shown in Fig. 1.

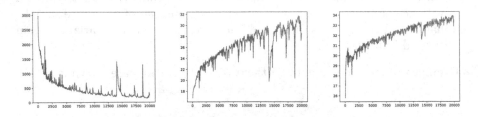

Fig. 1. Loss function (first column), PSNR for RGB channel (second column) and masking channel (third column) for scenario 1.

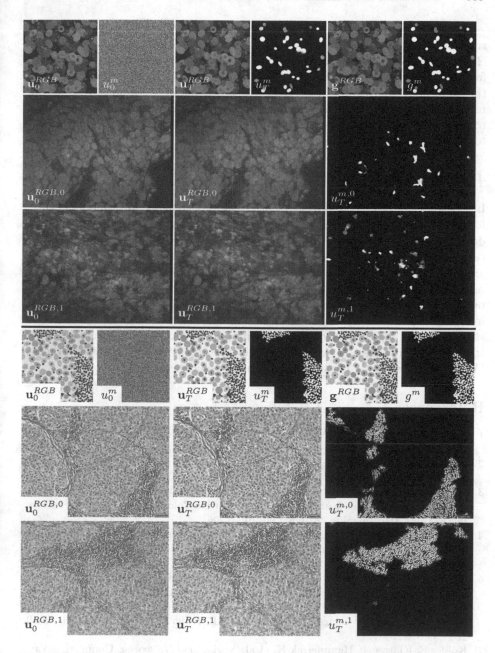

Fig. 2. Training data (pairs of image and mask of input, output and ground truth) for 2 scenarios. $\mathbf{u}_0^{RGB,i}$, $\mathbf{u}_T^{RGB,i}$ and $u_T^{m,i}$ ($i = 0, 1$) for histological sections in scenario 1 (second/third row) with two representative images of immunofluorescent stains of melanoma: with blue (DAPI, cell nuclei), red (CD45, immune cell marker), green (gp100, melanocyte marker), and scenario 2 (fifth/sixth row) H&E stains of melanoma.

Fig. 2 depicts pairs of RGB images and associated masking channels for training input data (first pair), computed pair of denoised image and estimated classification (second pair) and ground truth image and classification (third pair) for scenario 1 (first row) and scenario 2 (fourth row). In the remaining rows, the input data (first column), the denoised image (second column), and the corresponding classification (third column) are shown for scenario 1 (second/third row) and scenario 2 (fifth/sixth row). As an outcome, nearly all immune cells to be classified are actually detected.

4   Discussion

In this work, we investigated a deep learning approach using variational networks for joint image reconstruction and segmentation on melanoma tissue sections to detect direct interactions of immune cells with melanoma cells and patterns of tumor infiltrating immune cells. We were able to provide spatial localization and distribution of immune cells within the tumor microenvironment. Obvious limitations of the method are the restriction to ellipsoidal shaped cells and cell nuclei and the currently small number of cell or nuclei types, e.g. in the first image in Fig. 2 associated with scenario 2 small regions of extracellular matrix structures are erroneously classified as immune cells, probably because these structures are not treated explicitly as cell types in the data generation process. Future analyses should consider the complex heterogeneity of tumor cells.

References

1. Tumeh PC, Harview CL, Yearley JH, et al. PD-1 blockade induces responses by inhibiting adaptive immune resistance. Nature. 2014;515:568–571.
2. Jacquelot N, Roberti MP, Enot DP, et al. Predictors of responses to immune checkpoint blockade in advanced melanoma. Nat Commun. 2017;8.
3. Sirinukunwattana K, Raza SEA, Tsang YW, et al. Locality Sensitive Deep Learning for Detection and Classification of Nuclei in Routine Colon Cancer Histology Images. IEEE Trans Med Imaging. 2016;35(5):1196–1206.
4. Xu J, Luo X, Wang G, et al. A Deep Convolutional Neural Network for segmenting and classifying epithelial and stromal regions in histopathological images. Neurocomputing. 2016;191:214–223.
5. Janowczyk A, Madabhushi A. Deep Learning for Digital Pathology Image Analysis: A Comprehensive Tutorial with Selected Use Cases. J Pathol Inform. 2016;7.
6. Chen Y, Pock T. Trainable nonlinear reaction diffusion: A flexible framework for fast and effective image restoration. IEEE Trans Pattern Anal Mach Intell. 2017;39(6):1256–1272.
7. Kobler E, Klatzer T, Hammernik K, et al. Variational Networks: Connecting Variational Methods and Deep Learning. In: Ger Pattern Recognit Conf; 2017. p. 281–293.
8. Kingma DP, Ba JL. Adam: A Method for Stochastic Optimization. In: International Conference on Learning Representations; 2015.
9. Landsberg J, Kohlmeyer J, Renn M, et al. Melanomas resist T-cell therapy through inflammation-induced reversible dedifferentiation. Nature. 2012;490:412–416.

Frangi-Net

Weilin Fu[1], Katharina Breininger[1], Roman Schaffert[1], Nishant Ravikumar[1],
Tobias Würfl[1], Jim Fujimoto[3], Eric Moult[3], Andreas Maier[1,2]

[1]Pattern Recognition Lab, Department of Computer Science,
Friedrich-Alexander-University Erlangen-Nuremberg, Germany
[2]Erlangen Graduate School in Advanced Optical Technologies (SAOT)
[3]Department Electrical Engineering and Computer Science and Research Laboratory
of Electronics, Massachusetts Institute of Technology, USA
weilin.fu@fau.de

Abstract. In this paper, we reformulate the conventional 2-D Frangi
vesselness measure into a pre-weighted neural network ("Frangi-Net"),
and illustrate that the Frangi-Net is equivalent to the original Frangi
filter. Furthermore, we show that, as a neural network, Frangi-Net is
trainable. We evaluate the proposed method on a set of 45 high resolution fundus images. After fine-tuning, we observe both qualitative and
quantitative improvements in the segmentation quality compared to the
original Frangi measure, with an increase up to 17% in F1 score.

1 Introduction

Fundus imaging can help to diagnose and monitor a number of diseases, such
as diabetic retinopathy, glaucoma, age-related macular degeneration [1]. Visual analysis by a trained ophtamologist can be extremely time-consuming and
hinder broad clinical application. To support this workflow, automatic segmentation [2] of the retinal vessel tree has been studies for decades, among which
a vessel enhancement filter by Frangi et al. [3] is the most popular and forms
the basis to various other strategies [4]. However, this task is particularly challenging due to the complex structure of retinal vessels (e.g. branching, crossing)
and low image quality (e.g. noise, artifacts, low resolution). In recent years,
deep learning techniques have been exploited in the field of retinal vessel segmentation [5, 6]. These approaches are data-driven, and tend to share a similar
structure, where a classifier follows a feature extractor. For instance, Maji et
al. [5] use an auto-encoder as a feature extractor, and random forests as a classifier; Tetteh et al. [6] apply a convolutional neural network (CNN) inception
model for feature extraction and another CNN model for classification. These
novel, data-driven approaches perform comparably to conventional methods, but
do not yield significant improvements.

In this paper, we also investigate deep learning techniques on retinal vessel segmentation. To avoid an explicit separation into "feature extractor" and
"classification", we propose an alternative approach, which formulates the Frangi
filter as a pre-weighted network ("Frangi-Net"). The intuitive reasoning behind

341

such an approach is that, by representing the Frangi filter as a pre-weighted neural network, subsequent training of the latter should improve segmentation quality. We aim to utilize prior knowledge of tube segmentation as a basis, and further improve it using a data-driven approach.

2   Materials and methods

2.1   Frangi vessel enhancement filter

The Frangi vesselness filter [3] is based on the eigen-value analysis of the Hessian matrix in multiple Gaussian scales. Coarse scale structures are typically obtained by smoothing the image with a Gaussian filter g_σ where σ is the standard deviation. The Hessian matrix is a square matrix of second-order partial derivatives of the smoothed image. Therefore, it can be alternatively calculated by convolving the original image patch directly with the 3 2-D kernels, namely $\frac{\partial^2 g_\sigma}{\partial x^2}, \frac{\partial^2 g_\sigma}{\partial y^2}, \frac{\partial^2 g_\sigma}{\partial x \partial y}$, which are the second-order partial derivatives of the Gaussian filter g_σ.

$$G_\sigma = \begin{bmatrix} \frac{\partial^2 g_\sigma}{\partial x^2} & \frac{\partial^2 g_\sigma}{\partial x \partial y} \\ \frac{\partial^2 g_\sigma}{\partial x \partial y} & \frac{\partial^2 g_\sigma}{\partial y^2} \end{bmatrix} \tag{1}$$

The Hessian matrix at each pixel of image f is calculated as,

$$H_\sigma = G_\sigma * f = \begin{bmatrix} H_{xx} & H_{xy} \\ H_{xy} & H_{yy} \end{bmatrix} \tag{2}$$

The two eigenvalues of the Hessian matrix are denoted by λ_1 and λ_2 ($|\lambda_2| \geq |\lambda_1|$), which are calculated as

$$\lambda_{1,2} = \frac{(H_{xx} + H_{yy}) \pm \sqrt{(H_{xx} - H_{yy})^2 + 4H_{xy}^2}}{2} \tag{3}$$

A high vesselness response is obtained if λ_1 and λ_2 satisfy the following conditions: $\|\lambda_1\| \approx 0$, and $\|\lambda_2\| \gg \|\lambda_1\|$. A mathematical description of the vesselness response is presented in [3],

$$V_0(\sigma) = \begin{cases} 0, & \text{for dark tubes if } \lambda_2 < 0 \\ \exp(-\frac{R_B^2}{2\beta^2})(1 - \exp(-\frac{S^2}{2c^2})), & \text{otherwise} \end{cases} \tag{4}$$

where $S = \sqrt{\lambda_1^2 + \lambda_2^2}$ is the second order structureness, $R_B = \frac{\|\lambda_1\|}{\|\lambda_2\|}$ is the blobness measure, and V_0 stands for the vesselness value. β, c are image-dependent parameters for blobness and structureness terms, and are set to 0.5, 1, respectively.

When using a Gaussian kernel with a standard deviation σ, vessels whose diameters equal to $2\sqrt{2}\sigma$ have the highest vesselness response. The diameter of retinal vessels in this work range from 6 to 35 pixels. Hence we choose a series of σ as $3, 6, 12$ pixels accordingly. Instead of convolving a patch with three different kernels (i. e., $G_3, G_6,$ and G_{12}), we create a three-level resolution hierarchy [4], and convolve each level with G_3 only. The resolution hierarchy consists of the original patch and two downsampled versions, using factors 2 and 4, respectively.

2.2   Pre-weighted Frangi-Net

Inspired by [7], we implement the multi-scale Frangi filter as a neural network called Frangi-Net on the basis of the previous section. The architecture of Frangi-Net is described in Fig. 1. The proposed method is used to analyze image patches, with an output size set to 128×128 pixels. Input patches for the three sub-nets are cropped as in Fig. 1 (a).

For a single-scale sub-net, we first use a resize layer to downsample images to the corresponding size. Secondly, we use a 2-D convolution layer with three filters to get the Hessian matrix. These filters are initialized as second partial derivatives of the two-dimensional Gaussian function with $\sigma = 3$. After that, a combination of mathematic operation layers are applied, based on Eqs. 3 and 4 to calculate eigen-values and vesselness responses of this scale.

The raw vesselness scores from Frangi-Net typically range from 0 to roughly 0.4. To create a binary vessel mask, a threshold t is used, which is manually set to 10^{-3} in this work. This means that most background pixels are squashed inbetween $[0, t)$, and the rest few vessel pixels spread along $(t, 0.4)$. To obtain a probability map, we subtract the data with the threshold t, and asymmetrically scale it, so that raw scores are more evenly redistributed. Positive values are multiplied with scale s_{pos} and negative values with s_{neg}, where s_{pos}, s_{neg} are set to 2000 and 20,000 in this work. In this way, raw scores are redistributed to $[-20, 80)$ and after a sigmoid layer, raw vesselness values of $0, t,$ and 0.4 are converted to $0, 0.5,$ and 1, respectively.

2.3   Trainable Frangi-Net

With the proposed network structure, we observe two sets of trainable parameters in the network: first, the covolution kernels responsible for the computation of the Hessian matrix; second, the parameters $\beta, c,$ that control the influence of structureness and blobness features. For each scale, this results in three trainable convolution kernels and two additional parameters that can be adapted during training. In Frangi-Net, single-scale nets are structured in parallel and updated independently, which means in total we have nine kernels and six parameters to update during training.

A high resolution fundus (HRF) image database [8] is used in this work. The dataset includes 15 images of each healthy, diabetic retinopathy, and glaucomatous subjects. The HRF images are high resolution 3504×2336 pixel RGB fundus photographs. Only the green channels are used where vascular structures manifest a good contrast [9]. The intensity values are normalized to $[0, 1]$. We train Frangi-Net on each cartegory independently, randomly dividing from the

15 images 10 for training, 2 for validation and 3 for testing. We also train the network with all 45 images, randomly taking 30 for training, 6 for validation and 9 for testing. As segmentation of retinal vessels from fundus images is an unbalanced classification problem, where the background pixels outnumber vessel pixels by approximately 10 to 1, dice coefficient loss [10] instead of the common cross entropy loss is used. The optimizer we utilize here is gradient descent with learning rate 10^{-6} and momentum 0.5. 1000 steps are used for training on each category independently, while 3000 steps are used for training on the whole database. Batch size is chosen as 250. We use python and tensorflow framework for the whole implementation.

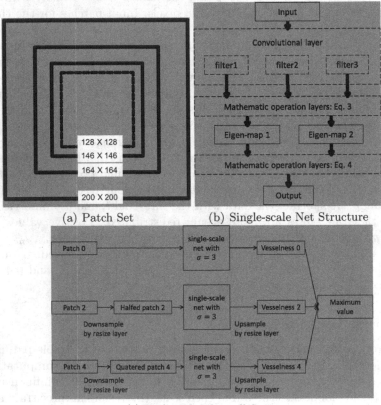

(a) Patch Set   (b) Single-scale Net Structure

(c) Frangi-Net Overall Structure

Fig. 1. The Frangi-Net architecture: In (a), dash line represents output patch size 128×128; solid lines represent the patch set in the resolution hierarchy. (b) describes the dataflow through the framework of a single-scale net, where eigen-map 1 and 2 are maps of λ_1, λ_2 respectively; (c) describes the overall structure of Frangi-Net, where patch 0, patch 2, patch 4 correspond to size 146×146, 164×164, 200×200 in (a).

Table 1. Segmentation quality before and after training.

Dataset	F1 score before	after	Accuracy before	after	Precision before	after	Recall before	after
Healthy	0.669	**0.712**	0.836	**0.843**	0.606	**0.675**	0.746	**0.753**
Diabetic retinopathy	0.495	**0.532**	0.819	**0.822**	0.524	**0.588**	0.468	**0.486**
Glaucomatous	0.495	**0.584**	0.838	**0.841**	0.477	**0.562**	0.608	**0.618**
Whole dataset	0.612	**0.672**	0.847	**0.855**	0.603	**0.675**	0.623	**0.670**

3   Results

A quantitative comparison of the trained Frangi-Nets with the original Frangi filter is summarized in Tab. 1. Each quality metric is calculated as an average of that of the testing datasets. After fine-tuning with four different training datasets, the F1 score, accuracy, precision and recall of the segmentation results on the testing datasets all get improved. Segmentation of heathy fundus images performs best, achieving a highest post-training F1 score as 0.712. Comparing the diseased cases to the healthy cases, the F1 score has a more significant improvement after training, up to 17%.

A comparison of the segmentation results before and after training using the healthy datasets is shown in Fig.2. Fig. 2(a) displays that Frangi-Net can segment main vessels well before training. However, it only partially segments the middle-sized vessels and fails to recognize most of the tiny ones. In contrast, after training, Frangi-Net is able to detect the middle-sized vessels well, and it also detects most of the tiny ones (Fig. 2(b)).

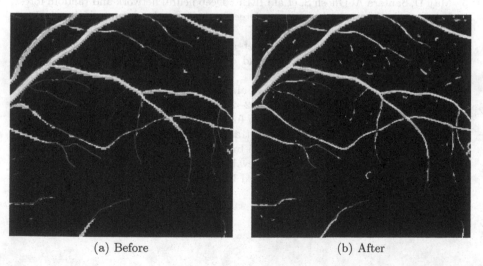

(a) Before   (b) After

Fig. 2. Vessel segmentation results before and after training. The red, green and yellow colors represent the manual labels, the segmentation results and the overlaps between them, respectively.

346   Fu et al.

4 Discussion

In this work, we proposed to combine the prior knowlegde about retinal vessel that is encoded in the Frangi-Filter with the data-driven capabilities of neural networks. We constructed a net that is equivalent to the multi-scale Frangi filter. We identified the trainable parts of Frangi-Net as convolutional kernels and parameters when computing vesselness. We redistributed the raw output vesselness values into a probability map and trained the net by optimizing dice coefficient loss. In experiments with high resolution fundus images of healthy and diseased patients, the trained Frangi-Net performs better than the original formulation both quantitatively and qualitatively.

Future work will investigate on different network architectures for Frangi-Net, or the combination of Frangi-Net with other networks. We will also evaluate Frangi-Net with other datasets.

References

1. Maji D, Santara A, Mitra P, et al. Ensemble of deep convolutional neural networks for learning to detect retinal vessels in fundus images. arXiv. 2016.
2. Kirbas C, Quek F. A review of vessel extraction techniques and algorithms. ACM Comput Surv. 2004;36(2):81–121.
3. Frangi AF, Niessen WJ, Vincken KL, et al.; Springer. Multiscale vessel enhancement filtering. Proc MICCAI. 1998; p. 130–137.
4. Budai A, Bock R, Maier A, et al. Robust vessel segmentation in fundus images. Int J Biomed Imaging. 2013.
5. Maji D, Santara A, Ghosh S, et al.; IEEE. Deep neural network and random forest hybrid architecture for learning to detect retinal vessels in fundus images. Proc EMBC. 2015; p. 3029–3032.
6. Tetteh G, Rempfler M, Zimmer C, et al.; Springer. Deep-FExt: deep feature extraction for vessel segmentation and centerline prediction. Int Worksh Mach Learn Med Imaging. 2017; p. 344–352.
7. Würfl T, Ghesu FC, Christlein V, et al.; Springer. Deep learning computed tomography. Proc MICCAI. 2016; p. 432–440.
8. Budai A, Odstrcilik J. High resolution fundus image database; 2013.
9. Yin B, Li H, Sheng B, et al. Vessel extraction from non-fluorescein fundus images using orientation-aware detector. Med Image Anal. 2015;26(1):232–242.
10. Taha AA, Hanbury A. Metrics for evaluating 3D medical image segmentation: analysis, selection, and tool. BMC Med Imaging. 2015;15(1):29.

Lung Vessel Enhancement in Low-Dose CT Scans
The LANCELOT Method

Nico Merten[1,2], Kai Lawonn[3], Philipp Gensecke[4],
Oliver Großer[4], Bernhard Preim[1,2]

[1]Research Campus STIMULATE
[2]Department of Simulation and Graphics, Otto-von-Guericke University
[3]Institute for Computational Visualistics, University of Koblenz-Landau
[4]Department of Radiology and Nuclear Medicine, University Hospital Magdeburg
nmerten@isg.cs.uni-magdeburg.de

Abstract. To reduce the patient's radiation exposure from computed tomography scans (CT), low-dose CT scans can be recorded. Several image processing methods exist to segment or enhance the lung blood vessels from contrast-enhanced or high resolution CT scans, but the reduced contrast in low-dose CT scans leads to over- or under-segmentation. Our LANCELOT method combines maximum response and stick filters to enhance lung blood vessels in native, low-dose CT scans. We compare our method with the vessel segmentation and enhancing methods from Frangi and Sato et al. Our method has two advantages that were confirmed in an evaluation with two clinical experts: First, our method enhances small vessels and vessel branches more clearly and second, it connects vessels anatomically correct, while the others create discontinuities.

1 Introduction

For a long time, the most important imaging methods for the detection of lung nodes were chest radiographs (CXRs). Compared to computed tomography scans (CTs), CXRs suffer from occlusion problems and are not able to reproduce as much contrast as CT scans are able to [1]. On the other hand, the radiation exposure during CT examinations is significantly higher. One way of reducing the patient's exposure to radiation is to take low-dose CT scans instead of diagnostic CTs, which leads to lower image contrast. Another possibility is the administration of contrast agent to emphasize blood vessels.

Several image processing methods are available for segmentation or enhancement of blood vessels from CT angiography (CTAs) diagnostic CT scans. Sato and Frangi et al. combine an evaluation of the Hessian matrix eigenvalues and a priori knowledge about the vessel and background brightness to enhance vessel-like structures in angiography scans [2, 3]. Alternatively, if high resolution CT scans are available, 3D region growing allows the extraction of blood vessels [4]. We refer to the VESSEL12 Study by Rudyanto et al. [5] for a detailed comparison of automated lung vessel segmentations in CT scans.

The aforementioned approaches produce convincing results for the image scans they were applied to, but we were not able to reproduce comparable results when applying them to low-dose CT scans. Using thresholding or region growing leads either to over- or under-segmentation and evaluating the Hessian Matrix is also not sufficient. While larger vessels are enhanced, many medium and small vessels are not. Furthermore, although visibly connected in the original scan, some vessels are separated since the contrast between them and parenchyma is too low in low-dose CT recordings. For that reason, we present our lung vessel enhancement method for *low*-dose *CT* scans, LANCELOT in short.

2   Materials and methods

In the following we abbreviate image coordinates, e.g., $I(x, y, z)$, by $I(\mathbf{x})$. Sato and Frangi et al. use multi-scale line enhancement filters to segment blood vessels in contrast-enhanced and native CT scans [2, 3]. First, a Gaussian convolution $G(\mathbf{x}; \sigma)$ is applied to reduce image noise. Then, the Hessian matrix $H(\mathbf{x})$ is set up for $I(\mathbf{x})$ and its eigenvalues λ_1, λ_2, and λ_3 are evaluated. This yields

$$H(\mathbf{x}; \sigma) = H(I(\mathbf{x}) * G(\mathbf{x}; \sigma)) \tag{1}$$

To find the brighter blood vessels in the dark parenchyma, the conditions

$$(\lambda_1 \approx 0) \wedge (\lambda_2 \approx \lambda_3 \ll 0) \tag{2}$$

must hold. To separate lines from sheet-like and blob-like shapes such as skin and noise components, respectively, a vesselness function evaluates how good these conditions are fulfilled. This function is called $\lambda_{123}(\mathbf{x}; \sigma)$.

These conditions are combined with 3D multi-scale filters. When multi-scale filters are applied, individual filter responses are first normalized and then the maximum response is added to $I(\mathbf{x})$. The result image $I'(\mathbf{x})$ is given by

$$I'(\mathbf{x}) = I(\mathbf{x}) + \max_{1 \leq i \leq n} (\sigma_i^2 \cdot \lambda_{123}(\mathbf{x}; \sigma_i)) \tag{3}$$

where n donates the number of multi-scale filters. For each multi-scale filter the vesselness measure is normalized with σ_i^2 from the Gaussian convolution.

We combine this maximum response approach with the Stick kernels from Czerwinski et al. [6]. To create filter kernels of varying sizes, we use the Bresenham algorithm [7]. This results in a filter radius $r_F \times 4$ individual filter kernels. As presented in Figure 1, for $r_F = 2$ this results in 8 individual kernels. In the following we abbreviate $r_F \times 2 + 1 = m$. For every image pixel $I(\mathbf{x})$ and kernel $(K_i)_m$, δ_i is computed with

$$\max \delta_i = \max_{K_i} |\mu((I(\mathbf{x})_m * (K_i)_m)) - \mu(I(\mathbf{x})_m)| \tag{4}$$

Each δ_i is the absolute distance between an averaged image region $I(\mathbf{x})_m$ and the averaged response of kernel $(K_i)_m$. The enhanced image values I_{enh} are computed with

$$I(\mathbf{x})_{enh} = \begin{cases} I(\mathbf{x}) + \max \delta_i & \text{if } I(\mathbf{x}) \geq \mu(I(\mathbf{x})_m) \\ I(\mathbf{x}) - \max \delta_i & \text{else} \end{cases} \tag{5}$$

This increases the contrast, because the difference of image values and their neighborhood's average is further increased or decreased. We defined $\sigma = m$ to adjust the Gaussian convolution to the stick kernel's width.

In summary, to enhance lung blood vessels in native, low-dose CT scans, the slices are first smoothed with a Gaussian convolution and then the aforementioned maximum response approach is combined with stick filter kernels. Formally, this yields

$$I(\mathbf{x})_{enh} = I(\mathbf{x}) \pm \max \delta_i(I(\mathbf{x}) * G(\mathbf{x}; \sigma)). \tag{6}$$

We implemented our method in MATLAB and used the Vesselness (Sato et al.) and HessianFilter (Frangi et al.) modules in MeVisLab 2.8.2 [8].

3   Results

Figure 2 shows two image series. This overview depicts the original image, the results of Sato and Frangi et al.'s methods, and the results of our method. The orange-framed image regions are magnified to show the results of all methods in more detail. Additionally, Figure 3 shows two enhanced vessel branchings from the second series in more detail. All our results were obtained with $m = 7$.

All methods were tested on five datasets and the respective processing times are listed in Table 1. We measured them with an i5-2500 processor with 3.70 GHz. Although our method can only be applied on single slices, the methods of Sato and Frangi et al. can be used on image stacks, too. Therefore, all results were acquired using implementations that process single images. We did not use parallel programming methods for any method.

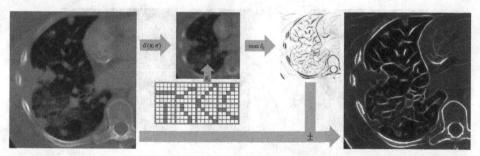

Fig. 1. The image processing pipeline of our method. First, the image is blurred with a Gaussian convolution $G(\mathbf{x}, \sigma)$ and then the Stick kernels $(K_i)_m$ are applied with $\sigma = m = 5$. Finally, the enhanced vessels are added to the input image. We inverted the enhanced vessels' visualization for presentation purposes.

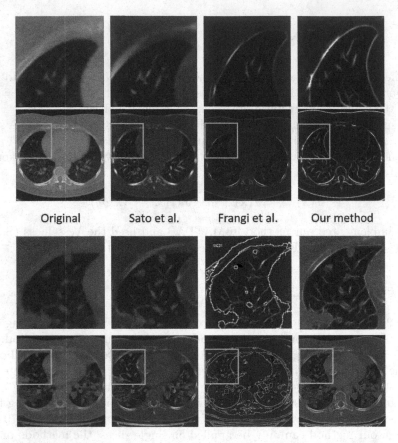

Fig. 2. These series show the original images and the results of the aforementioned methods. The framed image regions were magnified for presentation purposes. We used 7×7 filter kernels for our results.

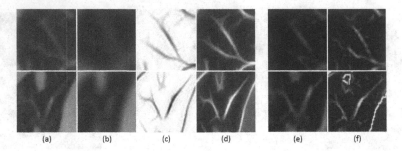

Fig. 3. This figure shows the (a) original input image and the interim results after (b) Gaussian convolution, (c) computation of $\max \delta_i$, and (d) when the enhanced vessels were merged with the original image. The last two images show emphasized image regions after the methods from (e) Sato and (f) Frangi et al. were applied.

Dataset Slices	Execution Time (s) Sato et al.	Frangi et al.	Our method
No. 1 117	6.45	3.25	34.49
No. 2 117	6.84	3.24	34.10
No. 3 108	5.83	2.98	31.25
No. 4 107	5.81	2.97	31.89
No. 5 63	3.44	1.75	18.65
Time per Slice (s)	0.05	0.03	0.29

Table 1. The processing times of the aforementioned methods for each data set. Each slice has the dimensions of 512 × 512 pixels. The times were averaged for five executions.

We applied all methods on five datasets. They all have a kilovoltage Peak of 120 kVp and an X-ray tube current between 40 and 80 mA. The acquisition parameters from the low-dose CT scans that were used in the National Lung Screening Trial lie in the same range [1].

4 Discussion

We evaluated our method by interviewing two clinical experts. The first interviewee is a Medical Technical Assistant (MTA) with 21 years of working experience in multiple clinical and technical environments. Eight years of that time she worked with CT scans and two years of that time she specifically worked with lung CT scans. When asked, she assessed her anatomical knowledge about the human lung to be fair. Our second interviewee is an assistant doctor with four years of clinical experience. Three and a half years of that time with CT scans and three years of that time specifically with lung CT scans. He reported his anatomical knowledge about the lung to be very good.

They were asked to compare all methods' results and to assess our method's clinical feasibility and possible application areas. We developed a software tool to enable them to explore the original scan and all result images. To support the comparison of multiple image data sets, the zooming, translation, and slicing features and the cursor position were synchronized for multiple views. We did not synchronize the transfer function, because, in general, the value ranges of the original and result images are different.

They stated that the enhancement of large vessels, vessel branches, and lesions is comparable, but our method enhanced mid-size and small vessels more clearly (Fig. 3). Furthermore, they assessed that although small and very thin vessels are visible in the original images, Sato and Frangi et al.'s methods split them while our method connects and enhances them anatomically correct. In summary, they assessed our method to be more suitable to separate blood vessels from surrounding parenchyma. Because of the different processing times (Tab. 1), we prepared our method's results beforehand. We asked them to evaluate the execution times and both stated that they are sufficient.

Both experts stated that our method improves the diagnostic and therapy planning value for low-dose CT scans. Finally, the MTA reported that our method would be beneficial for manual segmentations of lung vessels.

4.1   Limitations and future work

We introduced the LANCELOT method that can enhance smaller vessels than Sato and Frangi et al.'s methods, but if σ and m is small, it also enhances image noise (Fig. 2). Our method also enhances the edges of nodules, but they can be distorted (Fig. 3). This could be a problem for nodule detection and segmentation algorithms [9]. Therefore, they should be applied to the original images rather than our result images to prevent artifacts.

In the future we want to work on three extensions. First, the stick filter kernels should be extended to 3D to include spatial information about blood vessels and second, the processing times can be improved via parallel programming, e. g. on the GPU. Finally, our method computes the max δ_i for multiple stick kernels of the same size m and it would be interesting to see which results can be achieved when a multi-scale approach is used, where kernels of different sizes are included, too.

Acknowledgement. This work is partly funded by the Federal Ministry of Education and Research within the Forschungscampus STIMULATE (13GW0095A). We thank Cindy Lübeck and Sylvia Saalfeld for fruitful discussions and for providing us with valuable feedback for our method and results.

References

1. National Lung Screening Trial Research Team. The national lung screening trial: overview and study design. Radiology. 2011.
2. Sato, Y and Nakajima, S and Atsumi, H et al ; Springer. 3D Multi-scale line filter for segmentation and visualization of curvilinear structures in medical images. Proc CVRMed-MRCAS. 1997; p. 213–222.
3. Frangi, A F and Niessen, W J and Vincken, K et al ; Springer. Multiscale vessel enhancement filtering. Proc MICCAI. 1998; p. 130–137.
4. Kuhnigk, J-M and Hahn, H and Hindennach, M et al . Lung lobe segmentation by anatomy-guided 3D watershed transform. In: Proc SPIE. vol. 5032; 2003. p. 1482–1490.
5. Rudyanto, R D and Kerkstra, S and Van Rikxoort, E M et al . Comparing algorithms for automated vessel segmentation in computed tomography scans of the lung: the VESSEL12 study. Med Image Anal. 2014;18(7):1217–1232.
6. Czerwinski, R N and Jones, D L and O'brien, W D. Line and boundary detection in speckle images. IEEE Trans Image Process. 1998;7(12):1700–1714.
7. Bresenham, J E. Algorithm for computer control of a digital plotter. IBM Systems Journal. 1965;4(1):25–30.
8. Ritter, F and Boskamp, T and Homeyer, A et al . Medical image analysis. IEEE Pulse. 2011;2(6):60–70.
9. Kuhnigk, J-M and Dicken, V and Bornemann, L et al . Morphological Segmentation and Partial Volume Analysis for Volumetry of Solid Pulmonary Lesions in Thoracic CT Scans. IEEE Trans Med Imaging. 2006;25(4):417–434.

Whole Heart and Great Vessel Segmentation with Context-aware of Generative Adversarial Networks

Mina Rezaei, Haojin Yang, Christoph Meinel

Hasso-Plattner Institute for Digital Engineering
mina.rezaei@hpi.de

Abstract. Automatic segmentation of cardiac magnetic resonance imaging (CMRI) is an important application in clinical tasks. However, semantic segmentation of the myocardium and blood pool in CMR is a challenge due to differentiating branchy structures and slicing fuzzy boundaries. In this paper, we propose an automatic deep architecture for simultaneous myocardium and blood pool segmentation on patients with congenital heart disease (CHD). Inspired by vanilla generative adversarial networks (GANs), we propose a cascade of conditional GANs for semantic segmentation. The proposed cascade has three stages that are designed to share convolutional features and weights. Each stage has a conditional generative adversarial network with a unique loss function and trains on different images from the same patients. We further apply AutoContext Model to implement a context-aware generative adversarial network. The proposed method evaluated on the HVSMR dataset and the experimental results demonstrated the superior performance of our approach.

1 Introduction

Cardiac image segmentation plays an important role in heart disease diagnosis, treatment planning, and clinical monitoring. Cardiac Magnetic Resonance Imaging (CMRI) can provide rich information for premedication and surgery medication, which is extremely helpful for evaluating the treatment regimen. However, it is difficult to apply the raw data extracted from CMR images for diagnosis due to the large amount of the data. An accurate automatic whole-heart segmentation algorithm based on MR images might help to improve prediction accuracy and efficiency, which would enable better treatment planning and optimize the diagnostic progress.

Over the last few years, numerous automatic approaches have been developed to speed up medical image segmentation using deep neural networks (DNNs). DNNs are powerful models that have achieved excellent performance for learning a hierarchical representation of image data without any handcrafted features [1].

Of late, generative adversarial networks,-or GANs for short-, have gained so much momentum in the research fraternity, with many works having focused on image generation [2, 3]. A GAN comprises two models: a generative model and a discriminative model. The discriminator model is a classifier that determines whether a given image looks like a real image from the dataset, or like an artificial image created by the generator. The generator model takes random input values and transforms them into images through a deconvolutional neural network. In a conditioned generative model, there is a control on the modes of the data being generated. Notably, conditional GANs (cGANs)have been explored in various computer vision problems, e.g. classification [3], object detection [4], and image segmentation [5]. Xue *et al.* [6] have offered a cGAN, namely SegAN, for medical image segmentation with the idea of a multi-scale loss function for a generative network where the generative model is U-Net [7] and the multi-layer CNN is the discriminator. Moeskops *et al.* [8] have used dilated convolution as generator network and fully convolutional networks (FCNs) as discriminator for brain MRI segmentation. Adversarial networks have achieved notable results even on small data set for prostate cancer detection [9] and mammography mass segmentation [10].

In this paper, we address the semantic segmentation of blood pool and myocardium with the context aware of cGANs. Semantic segmentation is the task of classifying parts of images together that belong to the same object class. Inspired by cGAN networks [10, 5], we propose a fully automatic trainable adversarial cascade to perform whole-heart and great vessel segmentation.

2   Methodology

The proposed method has three stages with three individual cGAN models. These three stages are designed to share convolutional features and weights, where the later stages use the shared convolution features from the previous stage and transfer the learned convolutional features and weights to the next stage. Each stage involves a cGAN with an adversarial loss and individual parameters.

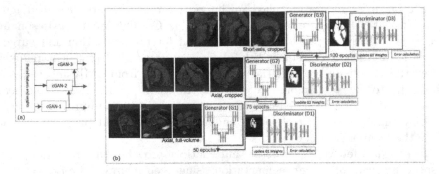

Fig. 1. The proposed method for CMR images segmentation with context-aware GANs in three stages (a). The proposed architecture is context-aware where the later stages use the shared convolution features plus the probability map obtained from previous stages and transfer the learned convolutional features to the next (b).

The cGAN architecture in each step has two networks of a generator and a discriminator. We train the discriminator model (D) and the generator model (G) simultaneously in single network. The generator model (G) maps the pixel's label of certain image and (D) tries to distinguish this certain boundary regions comes from the reference distribution or the generative network.

$$\mathcal{L}_{GAN}(G, D) = E_y \, pdata(y)[logD(y)] + E_x \, pdata(x), z \, p_z(z)[log1 - D(x, z)] \quad (1)$$

2.1 Generator

As Fig 1 shows, our generator is a fully convolutional encoder-decoder structure like a U-net with skip connections between corresponding layers in the encoder and the decoder. We use the convolutional layer with kernel size 4 *in* 4 and stride 2 for down-sampling, and perform up-sampling by image re-size layer with a factor of 2 and the convolutional layer with kernel size 3 × 3 stride 1.

2.2 Discriminator

The discriminator is a fully convolutional neural network. Hierarchical features are extracted from multiple layers of convolution and used to compute the $\mathcal{L}1$ loss function. We confirmed the solution suggested by Isola et al. [11] for using $\mathcal{L}1$ distance rather than $\mathcal{L}2$ as $\mathcal{L}1$ encourages less blurring. $\mathcal{L}1$ loss can capture long- and short-range spatial relations between pixels by using the hierarchical features.

Both the generator (G) and the discriminator (D) are trained through back-propagation from the proposed $\mathcal{L}1$ loss. The training of the generator and the discriminator is like playing a mini-max game Eq.(1): While the goal (G) is to maximize the discriminator loss, (D) tries to minimize it. This training process makes both networks increasingly powerful.

2.3 Context-aware cGAN

As shown in Fig. (1-a), in the cascade cGAN, later stages use the shared convolution features plus the probability map obtained from previous stages and transfer the learned convolutional features to the next. We train iteratively several GANs that take as input MRI patches and estimate corresponding segmented binary patches. These patches are concatenated as a second channel in the MRI patches, and this new data is used as input during the training of the next GAN. An illustration of this scheme is shown in Fig. (1-b).

3 Experiments and results

In the experiment, we applied real patient data provided by the HVSMR-2016 [1] on Whole-Heart and Great Vessel Segmentation from Cardiovascular MRI in Congenital Heart Disease.

---

[1] http://segchd.csail.mit.edu/data.html

Table 1. The evaluation result of the semantic segmentation network from single cGAN compared to cascade cGANs in the first two rows that demonstrates the performance gains by using cascade of cGANs. We compared our results with the third top approach from the HVSMR-2016. Performance of our method (CcGAN) on the testing datasets in terms of average distance of boundaries (Adb) and Dice. Label 1 indicates the myocardium tissue while label 2 stands for the blood pool.

Method	Adb1	Adb2	Dice1	Dice2	Sen1	Sen2	Spec1	Spec2
Cascade cGAN	1.02	0.87	0.80	0.93	0.87	0.90	0.96	0.99
single cGAN	1.19	1.07	0.72	0.89	0.82	0.88	0.94	0.99
U-Net(2D)	2.04	1.82	0.68	0.81	0.78	0.74	0.91	0.99
Shahzad et al. [12]	1.10	1.55	0.75	0.89	-	-	-	-
Yu et al. [13]	0.99	0.86	0.78	0.93	-	-	-	-
Wolterink et al. [14]	0.89	0.96	0.80	0.93	-	-	-	-

3.1   Dataset

Thirty training CMR scans from 10 patients were provided by the organizers of the HVSMR-workshop in MICCAI conference. Three images have provided for each patient: a complete axial CMR image, the same image cropped around the heart and thoracic aorta, and a cropped short axis reconstruction. In the present work, we use the axial full volume from all patients as an input for the first stage. The second stage takes the cropped image around the heart and thoracic aorta as input, and the same image cropped short axis is served as the input of third stage.

3.2   Preprocessing

Because the MRI volumes in the HVSMR does not possess an isotropic resolution, we prepared 2D slices in sagittal, axial, and coronal views. We applied a bias field correction on the MR images to correct the intensity non-uniformity in the MR images by using N4ITK. In the next preprocessing step, we applied histogram matching normalization.

3.3   Train and test

The proposed approach is trained on 80% training data released by the HVSMR-2016 benchmark, which consists of 24 CMR images. We used all provided images (full, axial crop, and axial short) from three axes of x, y, and z for training and testing. We achieved better results when the mini-batch consists of images from same patients and same acquisition plane. From Table 1, we can also infer that the cascade of GANs can improve training accuracy in the term of Dice by up to 8%. Qualitative results are shown in Figures 2. The training takes around three days for a total of 100 epochs on parallel Pascal Titan X GPUs for semantic segmentation tasks. We train three GANs iteratively where each GAN is trained not only with the feature data, but also with the probability map obtained from the previous GANs, which gives to the GAN additional context information. At testing time, the features will be processed for each GAN one after the other, concatenating the probability map to the input features. The proposed network provides two predicted masks of blood pool and myocardium for each 2D image in less than 30 ms.

4   Discussion

The results show good relation to the ground truth for the blood pool. The average value of the Dice index is around 0.93, which is the same as the result of the HVSMR-2016 challenge winner [13]. The main source of error here is the inability of the method to completely segment all the great vessels where the average Dice score is 0.80. Regarding the results Table 1, we have achieved better results when the network is a cascade of GANs. Higher accuracy is expected while each stage trains on shared extracted features and weights from the previous stage.

5   Conclusion

In this paper, we propose a context-aware cGAN for automated whole heart and great vessel segmentation from cardiovascular magnetic resonance (CMR) images. Our network performs accurate, efficient, and volume-to-volume prediction with three generators and three discriminators. More importantly, our

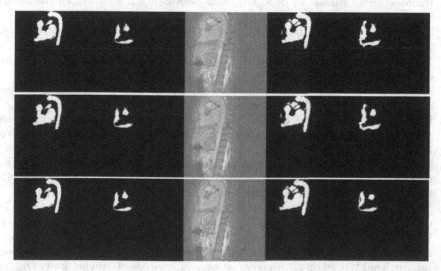

Fig. 2. The visualization results from three stages: The first two columns show the ground truth annotated by medical experts from the HVSMR2016, and the third column shows the z plan of CMR data, which is the input of context-aware cGAN. The fourth and fifth column show the predicted results by cascade-cGAN in different stages. The first row shows the output from the first stage after 50 epochs; the second and third rows are the output after 75 and 100 epochs from the second and third stages.

cascade uses transfer learning mechanism to alleviate the vanishing gradient problem and improves the training efficiency on a small medical image dataset. These networks learn a loss adapted to the task and data at hand, which makes them applicable in a wide variety of medical image segmentation. Experimental results on the MICCAI 2016 HVSMR Challenge dataset demonstrated the superior performance of our proposed method in handling large shape variation and delineating branchy structures. In the future, our method can be further improved by using LSTM between auto-encoder FCN in a generator network.

References

1. LeCun Y, Bengio Y, Hinton G. Deep learning. Nature. 2015;521(7553):436–444.
2. Mirza M, Osindero S. Conditional generative adversarial nets. Comp Res Rep. 2014;abs-1411.1784.
3. Reed SE, Akata Z, Mohan S, et al. Learning what and where to draw. In: Lee DD, Sugiyama M, Luxburg UV, et al., editors. Advances in Neural Information Processing Systems 29; 2016. p. 217–225.
4. Wang X, Shrivastava A, Gupta A. A-fast-rcnn: hard positive generation via adversary for object detection. arXiv preprint arXiv:170403414. 2017.
5. Isola P, Zhu J, Zhou T, et al. Image-to-image translation with conditional adversarial networks. Comp Res Rep. 2016;abs/1611.07004.
6. Xue Y, Xu T, Zhang H, et al. SegAN: adversarial network with multi-scale Loss for medical image segmentation. Comp Res Rep. 2017;abs/1706.01805.
7. Ronneberger O, Fischer P, Brox T. U-net: Convolutional networks for biomedical image segmentation. Proc MICCAI. 2015; p. 234–241.
8. Moeskops P, Veta M, Lafarge MW, et al. Adversarial training and dilated convolutions for brain MRI segmentation. Comp Res Rep. 2017;abs/1707.03195.
9. Kohl S, Bonekamp D, Schlemmer H, et al. Adversarial networks for the detection of aggressive prostate cancer. Comp Res Rep. 2017;abs/1702.08014.
10. Zhu W, Xie X. Adversarial deep structural networks for mammographic mass segmentation. Comp Res Rep. 2016;abs/1612.05970.
11. Radford A, Metz L, Chintala S. Unsupervised representation learning with deep convolutional generative adversarial networks. Comp Res Rep. 2015;abs/1511.06434.
12. Shahzad R, Gao S, Tao Q, et al. In: Automated cardiovascular segmentation in patients with congenital heart disease from 3D CMR scans: combining multi-atlases and level-sets. Springer International Publishing; 2017. p. 147–155.
13. Yu L, Yang X, Qin J, et al. In: 3D FractalNet: dense volumetric segmentation for cardiovascular MRI volumes; 2017. p. 103–110.
14. Wolterink JM, Leiner T, Viergever MA, et al.; Springer. Dilated convolutional neural networks for cardiovascular MR segmentation in congenital heart disease. International Workshop on Reconstruction and Analysis of Moving Body Organs. 2016; p. 95–102.

Impact of Gradual Vascular Deformations on the Intra-aneurysmal Hemodynamics

Samuel Voß[1,2], Patrick Saalfeld[3], Sylvia Saalfeld[1,3], Oliver Beuing[1,4],
Gabor Janiga[1,2], Bernhard Preim[1,3]

[1]STIMULATE Research Campus, University of Magdeburg
[2]Department of Fluid Dynamics and Technical Flows, University of Magdeburg
[3]Department of Simulation and Graphics, University of Magdeburg
[4]Institute of Neuroradiology, University Hospital Magdeburg
samuel.voss@ovgu.de

Abstract. The treatment of intracranial aneurysms based on stent-assisted coiling often leads to local vascular deformations. Patient-specific data of an aneurysm in the pre interventional and follow-up state is used to interpolate intermediate vessel-aneurysm configurations. Computational Fluid Dynamics simulations are performed in order to quantify the effect of vessel deformation on the blood flow. Results reveal gradual changes in the blood flow patterns shifting the load on the aneurysm wall from the dome to the neck region. Based on this novel concept, it is possible to virtually evaluate how different types of stents can improve or impair the treatment goal of reducing the intra-aneurysmal blood flow.

1 Introduction

Stent-assisted coiling therapy has become an established treatment strategy to prevent intracranial aneurysm rupture in order to avoid subarachnoid hemorrhage associated with severe clinical outcome. Within the endovascular treatment process, a stent is placed in front of the aneurysm. This stabilizes the parent artery and later prevents the coils from leaving the aneurysm through the aneurysms ostium, i.e., the aneurysm neck.

However, the placement of stents can cause local modifications of the vasculature ([1, 2] or see Fig. 1 left and right). Furthermore, this deformation depends on the aneurysm location [1, 2] and the stent design [1].

In order to evaluate the effect of the observed vascular deformation on the intra-aneurysmal hemodynamics, Computational Fluid Dynamics (CFD) can be performed. Gao et al. [3, 4] virtually removed the aneurysms in pre and post interventional datasets and investigated the hemodynamic effects. Thus, significant alteration of the flow at the bifurcation apex was found, including a narrowing and migration of the flow impingement zone. Jeong et al. [5] did not exclude the aneurysm in their study but only considered simplified artificial vasculature models. In addition, effects of a stent and simplified coils were included. Hence, the vessel straightening leads to reduced values of velocity, kinetic energy, wall shear stress (WSS), and vorticity.

In a recent study from Voß et al. [6], the investigations were extended by combining 1) a patient-specific anatomy with 2) retaining the aneurysm itself. CFD analysis leads to the conclusion that vessel straightening causes a blood flow redirection resulting in a decreased aneurysm neck inflow rate.

Within the present study, we examine the intermediate states of the vascular deformation based on geometrical interpolation. For the clinical practice, this can be interpreted as employment of different stent types associated with different bending stiffnesses. By determining the gradual effect on hemodynamics, we expect a better understanding of the relation between local deformation and flow patterns. First, the progress of change of the time-dependent simulated blood flow induced by the stent can be examined. Second, important information can be virtually gathered concerning the required stent stiffness, which could support clinicians in treatment planning.

2   Material and methods

2.1   Case description and preparation

This study is based on the image data of a 62 year old intracranial aneurysm patient. The patient was successfully treated with stent-assisted coiling therapy. Since follow-up image data revealed anatomical deformations of the parent artery harboring the aneurysm, an analysis of the pre, post and intermediate configurations was required to examine the deformation-induced changes in internal blood flow. This work extends the study presented in [6], where pre and post stent configurations but no intermediate deformations were compared.

2.2   Geometrical interpolation of intermediate configurations

Obtaining intermediate states between the pre and post configuration is difficult since both meshes were segmented independently and their topologies (number of vertices and their connectivity) differ. To align both topologies an approach from character modeling named *conforming* is used with the modeling software 3ds Max (Autodesk, San Rafael, USA). This techniques is also used, e.g., to deform vascular structures into flattened shapes [7]. One mesh is semi-automatically mapped onto another mesh by projecting vertices along their normal direction inwards or outwards until they hit the surface of the other mesh. Doing this semi-automatically is time-consuming (approx. four hours in our case) but it allows

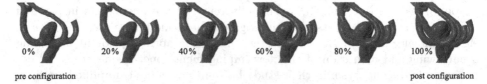

pre configuration   post configuration

Fig. 1. The six configurations of our approach, 0 % and 100 % corresponds to the pre and post configuration, respectively.

controlling deformations and artifacts that would be produced with automatic projection approaches. Fig. 1 shows the six created states, i.e., 0 %, 20 %, 40 %, 60 %, 80 %, and 100 % where 0 % corresponds to the pre configuration and 100 % corresponds to the post configuration. The intermediate states are created with linear interpolation applied to each vertex.

2.3   Hemodynamic simulation

The surface meshes are imported into the simulation software STAR-CCM+ 10.04 (Siemens Product Lifecycle Management Software Inc., Plano, TX, USA) which is used to solve the Navier-Stokes equations numerically. The simulation domain is spatially discretized based on finite volume polyhedral and prism cells. An unsteady mass inflow rate is used [8]. Further, no-slip wall conditions and a flow split outlet based on the outlet area is defined. Blood is modeled as non-Newtonian fluid [6]. The CFD simulations were run on 3 nodes each with 16 cores (2x Intel Xeon E5-2630 v3). Wall-clock CPU times per case was approx. one day.

2.4   Extraction of morphological parameters

For an assessment of the plausibility of the intermediate interpolation steps, we analyzed the aneurysms shape based on the morphological parameters: S_A - aneurysm surface area, V_A - aneurysm volume, D_{Max} - maximum diameter parallel to ostium plane, H_{Max} - maximum distance from aneurysm to ostium, H_{Ortho} - maximum distance perpendicular to ostium plane, N_{Max} - maximum diameter of ostium, and AR - aspect ratio of the aneurysm, i.e., H_{Ortho}/N_{Max} [9]. For the extraction of morphological parameters, we separated the aneurysm from the parent vessel with the method presented in [10]. To obtain V_A and S_A, the ostium contour is closed by connecting it with its center point. The parameter values for all datasets are provided in Tab. 1, where σ denotes the standard deviation and p_σ its percentual amount w.r.t. the mean μ, i.e. $p_\sigma = \sigma/\mu \cdot 100 \%$.

3   Results

For an evaluation of our method, we first analyzed the morphological parameter variations of the pre, post, and intermediate configurations, recall Tab. 1. As a result, we obtain very low values for σ indicating a high correspondence between the different configurations especially for the aneurysm's aspect ratio. Analyzing p_σ further confirms this finding with a maximum value of approx. 4 % for the aneurysm height.

Fig. 3 indicates clear differences in the qualitative comparison of all six configurations. Due to the vascular deformation, the blood flow is redirected from the aneurysm dome (a) towards the neck region (f) according to streamlines (Fig. 3-1) and velocity iso-surfaces (Fig. 3-2). This change of flow patterns moves the impact zone and results in modified wall loads, represented by the time averaged

Table 1. Extracted morphological parameters based on [9] for all datasets, 0 % refers to the pre, 100 % to the post configuration.

	Morphological parameters						
Dataset	S_A[mm^2]	V_A[mm^3]	D_{Max}[mm]	H_{Max}[mm]	H_{Ortho}[mm]	N_{Max}[mm]	AR
0 %	65.97	53.37	6.76	5.17	4.37	4.30	1.02
20 %	64.61	51.31	6.54	4.98	4.38	4.30	1.02
40 %	64.18	53.78	6.28	4.87	4.44	4.32	1.03
60 %	64.00	53.10	6.25	4.98	4.58	4.32	1.06
80 %	65.24	52.57	6.39	5.13	4.70	4.45	1.06
100 %	66.85	55.82	6.72	5.27	4.68	4.65	1.03
σ	1.11	1.49	0.22	0.15	0.18	0.14	0.02
p_σ	1.70 %	2.80 %	3.41 %	2.80 %	3.99 %	3.17 %	1.84 %

wall shear stress (AWSS), see Fig. 3-3. Furthermore, the flow is more stable in the post configuration, the oscillatory shear index (OSI) decreases with increasing deformation (Fig. 3-4). This finding is supported by Fig. 2, showing more similar flow patterns over time in the post configuration. Overall, a smaller amount of blood enters the aneurysm over the cardiac cycle in the case of higher deformations, a total reduction of more than 50 % is calculated.

4   Discussion

The concept of intermediate states of pre interventional and follow-up aneurysm anatomy is motivated by the varying bending stiffnesses of stents in clinical use. Accordingly, this method can be used to better understand the relation between stent related vascular deformation and hemodynamics without any risk for the patient. In addition, within a semi-automatized workflow, different scenarios can be virtually compared in order to 1) assess different treatment options or devices and 2) consider possible uncertainties due to individual mechanical properties of the vessel wall, potential pathologies and surrounding structures.

Our evaluation showed errors less than 4 % for morphological parameters due to the geometrical interpolation. From the computed blood flow, we observe clear differences in the inflow rates, which is important for thrombus formation

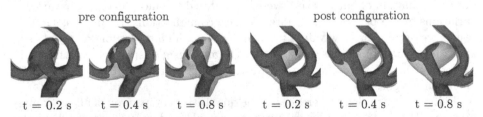

pre configuration   post configuration

t = 0.2 s   t = 0.4 s   t = 0.8 s   t = 0.2 s   t = 0.4 s   t = 0.8 s

Fig. 2. Iso-surfaces of the velocity field at 0.5 m/s for different time steps: In the pre interventional configuration (left) the flow patterns vary over time, while in the post interventional configuration (right) the flow is rather constant.

and aneurysm occlusion. In our case, vascular deformation leads to changes that can be expected to have a positive effect on the clinical outcome. However, in other patients such high grades of deformation may have the opposite effect and impair the flow conditions.

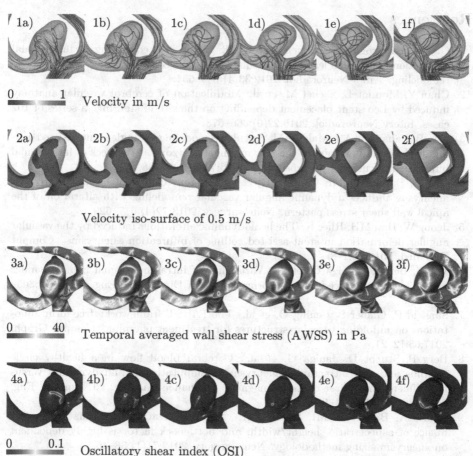

Velocity in m/s

Velocity iso-surface of 0.5 m/s

Temporal averaged wall shear stress (AWSS) in Pa

Oscillatory shear index (OSI)

Fig. 3. The different deformation configurations are shown from the pre (a) to the post (f) interventional state from left to right, respectively. First row: The deformation affects the intra-aneurysmal blood flow, visualized using velocity-coded streamlines of the time averaged flow field. Second row: Iso-surfaces of the velocity field at 0.5 m/s show a gradual migration of the flow impingement zone from the aneurysm dome (a) towards the neck region (f). This redirection of the blood flow is caused only by changes of the local vasculature. Third row: Local time averaged wall shear stress (AWSS) values vary according to the redirected blood flow. While the more pre configurations (a) to (c) show higher values at the aneurysm dome, in the more post configurations (d) to (f) values are higher in the neck region. Fourth row: Vascular deformations cause considerable changes in the oscillatory shear index (OSI). High values in configurations (a) and (b) indicate fluctuations in the time dependend flow patterns.

Acknowledgement. This work is partly funded by the European Regional Development Fund under the operation number ZS /2016/04/78123 as part of the initiative Sachsen-Anhalt WISSENSCHAFT Schwerpunkte.

References

1. Gao B, Baharoglu MI, Cohen AD, et al. Stent-assisted coiling of intracranial bifurcation aneurysms leads to immediate and delayed intracranial vascular angle remodeling. Am J Neuroradiol. 2012;33(4):649–654.
2. Chau Y, Mondot L, Sachet M, et al. Modification of cerebral vascular anatomy induced by Leo stent placement depending on the site of stenting: a series of 102 cases. Interv Neuroradiol. 2016;22(6):666–673.
3. Gao B, Baharoglu MI, Malek AM. Angular remodeling in single stent-assisted coiling displaces and attenuates the flow impingement zone at the neck of intracranial bifurcation aneurysms. Neurosurgery. 2013;72(5):739–748.
4. Gao B, Baharoglu MI, Cohen AD, et al. Y-stent coiling of basilar bifurcation aneurysms induces a dynamic angular vascular remodeling with alteration of the apical wall shear stress pattern. Neurosurgery. 2013;72(4):617–629.
5. Jeong W, Han MH, Rhee K. The hemodynamic alterations induced by the vascular angular deformation in stent-assisted coiling of bifurcation aneurysms. Comput Biol Med. 2014;53:1–8.
6. Voß S, Berg P, Janiga G, et al. Variability of intra-aneurysmal hemodynamics caused by stent-induced vessel deformation. Curr Dir Biomed Eng. 2017;3(2):305–308.
7. Saalfeld P, Glaßer S, Beuing O, et al. The FAUST framework: free-form annotations on unfolding vascular structures for treatment planning. Comput Graph. 2017;65:12–21.
8. Berg P, Stucht D, Janiga G, et al. Cerebral blood flow in a healthy circle of willis and two intracranial aneurysms: computational fluid dynamics versus four-dimensional phase-contrast magnetic resonance imaging. J Biomech Eng. 2014;136(4):041003/1–9.
9. Lauric A, Baharoglu MI, Malek AM. Ruptured status discrimination performance of aspect ratio, height/width, and bottleneck factor is highly dependent on aneurysm sizing methodology. Neurosurgery. 2012;71(1):38–46.
10. Neugebauer M, Diehl V, Skalej M, et al. Geometric reconstruction of the ostium of cerebral aneurysms. Proc VMV. 2010; p. 307–314.

Myocardial Twist from X-ray Angiography

Can we Observe Left Ventricular Twist in Rotational Coronary Angiography?

Tobias Geimer[1,2,*], Mathias Unberath[1,2,*], Johannes Höhn[1],
Stephan Achenbach[3], Andreas Maier[1,2]

[1]Pattern Recognition Lab, Friedrich-Alexander-Universität Erlangen-Nürnberg
[2]Erlangen Graduate School of Advanced Optical Technologies
[3]Department of Cardiology, Friedrich-Alexander-Universität Erlangen-Nürnberg
*Both authors contributed equally.
tobias.geimer@fau.de

Abstract. We present preliminary evidence that left ventricular twist can be observed and thus estimated from rotational coronary angiography. Our method is based on an ellipsoidal parametric model initially developed for functional analysis of cardiac tagged MRI. First, we fit the model to 3D coronary artery centerlines reconstructed from rotational angiography and then use 3D/2D registration to optimize for the functional parameters driving the model. On two clinical acquisitions, we show that our method is able to recover cardiac motion indicated by an average reduction in reprojection error of 28.1±3.0 %. Analysis of the functional progression of the functional parameters over time reveals radial and longitudinal contraction, and left ventricular twist. We believe that these results are exciting and encourage improvement of the proposed method in future work.

1 Introduction

X-ray angiography using C-arm cone-beam systems is the clinical gold standard imaging modality for diagnostic assessment and interventional guidance of coronary artery disease [1]. Recently, rotational angiography has received considerable attention. In this imaging protocol, the X-ray source rotates around the patient on a circular source trajectory acquiring images with high spatial and temporal resolution while contrast agent is administered to selectively contrast the coronary arteries. These acquisitions allow for 3D and 3D+t reconstruction of the vascular tree that are associated with increased diagnostic value [1, 2]. In contrast to static 3D reconstructions, dynamic 3D+t models further offer the possibility to recover functional parameters of the myocardium [3, 4], as the coronary arteries are directly attached to the outer wall of the heart muscle [5]. One potentially exciting application is the estimation of left ventricular twist from rotational angiography, a functional parameter that has so far not be considered in X-ray-based imaging due to the uniformity of the myocardial tissue in the X-ray spectrum [4]. In order to derive functional heart parameters from

365

rotational angiography, surface models can be fitted to the imaging data. Until now, bicubic hermite splines [6] and superquadrics [7] have been used, however, in virtually all models functional parameters, such as longitudinal contraction of ventricular twist, have to be derived rather than being integral part of the model representation. On the contrary, Park et al. [8] proposed a left ventricular (LV) heart model for the functional analysis of cardiac tagged MRI. The left ventricle is modeled as a deformable ellipse and otherwise global ellipsoid parameters are replaced by parameter functions that vary over both the apical-basal axis and time to express shape and deformations, respectively. Moreover, these regional parameters are directly related to functional parameters of the heart [8]. Based on our previous work that described fitting a static parameter ellipsoid to a 3D coronary artery model [9], we present preliminary evidence that LV twist can be recovered from rotational coronary angiography. Our method estimates parameter functions of the LV model over time via 3D/2D registration of the parametric model to the rotational angiography sequence to recover physiologically meaningful parameters of the left ventricle.

2   Material & methods

In the following, the formulation of the parametric ellipsoid model is introduced. We then briefly review prior work on fitting a static model to 3D coronary artery centerlines. Finally, our contribution is the dynamic fitting process over the cardiac cycle in a 3D/2D registration approach. The section is concluded by an overview of test data and evaluation methods.

2.1   Parametric ellipsoid model

Park et al. modeled the left ventricle as a parameter function ellipsoid (PFE) cut off at $u = \frac{\pi}{4}$ [8]. $f_{\mathbf{t},\mathbf{a}_x,\mathbf{a}_y,\mathbf{a}_z,\mathbf{e}_x,\mathbf{e}_y}(u,v)$

$$
= \underbrace{\begin{pmatrix} \cos\tau(u) & -\sin\tau(u) & 0 \\ \sin\tau(u) & \cos\tau(u) & 0 \\ 0 & 0 & 1 \end{pmatrix}}_{\text{twisting}} \underbrace{\begin{pmatrix} a_x(u)\cos u \cos v \\ a_y(u)\cos u \sin v \\ a_z(u)\sin u \end{pmatrix}}_{\text{ellipsoid and scaling}} + \underbrace{\begin{pmatrix} e_x(u) \\ e_y(u) \\ 0 \end{pmatrix}}_{\text{axis offset}}
$$

with $u \in [\frac{-\pi}{2}; \frac{\pi}{4}]$ and $v \in [-\pi; \pi]$. The ellipsoid parameters are described in terms of functions $\tau(u)$, $a_x(u)$, $a_y(u)$, $a_z(u)$, $e_x(u)$, $e_y(u)$: $[u_{\min}; u_{\max}] \rightarrow \mathbb{R}$ along the apical-basal u-axis, which coincides with the z-axis in the PFE's reference system. Changes in $a_x(u)$ and $a_y(u)$ ($a_z(u)$) lead to contraction and elongation across (along) the apical-basal axis. $e_x(u)$ and $e_y(u)$ describe bent shape of the left ventricle by an offset from the principal axis. Lastly, the twist $\tau(u)$ rotates the model around the long axis. The impact of the different parameters is illustrated in Fig. 1.

2.2 Centerline reconstruction and static model fitting

Coronary artery centerlines are segmented in all 2D fluoroscopy images and then reconstructed in 3D at an end-diastolic heart phase using a symbolic reconstruction algorithm based on the epipolar geometry [2]. Fitting the static parametric model to the 3D centerlines at end-diastole is a two step process, the details of which are provided in [9]. Put concisely, we first estimate the long axis of the LV using projection domain annotations of the user (apex and mid-basal points in two images) and, using this data to initialize the principle axis, fit a regular ellipsoid to the centerline points. Second, we replace the global parameters by parameter functions and refine the initial fit in a coarse-to-fine scheme. In this stage, the twist is set to zero. Once converged (Fig. 2), we associate each centerline point with its closest point on the model for further optimization.

2.3 Estimating a dynamic model

The static parameter function map retried in Sec. 2.2 is extended by a temporal dimension and initialized using the static result. Each projection image is associated with a normalized cardiac time $[0, 1[$, such that the dynamics can be recovered via 3D/2D registration. We seek to optimize

$$\operatorname*{arg\,min}_{\mathbf{T}_x, \mathbf{A}_x, \mathbf{A}_y, \mathbf{A}_z \mathbf{E}_x, \mathbf{E}_y} \sum_{\mathbf{u}}^{U} \sum_{i}^{I} \Gamma_i(proj(f_{\mathbf{T}_x, \mathbf{A}_x, \mathbf{A}_y, \mathbf{A}_z \mathbf{E}_x, \mathbf{E}_y}(\mathbf{u}, t_i), \mathbf{P}_i)) \qquad (1)$$

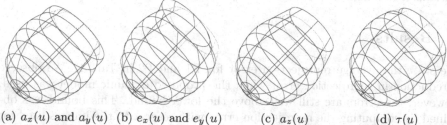

(a) $a_x(u)$ and $a_y(u)$ (b) $e_x(u)$ and $e_y(u)$ (c) $a_z(u)$ (d) $\tau(u)$

Fig. 1. Effects of changed parameters of the parameter function ellipsoid at the basis.

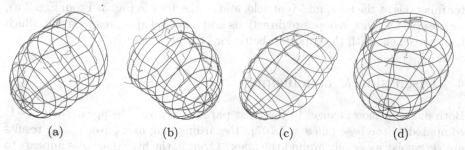

       (a)   (b)   (c)   (d)

Fig. 2. Static PFE fitting result for P1 (a,b) and P2 (c,d) in two views each.

Table 1. Average reprojection error over all projections for the static (Sec. 2.2) and dynamic model (Sec. 2.3).

	P1 [mm]	P2 [mm]
Static	2.67	2.67
Dynamic	2.12	2.05

where I is the number of projection images, U is the set of centerline points on the PFE, and Γ_i is the distance transform of the 2D centerline used to read out the reprojection error in view i. Further, uppercase letters $\mathbf{T}, \mathbf{A}, \mathbf{E}$ denote the dynamic versions of the parameter maps introduced in Sec. 2.1, and $proj((u), \mathbf{P}_i)$ describes the projective mapping of a 3D point $\mathbf{u}$ to 2D image coordinates of image i using the projection matrix $\mathbf{P}_i$. Eq. 1 is optimized in a coarse-to-fine scheme using a line-search algorithm.

2.4 Data and experiments

We evaluate the proposed method on two clinical rotational angiography acquisitions referred to as P1 and P2, respectively. The data was acquired on a Siemens Artis Zee (Siemens Healthcare GmbH, Forchheim) and consists of 133 projections over 5 seconds. Coronary arteries centerlines were segmented and reconstructed, and the static model fitted as described in Sec. 2.2. We then adapt the dynamic model to the 2D projections by optimizing Eq. 1. On the finest resolution, 5 time steps are defined and parameters are interpolated in between. Finally, we state the average reprojection error before and after 3D/2D registration to quantify the effectiveness of motion compensation and plot the parameter functions over time to review whether LV twist could be retrieved.

3   Results

We state the average reprojection error for P1 and P2 in Tab. 1. We observe a reduction in reprojection error when the proposed dynamic model was used, however, the errors are still well above the lower bound. This bound was obtained by computing the reprojection error with respect to the images used for reconstructing the 3D centerlines only and is 1.13 mm and 1.01 mm for P1 and P2, respectively. Additionally, we show the temporal progression of the parameter functions at the base, mid-ventricle, and at the apex in Fig. 3. From Fig. 3(a), we observe LV twist in opposite directions and base and apex, respectively, which is in agreement with the expected behavior [4].

4   Discussion & conclusion

Both datasets show changes in the twist parameter w.r.t. the apex ($\sin u = -1$) compared to the base ($\sin u = 0.707$). Regarding long axis offset e_x, e_y, results are very noisy especially around the apex. Overall, the fitting process appears to be unable to fully recover the heart motion, which can be attributed to several factors. Very sparse sampling of coronary arteries at the apex does not allow for robust estimation of all functional parameters in that region. Further, erroneous segmentation have a two-fold effect on the results. First, it leads to discontinuities in the reconstructed artery tree of the reference phase, further affecting the sparsity problem. Second, wrongly segmented pixels in the other views can severely increase the reprojection error in the dynamic case.

In conclusion, we presented preliminary indication that LV twist can be estimated from rotational coronary angiography. We used an ellipsoidal parametric model initially developed for cardiac tagged MRI to estimate the LV surface based on coronary artery centerlines. We then recovered the parameters of

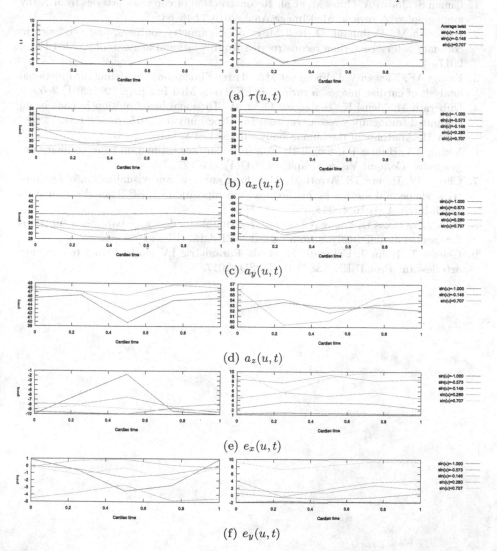

Fig. 3. Temporal progression of the functional parameters for P1 and P2 in the left and right column, respectively.

a dynamic model using 3D/2D registration to the projections. The proposed approach was able to compensate for cardiac motion and retrieves functional parameters, such as LV twist. While improvements to the method are necessary to draw more resilient conclusions, we believe that the results encourage future work.

References

1. Çimen S, Gooya A, Grass M, et al. Reconstruction of coronary arteries from X-ray angiography: A review. Med Image Anal. 2016;32:46–68.
2. Unberath M, Taubmann O, Hell M, et al. Symmetry, outliers, and geodesics in coronary artery centerline reconstruction from rotational angiography. Med Phys. 2017.
3. Frangi AF, Niessen WJ, Viergever MA. Three-dimensional modeling for functional analysis of cardiac images, a review. IEEE Trans Med Imaging. 2001;20(1):2–5.
4. Unberath M, Mentl K, Taubmann O, et al. Torsional heart motion in cone-beam computed tomography reconstruction. In: Proc Fully3D; 2015. p. 651–654.
5. Gray H. Anatomy of the human body. vol. 8. Lea & Febiger; 1878.
6. Young AA, Hunter PJ, Smaill B. Epicardial surface estimation from coronary angiograms. Comput Vision Graph. 1989;47(1):111–127.
7. Chen CW, Huang TS, Arrott M. Modeling, analysis, and visualization of left ventricle shape and motion by hierarchical decomposition. IEEE Trans Pattern Anal Mach Intell. 1994;16(4):342–356.
8. Park J, Metaxas D, Young AA, et al.. Deformable models with parameter functions for cardiac motion analysis from tagged MRI data. IEEE; 1996.
9. Geimer T, Höhn J, Unberath M, et al. Parametric LV model fitting to coronary arteries. In: Proc IEEE NSS/MIC/RTSD; 2017.

Abstract: Retrieval of Attenuation Values by the Augmented Likelihood Image Reconstruction in the Presence of Metal Artefacts

Maik Stille[1], Christian Ziemann[2], Florian Cremers[2], Dirk Rades[2], Thorsten M. Buzug[1]

[1]Institute of Medical Engineering, University of Luebeck
[2]Department of Radiotherapy, University Hospital Schleswig-Holstein, Campus Luebeck

stille@imt.uni-luebeck.de

Metal implants are able to cause severe artefacts in CT images due to physical effects such as scattering, total absorption, noise, or beamharding. Typically, the reconstructed images feature dark shadows around high-density objects as well as bright and dark streaks that may reduce the diagnostic value drastically. Within an extensive evaluation, the novel algorithm Augmented Likelihood Image Reconstruction has proven to reduce occurring artefacts accurately [1]. Moreover, the quality of artefact reduction should not only be based on the ability to reconstruct the shape of anatomical structures but on the resulting attenuation values as well. A commercially available phantom, Gammex Electron Density CT Phantom Model 465, Radiation Measurements Inc, is used to investigate the ability to retrieve attenuation values of various tissue classes [2]. The phantom is equipped with two steel inserts that cause strong artefacts similar to metal implants. On a position between the two metal rods where the manifestation of artefacts is strongest, 12 different inserts with tissue equivalent attenuation values were placed. The investigated attenuation values cover a range from lung tissue with -700 HU to cortical bone with 1336 HU. For each insert, mean value and standard deviation are compared to reference values, which are gained from a scan with removed metal rods. The evaluation shows that the HU-values of the different tissue classes could be retrieved with errors below the standard deviation of the reference images. The lowest error could be achieved for cortical bone with a difference in the mean value of only 5 HU and a standard deviation of 67 HU. Notably, the evaluation shows an overall drop in the standard deviation compared to the reference values. While the shape of the inserts was reconstructed accurately, this indicates an ability to reduce noise in the images.

References

1. Stille M, Kleine M, Buzug TM, et al. Augmented Likelihood Image Reconstruction. IEEE Transactions on Medical Imaging. 2016;35(1):158–173.
2. Ziemann C, Stille M, Cremers F, et al. The effects of metal artifact reduction on the retrieval of attenuation values. Journal of Applied Clinical Medical Physics. 2017;18(1):243–250.

Abstract: Efficient Epipolar Consistency

André Aichert, Katharina Breininger, Thomas Köhler, Andreas Maier

Pattern Recognition Lab, Friedrich Alexander-Universität Erlangen-Nürnberg
andre.aichert@fau.de

Epipolar consistency (EC) is one of the simplest consistency conditions in cone-beam computed tomgraphy. It describes redundant line integrals between any two projection images. Its simplicity is an advantage for practical implementation and applications for calibration and motion correction in FDCT. Not only is this consistency metric efficient to compute, it was also shown to be applicable to any set of X-ray projections, no matter the type and shape of trajectory, as long as no major structures are truncated in the projection images. In addition, EC has been applied to tracking in fluoroscopy, tomosynthesis, as well as rotational angiography of the heart. Aichert et al. [1] present both pseudo-code and a MATLAB demo to estimate the relative geometry between two X-ray projections. The algorithm is simplified analytically, to break down the problem for two source positions into two 3×2 matrices. A researcher who wishes to implement EC for their own application only needs to add computation the Radon intermediate function $\frac{\partial}{\partial t}\rho(\alpha, t)$, with angle to the image u-axis α and distance to the center of the image t. It is the Radon transform of each projection image, followed by a derivative in the t-direction. On high-end mobile hardware, our GPU implementation evaluates the EC metric in 44 ms for a scan with 133 projections (i.e. $8,778$ pairs of projections), excluding the time to pre-compute Radon transforms of the projection images with 512×512 bins each. The metric can be used as an objective function in a non-linear optimization, to correct, for example, parameters of detector misalignment or patient motion. As supplementary material, an open-source example[1] of the ECC algorithm is provided. We hope that this work allows other groups interested in epipolar consistency to quickly adapt an efficient solution.

Acknowledgement. We are supported by the German Research Foundation; DFG MA 4898/3-1 "Consistency Conditions for Artifact Reduction in Cone-beam CT".

References

1. Aichert A, Breininger K, Köhler T, et al. Efficient epipolar consistency. In: Kachelriess M, editor. Proceedings of the 4th CT Meeting. Proc 4th CT Meeting; 2016. p. 383–386.

---

[1] https://www5.cs.fau.de/research/software/epipolar-consistency

Magnetic-Particle-Imaging mit mehreren Gradientenstärken

Patryk Szwargulski[1,2], Nadine Gdaniec[1,2], Tobias Knopp[1,2]

[1] Abteilung für Biomedizinische Bildgebung, Universitätsklinikum
Hamburg-Eppendorf
[2] Institut für Biomedizinische Bildgebung, Technische Universität Hamburg
p.szwargulski@uke.de

Die Magnetpartikelbildgebung (engl. Magnetic-Particle-Imaging, MPI) ist ein tomografisches Bildgebungsverfahren mit dem super-paramagnetische Nanopartikel mit einer hohen zeitlichen Auflösung visualisiert werden können [1]. Die räumliche Auflösung und die Größe des Bildgebungsbereiches hängen direkt mit der genutzten Gradientenfeldstärke zusammen. Bei einer hohen Gradientenfeldstärke kann zwar eine sehr gute räumliche Auflösung erreicht werden, gleichzeitig verringert sich allerdings der Bildgebungsbereich. Um ein größeres Volumen mit einer hohen räumlichen Auflösung vermessen zu können werden multi-patch Ansätze verwendet bei denen der Bildgebungsbereich mithilfe weiterer Felder im Raum verschoben wird [2]. Da die gesamte Messzeit mit der Anzahl der zu messenden Patches linear zunimmt wird die zeitliche Auflösung dabei aber reduziert. In dieser Arbeit wird eine Methode vorgestellt, bei der zuerst ein schneller niedrig aufgelöster Übersichtsscann aufgenommen wird. Dieser wird anschließend dazu genutzt efine geringe Anzahl von hoch aufgelösten Messungen zu planen. Dabei werden nur solche Bereiche abgetastet die überhaupt Magnetpartikel enthalten. Gerade bei angiographischen Messungen kann so ein großes Volumen mit einer anisotropen räumlichen Auflösung in einem Bruchteil der Zeit aufgenommen werden, die bei der konventionellen Methode notwendig wäre. Die Rohdaten der verschiedenen Messungen werden dazu in einem gemeinsamen linearen Gleichungssystem zusammengefasst und anschließend mittels iterativer Verfahren gelöst [3].

Literaturverzeichnis

1. Gleich B, Weizenecker J. Tomographic imaging using the nonlinear response of magnetic particles. Nature. 2005;435(7046):1214 – 1217.
2. Rahmer J, Gleich B, Bontus C, et al. Rapid 3D in vivo magnetic particle imaging with a large field of view. Proc Int Soc Magn Reson Med. 2011;19:3285.
3. Gdaniec N, Szwargulski P, Knopp T. Fast multiresolution data acquisition for magnetic particle imaging using adaptive feature detection. J Med Phys. 2017;44(12):6456–6460. Available from: http://dx.doi.org/10.1002/mp.12628.

3D Adaptive Wavelet Shrinkage Denoising while Preserving Fine Structures

Cosmin Adrian Morariu[1], Alice Eckhardt[1], Tobias Terheiden[1],
Stefan Landgräber[2], Marcus Jäger[2], Josef Pauli[1]

[1]Intelligent Systems, Faculty of Engineering, University of Duisburg-Essen
[2]Department of Orthopaedics and Trauma Surgery, University Hospital Essen
`adrian.morariu@uni-due.de`

Abstract. By this contribution we tackle the challenge of denoising
MRI image data while preserving fine structures. Log-Gabor wavelets
offer a good compromise between spatial and spectral resolution, thus allowing to extract the local phase at all image voxels. Shrinking only the
complex-valued wavelet response vectors at different scales and orientations leaves the essential phase information undistorted. We propose an
adaptive shrinking threshold based on supervoxels and also based on the
amount of texture in a particular image region. Therefore, the proposed
adaptive 3D technique preserves fine structures and outperforms existing methods in terms of peak signal-to-noise ratio (PSNR)/structural
similarity (SSIM) in cases of elevated noise perturbation.

1 Introduction

In order to maintain fine structures, article [1] introduced a region-homogeneity
criterion, based on which the degree of filtering will be adapted at any image
location. Thus, local object scale is aimed to preserve even low-gradient boundaries. Due to low-contrast and fuzzy edges in case of fine structures in medical
imaging, local image properties also other than the gradient need to be investigated. Related to wavelet denoising, this work strives to preserve fine structures
by reducing only filter response vectors not related to fine structures. The 2D
wavelet shrinking denoising algorithm introduced in [2] represents a promising
basis for preserving fine structures via phase preservation. However, the strong
modification of the image gray values by the proposed filter, in the form of a gray
value shift, exerts a strong, negative influence on the PSNR / SSIM evaluation.
This shift is very pronounced in homogeneous regions, so that the filtered image
reveals negative gray values (Fig. 1 c)). Positive gray values are displayed bright,
while dark regions represent negative gray values. Most gray value frequencies
now lie in the origin of the histogram. Compensating this gray-scale shift leads
to the result image depicted in Fig. 1 d).

2 Materials and Methods

Our spectral 3D filter $F^{3D}_{\omega_n, \varphi_m, \theta_m}$ encompasses a Log-Gabor component G_{ω_n} of
center frequency ω_n and a directional component R_{φ_m, θ_m}, both devised in spher-

ical coordinates:

$$
\begin{aligned}
F^{3D}_{\omega_n,\varphi_m,\theta_m}(\omega,\varphi,\theta) &= G_{\omega_n}(\omega) \cdot R_{\varphi_m,\theta_m}(\varphi,\theta) \\
&= e^{\frac{-log(\omega/\omega_n)^2}{2log(\sigma/\omega_n)^2}} \cdot e^{-(D_{\varphi_m,\theta_m}(\omega,\varphi,\theta))^2/2\sigma_\theta^2}
\end{aligned} \tag{1}
$$

The directional component $R_{\varphi_m,\theta_m}(\varphi,\theta)$ represents an intrinsic 2-manifold embedded in 3D space, which does not require the radial frequency ω in order to compute the angular differential

$$
D_{\varphi_m,\theta_m}(\omega,\varphi,\theta) = cos^{-1}[cos(\theta)cos(\theta_m) + sin(\theta)sin(\theta_m)cos(\varphi - \varphi_m)] \tag{2}
$$

between filter orientation (φ_m, θ_m) and spherical coordinates (φ, θ) of all points in 3D space. This differential represents the argument of a Gaussian function, which remains a Gaussian after spatial domain transformation. Hence, after convolving the image with $F^{3D}_{\omega_n,\varphi_m,\theta_m}$ only its amplitudes will be modulated by the angular component, while the phase information extracted by the Log-Gabor component will be preserved. We empirically establish by grid search on the same dataset as used in the evaluation $\sigma_\theta = 1.2$ in conjunction with $M = 13$ main orientations pertaining to the discrete 26-neighborhood of a voxel. In order to obtain undistorted phase information locally, i.e. at each voxel, for different frequency components, we employ 6 Log-Gabor quadrature filter pairs G_{ω_n} of center frequency $\omega_n = 1/(\lambda \cdot 2^{n-1})$ for the n-th filter. These frequencies are yielded by scaling of a minimal wavelength λ. They further influence the filter bandwidth $\sigma = 0.4 \cdot \omega_n$.

The spatial-domain quadrature filter pair $[F^e_{n,m}, F^o_{n,m}] = FFT^{-1}(F^{3D}_{\omega_n,\varphi_m,\theta_m})$ (even and odd, respectively real and imaginary part) is obtained by the Inverse Fourier Transform. Convolution with the 3D image $I(x)$ leads to the even and odd filter responses

$$
EO(x) = [e_{n,m}(x), o_{n,m}(x)] = [I(x) * F^e_{n,m}, I(x) * F^o_{n,m}]. \tag{3}
$$

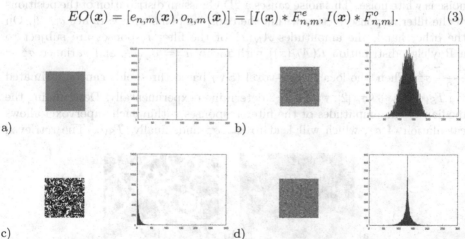

Fig. 1. a) Homogeneous image and its histogram. b) Image overlapped by additive gaussian noise. c) Denoising result using method in [2]. Negative-valued filter results displayed in black. d) Correction result after compensating the grayscale shift.

The amplitude of the filter responses at a given wavelet scale n and orientation m is given by $A_{n,m}(x) = \sqrt{e_{n,m}(x)^2 + o_{n,m}(x)^2}$ and the phase of the filter response vector will be described by $\Phi_{n,m}(x) = atan2(o_{n,m}(x), e_{n,m}(x))$.

Since the wavelet shrinkage process ensues in the same manner for all orientations, the notation will be simplified in the following by omitting the orientation index m. In order to preserve fine structures this work proposes a local adaptation of the noise threshold to gray value edges. To locate edges, the Canny algorithm is used, which is particularly suitable for the extraction of edges in noisy image data due to the hysteresis technique and non-maximum suppression [3]. We have employed the automatically determined MATLAB parameters for the Canny algorithm. The result of edge detection, for a single 2D slice from a 3D MRI dataset is a binary matrix. The matrix E containing edge pixels will be used later to apply a soft-threshold, which leads to a smaller amount of shrinking wavelet coefficients for edge voxels. In case of edge-free regions, a hard threshold is formed later, which shrinks the amplitude responses by the full amount of the noise threshold. The negated matrix $\neg E$ characterizes these hard-threshold regions.

Furthermore, the adaptive determination of the noise threshold takes place also via the subdivision of the medical 3D datasets into patches. Generation of patches (superpixels or supervoxels) ensues by means of the SLIC algorithm [4]. The compactness parameter of the SLIC algorithm controls the shape of superpixels. A higher value leads to equally large, quadratic superpixels. A lower value causes alignment of the superpixels along the structure boundaries, causing the superpixels to be irregular in shape. The alignment of superpixels along the structure boundaries can be clearly seen in Fig. 2 b).

After obtaining $EO(x)$ by equation 3, the noise component is estimated for each supervoxel. Extraction of the noise thresholds is made assuming that the noise is white noise. This noise causes a 2D Gaussian distribution of the positions of the filter response vectors within the complex plane with variance σ_g^2 [2]. On the other hand, the amplitudes $A_N(x)$ of the filter responses are subject to a Rayleigh distribution $R(A_N(x))$ with mean $\mu_r = \sigma_g\sqrt{\frac{\pi}{2}}$ and variance $\sigma_r^2 = \frac{4-\pi}{2}\sigma_g^2$. Then, the local, super-voxel (SV) based thresholds can be estimated via $T_{SV} = \mu_r + k\sigma_r$ [2], with $k = 2$ determined experimentally. Determining the median of the amplitudes of the filter responses within each supervoxel allows calculation of σ_g, which will lead to μ_r, σ_r^2 and, finally, T_{SV}. The retrieved

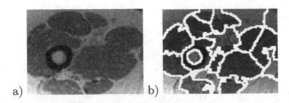

a)   b)

Fig. 2. a) Original 2D slice b) Superpixels determined by the SLIC algorithm.

noise thresholds are combined into a matrix so that the individual values can be assigned to the respective supervoxel.

Once the thresholds have been set, adaptive shrinkage processing is performed. The matrix $V(x)$ consists of the soft-threshold $V_{soft}(x)$ and the hard-threshold $V_{hard} = 1$. For computing $V(x)$, the amplitudes $A_N(x)$ are first compared with the $T_{SV}(x)$ matrix and those x are set to 1 as soon as they exceed the supervoxel-dependent noise thresholds, i.e. $validEO(x) = (A_N(x) > T_{SV}(x))$. The resulting binary matrix is named $validEO(x)$, due to the fact that the filter response contains also valid signal for the respective scale (i.e. not solely noise) at 1-valued positions. Computation of the soft threshold (see equation 4) is performed using the E matrix. The variable *softness* with values between 0 and 1 is used to set the percentage of how low the soft threshold is selected. The matrix

$$V_{soft}(x) = \frac{softness * T_{SV}(x) * E(x) * EO(x)}{A_N(x) + \varepsilon} \qquad (4)$$

is designed to provide a lower noise threshold at edges, with all regions without edges equaling zero in that matrix. Calculation of the V_{hard} matrix ensues by using the variable *hardness* = 1 and the binary $\neg E$ matrix (negated, see above). The resulting matrix is intended in the following calculation steps to shrink the amplitudes of the filter responses within edge-less regions, by the complete amount of the noise threshold.

$$V_{hard}(x) = \frac{hardness * T_{SV}(x) * \neg E(x) * EO(x)}{A_N(x) + \varepsilon} \qquad (5)$$

Adding the soft-threshold matrix to the hard-threshold matrix yields the matrix $V(x) = V_{soft}(x) + V_{hard}(x)$. The matrix V so far contains only noise thresholds of the filter responses, which consist of a noise and signal component. To eliminate filter responses with pure noise, the noise threshold matrix V must be adjusted. This is done by multiplying the negated $validEO(x)$ matrix, denoted as $\neg validEO(x)$, by the even and odd filter responses $EO(x)$. The term comprises all filter responses which are below the threshold T_{SV} and thus it is assumed to contain mainly noise. The product of $validEO(x)$ and V contains the filter responses which exhibit both noise and signal components and are provided with the soft or hard threshold:

$$V_{new}(x) = \neg validEO(x) * EO(x) + validEO(x) * V(x). \qquad (6)$$

Subsequently we subtract the V_{new} from the filter responses EO, i.e. $EO(x) = EO(x) - V_{new}(x)$. The generated matrix thus only consists of filter responses with a pure signal component. To reconstruct the pure signals, the determined $EO(X)$ are assembled from the six scales, yielding the local energy. Grayscale shifting is performed in the 2D and 3D adaptive shrinkage denoising method according to the same scheme presented in the beginning of this section.

In order to provide a quantitative assessment of the proposed method, 10 MRI datasets containing 40 to 208 slices with a slice spacing ranging from 2.4 to 3.6 mm will be utilized for evaluation. The within-slice resolution of the slices (each of 256×256 voxels) varies between 0.898 and 1.09 mm.

378   Morariu et al.

Table 1. PSNR and SSIM yielded by different denoising methods for low noise levels (variance 0.01) and elevated levels (variance 0.04). The adaptive 3D technique exhibits best results when the noise perturbation is high.

Method	V0.01: PSNR	V0.01: SSIM	V0.04: PSNR	V0.04: SSIM
No filtering	20.14 ± 0.10	0.42 ± 0.06	14.64 ± 0.22	0.20 ± 0.04
Orig. 2D	11.86 ± 1.39	0.23 ± 0.10	11.50 ± 1.36	0.15 ± 0.03
2D (scaled)	24.22 ± 1.51	0.69 ± 0.04	21.53 ± 0.92	0.49 ± 0.04
Adaptive 2D	23.75 ± 1.34	0.63 ± 0.05	20.05 ± 0.65	0.40 ± 0.05
3D (scaled)	23.23 ± 1.79	0.65 ± 0.03	21.80 ± 1.27	0.53 ± 0.03
Adaptive 3D	23.15 ± 1.74	0.64 ± 0.03	21.86 ± 1.25	0.53 ± 0.03

3 Results

The 10 MRI datasets are corrupted by additive gaussian distributed noise of various variances, ranging from 0.007 to 0.04. Table 1 encompasses the PSNR and SSIM for the unfiltered, noise-corrupted image, the original 2D wavelet denoising proposed by Kovesi [2], the 2D method improved by grayvalue-shift compensation, the adaptive 2D technique using superpixels and soft thresholding, as well as the adaptive / non-adaptive 3D techniques with / without supervoxels and soft thresholding. In 2D, the adaptive wavelet shrinkage denoising is defined in a similar manner. However, the spectral filter from eg. 1 possesses a more elementary directional component R_{φ_m,θ_m} as defined in [5]. The Log-Gabor component, which depends only on the frequency, remains unchanged, while replacing supervoxels by superpixels. The results of the adaptive 2D / 3D methods have been yielded by employing 10 - 25 superpixels/ supervoxels and a soft threshold *softness* between 0.8 - 1. Fig. 3 illustrates how the adaptive technique is more useful in preserving the fine boundaries of the femoral bone compared to the non-adaptive technique. As depicted in Fig. 4, the overall PSNR and SSIM values reveal higher values for the 3D techniques in case of elevated noise levels. When the noise perturbation is low, the PSNR/SSIM are higher for the shift-compensated 2D techniques. Only the original 2D method [2] yields much lower PSNR/SSIM values due to the grayscale modification, leading to a strong dismatch with the original image.

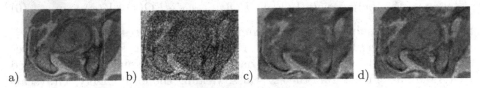

a)   b)   c)   d)

Fig. 3. a) Original MRI slice. b) Image corrupted by white noise of variance 0.02. c) Result after shift-compensated denoising. d) Result after adaptive shift-compensated denoising.

Fig. 4. a) PSNR and b) SSIM of various denoising methods for an MRI dataset plotted over several white noise variances. The 3D denoising methods yield best results for high noise corruption, i.e. high noise variance.

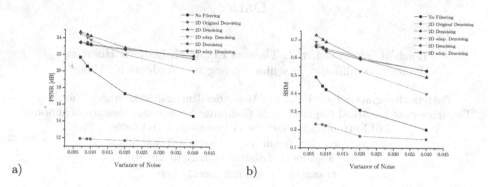

a)   b)

4   Discussion

This contribution contrives a genuine 3D denoising approach based on Log-Gabor quadrature filter pairs. It also introduces an adaptive wavelet shrinkage technique based on supervoxels. The threshold for shrinkage of wavelet coefficients is determined for each supervoxel separately. An additional soft threshold in edge-rich image regions enforces preservation of fine structures. The proposed adaptive 3D technique yields good PSNR/SSIM values when the noise levels are high. On the other hand, the 2D filter incorporates only slicewise information and, therefore, it changes the image to a reduced degree, which exposes a desired effect in the context of low noise levels.

References

1. Saha PK, Udupa JK. Scale-based diffusive image filtering preserving boundary sharpness and fine structures. IEEE Trans Biomed Eng. 2001;20(11):1140–1155.
2. Kovesi P. Phase preserving denoising of images. Austr Pat Recogn Soc Conf DICTA. 1999;4(3):212–217.
3. Canny J. A computational approach to edge detection. IEEE Trans Pattern Anal Mach Intell. 1986;(6):679–698.
4. Achanta R, Shaji A, Smith K, et al. SLIC superpixels compared to state-of-the-art superpixel methods. IEEE Trans Pattern Anal Mach Intell. 2012;34(11):2274–2282.
5. Morariu CA, Dohle DS, Tsagakis K, et al. Extraction of the aortic dissection membrane via spectral phase information. In: Proc BVM. Springer; 2015. p. 305–310.

Abstract: QuaSI – Quantile Sparse Image
A Prior for Spatio-Temporal Denoising of Retinal OCT Data

Franziska Schirrmacher[1,*], Thomas Köhler[1,*], Lennart Husvogt[1],
James G. Fujimoto[2], Joachim Hornegger[1], Andreas K. Maier[1]

[1]Pattern Recognition Lab, Friedrich-Alexander-Universität Erlangen-Nürnberg
[2]Department of Electrical Engineering & Computer Science and Research Laboratory
of Electronics, Massachusetts Institute of Technology
https://www5.cs.fau.de/en/research/software/idaa/
* These authors contributed equally to this work.
franziska.schirrmacher@fau.de

Optical Coherence Tomography (OCT) is a standard non-invasive imaging modality widely used in opthalmology. Due to its high spatial resolution OCT has become a standard imaging technique. However, speckle noise caused by photon interference during the acquisition is its major drawback. To this end, we propose a spatio-temporal denoising algorithm using the quantile sparse image (QuaSI) prior that is based on quantile filtering [1]. For OCT denoising, the median filter is used as it faciliates structure preservation and handles non-Gaussian noise. An energy minimization formulation is developed including the QuaSI prior coupled with the total variation prior. The proposed alternating direction method of multiplier scheme enables efficient optimization with the non-linear QuaSI prior. To tackle the non-linearity of the median filter, a linearization of the filter is computed. The median operator is replaced by a matrix-vector operation that can be optimized directly.

The proposed spatio-temporal denoising algorithm is evaluated on two data sets. We compare our method to the well known BM3D as well as current OCT noise reduction algorithms, namely Bayesian estimation denoising, averaging of registered B-scans, and wavelet-multi-frame denoising. The publicly available pig eye data set comprises 35 eye positions with 13 B-scans each. We also investigate denoising on clinical data from 14 human subjects. The proposed algorithm achieved the best denoising performance on both data sets in terms of all measures.

References

1. Schirrmacher F, Köhler T, Husvogt L, et al. QuaSI: quantile sparse image prior for spatio-temporal denoising of retinal oct data. Proc MICCAI. 2017;Part II:83–91.

Erratum zu: Bildverarbeitung für die Medizin 2018

Andreas Maier, Thomas M. Deserno, Heinz Handels, Klaus H. Maier-Hein,
Christoph Palm und Thomas Tolxdorff

Erratum zu:
A. Maier et al. (Hrsg.), *Bildverarbeitung für die Medizin 2018,*
Informatik aktuell, https://doi.org/10.1007/978-3-662-56537-7

Die Reihenfolge der Autoren war in der Orginalversion dieser Beiträge vertauscht.
Die korrekte Reihenfolge wird hier dargestellt:

An Open Source Tool for Creating Model Files for Virtual Volume Rendering in PDF
Documents
Julian Brandner, Axel Newe, Wolfgang Aichinger, Linda Becker

Segmentierung von Brustvolumina in Magnetresonanztomographiedaten unter der
Verwendung von Deep Learning
Thomas G. Jentschke, Katrin Hegenscheid, Henry Völzke, Florentin Wörgötter,
Tatyana Ivanovska

Effiziente Segmentierung trachealer Strukturen in MRI-Aufnahmen
Philip Dietrich, Catherine Schmidt, Henry Völzke, Achim Beule, Florentin Wörgötter,
Tatyana Ivanovska

Der Originalbeitrag wurde korrigiert.

Die aktualisierte Originalversion des Kapitels kann hier abgerufen werden
https://doi.org/10.1007/978-3-662-56537-7_43
https://doi.org/10.1007/978-3-662-56537-7_52
https://doi.org/10.1007/978-3-662-56537-7_54

Erratum zu: Amplitude of brain signals classify hunger status based on machine learning in resting-state fMRI

Arkan Al-Zubaidi, Alfred Mertins, Marcus Heldmann, Kamila Jauch-Chara, Thomas F. Münte

Erratum zu:
Kapitel 13 in: A. Maier et al. (Hrsg.), *Bildverarbeitung für die Medizin 2018,* Informatik aktuell, https://doi.org/10.1007/978-3-662-56537-7_13

An incorrect version of the article by Al-Zubaidi et al. was initially published. The original version has been retracted, and the correct version of the article has been published (under doi https://doi.org/10.1007/978-3-662-56537-7_13) online and in the print version of this book. The original version has been updated to indicate the retraction, and the correct version is now the version of record.

Die aktualisierte Originalversion des Kapitels kann hier abgerufen werden
https://doi.org/10.1007/978-3-662-56537-7_13

Autorenverzeichnis

Printed in the United States
By Bookmasters